PRACTICAL PEDIATRIC ENDOCRINOLOGY IN A LIMITED RESOURCE SETTING

PRACTICAL PEDIATRIC ENDOCRINOLOGY IN A LIMITED RESOURCE SETTING

Edited by

MARGARET ZACHARIN

The Royal Children's Hospital Melbourne, Parkville, Australia

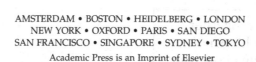

AMSTERDAM • BOSTON • HEIDELBERG • LONDON
NEW YORK • OXFORD • PARIS • SAN DIEGO
SAN FRANCISCO • SINGAPORE • SYDNEY • TOKYO

Academic Press is an Imprint of Elsevier

Academic Press is an imprint of Elsevier
32 Jamestown Road, London NW1 7BY, UK
225 Wyman Street, Waltham, MA 02451, USA
525 B Street, Suite 1800, San Diego, CA 92101-4495, USA

First edition 2013

Medicine is an ever-changing field. Standard safety precautions must be followed, but as new research and clinical experience broaden our knowledge, changes in treatment and drug therapy may become necessary or appropriate. Readers are advised to check the most current product information provided by the manufacturer of each drug to be administered to verify the recommended dose, the method and duration of administrations, and contraindications. It is the responsibility of the treating physician, relying on experience and knowledge of the patient, to determine dosages and the best treatment for each individual patient. Neither the publisher nor the authors assume any liability for any injury and/or damage to persons or property arising from this publication.

Permissions may be sought directly from Elsevier's Science & Technology Rights Department in Oxford, UK: phone (+44) (0) 1865 843830; fax (+44) (0) 1865 853333; email: permissions@elsevier.com. Alternatively, visit the Science and Technology Books website at www.elsevierdirect.com/rights for further information

Notice
No responsibility is assumed by the publisher for any injury and/or damage to persons or property as a matter of products liability, negligence or otherwise, or from any use or operation of any methods, products, instructions or ideas contained in the material herein.

Because of rapid advances in the medical sciences, in particular, independent verification of diagnoses and drug dosages should be made

British Library Cataloguing-in-Publication Data
A catalogue record for this book is available from the British Library

Library of Congress Cataloging-in-Publication Data
A catalog record for this book is available from the Library of Congress

ISBN: 978-0-12-810275-6

For information on all Academic Press publications visit our website at elsevierdirect.com

Typeset by TNQ Books and Journals
www.tnq.co.in

Printed and bound in United States of America

12 13 14 15 16   10 9 8 7 6 5 4 3 2 1

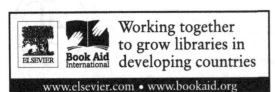

Contents

Contributors

Dr. Leena Patel spent her childhood in Uganda. She graduated and qualified as a pediatrician with an MD from Ahmedabad, India. Thereafter she gained subspecialty experience and broadened her academic interests in the UK, became a Fellow of the Royal College of Paediatrics and Child Health and obtained a Research MD (University of Manchester) as well as a Masters in Health Professionals Education (University of Maastricht). She is an honorary Consultant Pediatric Endocrinologist at the Royal Manchester Children's Hospital which provides a tertiary level service for the North West of England. Her research interests and publications are in clinical pediatric endocrinology and growth disorders. As Senior Lecturer in Child Health at the University of Manchester, she has made major contributions to undergraduate medical education, faculty development and postgraduate training.

Dr. Jaya Sujatha Gopal-Kothandapani graduated from Madras Medical College and Research Institute in 1999 and did her basic pediatric training at the Institute of Child Health, India. She moved to the UK in 2003 for further training in Pediatric Endocrinology. She became a member of Royal College of Paediatrics and Child Health (RCPCH) in 2007 and will complete her training in 2014 at the Royal Manchester Children's Hospital.

Dr. Indraneel Banerjee MD, FRCPCH is a consultant Pediatric Endocrinologist at the Royal Manchester Children's Hospital and an honorary senior lecturer in the University of Manchester in the United Kingdom. Dr Banerjee's basic training was in Kolkata, India. He moved to the UK and trained in pediatric endocrinology in Cardiff and then at Manchester, before his current consultant appointment. Dr Banerjee's main subspecialty interests are in delayed puberty and congenital hyperinsulinism. He is the clinical lead for the highly specialised Northern Congenital Hyperinsulinism (NORCHI) service providing clinical management for children with hypoglycaemia due to congenital hyperinsulinism in the north of the UK. Dr Banerjee's research interests are focused around mechanisms of delayed puberty and congenital hyperinsulinism. He has authored a number of publications in these areas and has contributed to several book chapters, including the Oxford Textbook of Medicine.

Associate Professor Margaret Zacharin is a pediatric and adult endocrinologist, a fellow of the Royal Australasian College of Physicians, associate professor at the University of Melbourne and adjunct Professor at the University of New England, NSW. She works at the Royal Children's Hospital, Melbourne, Australia and consults for the Peter McCallum Cancer Hospital, Melbourne. Her main clinical areas of interest and research include hormone replacement treatment, bone fragility disorders of childhood and adolescence and management of long-term endocrine effects of childhood cancer, with wide publication in these areas. She has a major commitment to education, with involvement in teaching programmes developed by the European Society for Pediatric Endocrinology for both winter school and the Pan African teaching programme, collaborative research in India and teaching with the Indian pediatric and adolescent society.

Dr. Anna Simon after her completion of training in general pediatrics from the Institute of Child Health, Chennai, India in 1994, joined the Pediatric Endocrinology unit of the Christian Medical College, Vellore, South India, a tertiary referral hospital of excellence in patient care, education and research. She has also spent three years of training in metabolic medicine and endocrinology at the Women's and Children's hospital, Adelaide, Australia. Her main area of interest is in clinical endocrinology services with care of diabetes and many diverse and complex endocrine disorders in a large cohort of children and adolescents. She has also been involved in a successful hospital-based neonatal thyroid screening program since 2001, which probably is the only ongoing thyroid screening project in India. She is committed to education and involved in training of undergraduate medical students and pediatric postgraduate trainees. She has contributed chapters to the ISPAE guidelines on Childhood Diabetes (2010) and IAP Speciality Series (2011) in Endocrinology and published in peer reviewed journals.

Professor Martin Ritzén is a professor emeritus in Pediatric Endocrinology at the Karolinska Institutet, Stockholm, Sweden. He has paid a lifelong interest in endocrine disorders in children, first with a focus on basic sciences, later on clinical matters. His research has focused on testicular and adrenal function, growth and puberty, resulting in over 300 published scientific articles. Among prestigious international prizes, he values the Andrea Prader Prize most, awarded by the European Society for Paediatric Endocrinology (ESPE) for outstanding contributions to pediatric endocrinology. Through leading an ESPE teaching team to Nigeria in 2005 and by being an active founding member of the ESPE group that started the Pan-African Paediatric Endocrinology Training Centre in Nairobi, he has gained insight into the needs for pediatricians who practice endocrinology in a resource poor environment.

Professor Syed Faisal Ahmed graduated from the University of Edinburgh and received his clinical and academic training mainly at the Royal Hospital for Sick Children, Edinburgh, University of Edinburgh and at Addenbrookes Hospital and the University of Cambridge. Currently, he is Professor of Developmental pediatrics and consultant at the Royal Hospital for Sick Children, Yorkhill, Glasgow, clinical lead for children's services R&D for Greater Glasgow & Clyde Health Board, Director of the Children's Clinical Research Facility at Yorkhill and holds an honorary chair at the University of Glasgow. At Yorkhill, he is the clinical lead for a comprehensive, multimodality bone densitometry service and a multidisciplinary pediatric metabolic bone service dedicated for children across Scotland.

In addition he is one of the founder members and former clinical lead of the Scottish Disorders of Sexual Development SD Network, a national managed clinical network for children with DSD, with an active research group with several collaborative links with other groups in Glasgow and beyond, with international recognition for his expertise. Professor Ahmed recently chaired a UK taskforce which developed national guidance for the initial approach to a child with DSD. In addition, he coordinates the International DSD Register which facilitates international research through initiatives such as EuroDSD. Professor Ahmed is an active member of the European Society of Paediatric Endocrinology. He was the ESPE lead for the Nairobi Training Centre between 2009 and 2011 and is currently the coordinator of the ESPE Summer School.

Dr. Iroro Yarhere started his medical career in the University of Port Harcourt Teaching Hospital Nigeria in 2004. He was among the first eight fellows to graduate from the ESPE-tutored pan-African pediatric endocrinology training centre in Nairobi in 2009 and has been working as a pediatric endocrinologist since then. He wishes to see an era where medical practice in Nigeria will be on par with that in most of Europe and America.

Dr. Orit Pinhas-Hamiel received her medical degree at Sackler School of Medicine, Tel Aviv University (1984). She was a Pediatric Endocrine Fellow at Children's Hospital in Cincinnati, Ohio (1992–1995). She is certified by the Israeli Board of Pediatrics and by the Subspecialty Board of Pediatric Endocrinology. She has been the director of the Pediatric Endocrinology and Diabetes Unit of Safra Children's Hospital, Sheba Medical Center since 2002 and is also the head of the Juvenile Diabetes Clinic in Maccabi health care services. Dr Pinhas-Hamiel is particularly interested in obesity, and associated comorbidities, specifically type-2 diabetes mellitus in children and adolescents.

Dr. Matthew Sabin trained at Guy's and St Thomas' Hospitals in London (UK) and undertook general paediatric training in England, before completing higher specialist training in pediatric endocrinology and diabetes in Melbourne, Australia.

He is a Consultant in the Department of Endocrinology and Diabetes at the Royal Children's Hospital in Melbourne, Senior Research Fellow at the Murdoch Children's Research Institute, Lecturer at the University of Melbourne, and an Adjunct Senior Lecturer in Physiology at Monash University.

His PhD investigated the links between childhood obesity and early Type 2 diabetes. Current clinical research endeavours involve investigation into the role of genetics vs. environment in the development of obesity-related disease. Laboratory research focuses on investigations into the role that early nutrition plays in altering susceptibility to later obesity and diabetes, as well as probing ways in which processes underlying these relationships can be altered by growth factors and modulators of inflammation. Dr Sabin is a current recipient of an NHMRC Postdoctoral Training Fellowship with international recognition for expertise in the clinical management of overweight and obese children. He is a member of the Royal College of Paediatrics and Child Health in the UK, and a fellow of the Royal Australasian College of Physicians.

Professor Vijayalakshmi Bhatia obtained her basic medical training and pediatric residency from the All India Institute of Medical Sciences, New Delhi. After she completed her pediatric endocrinology fellowship from the University of Massachusetts Medical Center, Worcestor, Massachusetts, USA, she has been on the faculty of the endocrinology department at the Sanjay Gandhi Postgraduate Institute of Medical Sciences, Lucknow, India. The department offers a formal training program in pediatric endocrinology. Dr Bhatia's research interests include vitamin D and calcium status in pregnancy, newborns and adolescents and type 1 diabetes. She has served as secretary of the Indian Society for Pediatric and Adolescent Endocrinology, and as a member of the Child Health Task Force of the Indian Council for Medical Research.

Dr. Abhishek Kulkarni obtained his basic medical degree from Grant Medical College, Mumbai and completed his masters in pediatrics from the Maharaja Sayajirao University, Baroda, India. He has been trained in pediatric endocrinology at Sanjay Gandhi Postgraduate Institute of Medical Sciences, Lucknow, India. He has authored a chapter on Hypocalcemia in Infants and Children, for the Indian Academy of Pediatrics Speciality Series and is a co-author of a textbook on Pediatric Toxicology. He currently runs a pediatric endocrine clinic at Mumbai, India and is a consultant pediatric endocrinologist at Seven Hills Hospital and Global Hospital and Research Centre, Mumbai, India.

Dr. Veena V. Nair completed her basic medical degree, as well as pediatric residency, from Medical College, Thiruvananthapuram, India. Her training in pediatric endocrinology was from Sanjay Gandhi Postgraduate Institute of Medical Sciences, Lucknow, India, during which period she was involved in research on type 1 diabetes as well as vitamin D deficiency in pregnancy and the newborn. She has served as an editorial assistant for clinical textbooks for pediatric students and practitioners. She is currently working as research officer in the department of endocrinology, Christian Medical College, Vellore, India.

Professor Ursula Kuhnle-Kral graduated from medical school at the University of Munich, Germany and the University School of Aberdeen, Great Britain between 1970–75. She then obtained her degree with distinction as Doctor of Medicine in 1979, with board Certification in Paediatrics in 1986. She was promoted to Professor of Pediatrics in 1997. Early appointments in Munich, Germany and at Cornell Medical School, New York, USA, were followed by appointments as Assistant Professor at the University Children's Hospital in Munich (1981–92), Associate professor and Consultant Pediatrician at the National University in Kuala Lumpur (1993–96), Consultant and Head of the Pediatric Policlinic and Consultant Pediatric Endocrinologist at the University Children's Hospital in Munich, Germany (1997–2002) and Consultant Pediatric Endocrinologist at the Private Centre for Child and Adolescent Health in Munich from 2003. She has been Lecturer at the PanAfrican Training Programme in Pediatric Endocrinology in Nairobi, Kenya in 2008 and 2010. She has published widely in several areas of pediatric endocrinology.

Dr. Joshua Kausman is a staff pediatric nephrologist and acting head of department of Nephrology at

Royal Children's Hospital, Melbourne. He has clinical experience and training in pediatric nephrology in Australia and the United Kingdom. Academic interests include renal tubular defects, including X-linked hypophosphataemic rickets, as well as immune-mediated kidney diseases, such as haemolytic-uraemic syndrome, vasculitis and transplantation. He has ongoing involvement in laboratory based research on the roles of dendritic cells and inflammatory mediators in the progression of kidney disease. Dr. Kausman is sub-editor for nephrology for the Journal of Paediatrics and Child Health and is a committee member and author of national nephrology practice guidelines by CARI (Caring for Australasians with renal Impairment).

Associate Professor Craig F. Munns is a Senior Staff Specialist in Bone and Mineral Medicine and Endocrinology at the Children's Hospital at Westmead and Conjoint Associate Professor in the Sydney Medical School at the University of Sydney, Australia. Following the completion of his Pediatric and Endocrinology training at The Royal Children's Hospital, Brisbane, Australia, A/Prof. Munns spent two years as a Clinical Associate in Genetic and Metabolic Bone Disorders at the Shriners Hospital for Children, Montreal, Canada. He was awarded his PhD on the effects of the SHOX gene on growth in 2004. Diagnosis and management of primary and secondary pediatric bone disorders is his area of expertise and his primary clinical and research interest, with numerous publications in this field.

Dr. Annemieke M. Boot is pediatric endocrinologist at University Medical Center Groningen — Beatrix Children's Hospital in Groningen in the Netherlands. Her research is focussed on bone mineral density and bone metabolism in children. She obtained her PhD in 1997. From 1989 to 1992 she worked as general medical doctor in Blantyre and Mangochi in Malawi, Africa. Her training in pediatrics and pediatric-endocrinology was in Sophia Children's Hospital — Erasmus MC in Rotterdam, the Netherlands. She is a member of The European Society of Paediatric Endocrinology (ESPE) and is active in the ESPE Bone and Growth Plate working group. In November 2009 she was a tutor in the

sub-Saharan pediatric endocrinology fellowship programme in Nairobi, Kenya.

Associate Professor Sonia Grover is director of the department of pediatric and adolescent gynaecology at the Royal Children's Hospital (RCH), Melbourne, Australia. She has been working in this field for 20 years and has played a key role in developing pediatric and adolescent gynaecology services not only at RCH, but around Australia and she is involved in supporting the training of others throughout the Asian region. Herresearch interests include disorders of sex development, the menstrual management of girls with disabilities and bleeding disorders in young women. She has published widely in these areas.

Dr. Amanda L. Ogilvy-Stuart (DM, BM, MRCPCH, FRCP) has been a consultant neonatologist at the Rosie Hospital, Cambridge University Hospitals NHS Foundation Trust, since 1998 and is currently the clinical director. She is also a senior member of St Edmund's college, University of Cambridge. She trained in pediatrics in Nottingham, Oxford, the Hospital for Sick Children, Great Ormond Street, New Zealand and Manchester. Although interested in all aspects of neonatal care, her main interest is neonatal endocrinology, having trained in pediatric endocrinology in Manchester whilst studying for her DM thesis. This was followed by a post as clinical lecturer in pediatrics at the University of Oxford where she commenced her research into the endocrinology of the newborn. She has written textbook, chapter publications, a number of commissioned reviews and original research articles on neonatal endocrinology. She also has an interest in medical education and ran the East of England regional registrar study days for five years before becoming one of the training programme directors for the Eastern Deanery for three years. She is the honorary treasurer of the British Association of Perinatal Medicine, and has previously been treasurer for the British Society for Paediatric Endocrinology and Diabetes.

Dr. Paula Midgley is a senior lecturer in Child Life and Health at the University of Edinburgh. She is a consultant on the Neonatal Unit at the Simpson Centre for Reproductive Health and at the Royal

Hospital for Sick Children in Edinburgh. She is a neonatal endocrinologist with a special interest in perinatal adrenal function. She is heavily involved in undergraduate and postgraduate education and has recently set up an online distance learning MSc Programme in Pediatric Emergency Medicine at the University of Edinburgh. She has published a handbook of neonatal endocrinology.

Professor Stuart Brink is the Senior Pediatric Endocrinologist at NEDEC (New England Diabetes and Endocrinology Center) in Waltham, Massachusetts, USA. He is an Associate Clinical Professor of Pediatrics at Tufts University School of Medicine and a Clinical Instructor in Pediatrics at Harvard Medical School. He is a Past-President of ISPAD (the International Society for Pediatric and Adolescent Diabetes) and has been ISPAD's Secretary-General twice in the past as well as ISPAD's current International Education Liaison Chair with current projects ongoing in Krasnoyarsk, Russia; Timisoara, Romania; and sub-Saharan Africa. He has served on the National Board of Directors of the American Diabetes Association (ADA) as well as been the ADA's National Chair for the Council on Diabetes and Youth. He was a co-investigator of the NIH-sponsored DCCT for ten years and also served on the American Academy of Pediatrics Endocrine Executive Committee and on the International Diabetes Federation's Youth Section Consultative Section as well as Youth Task Force. In addition to the AAP, ADA, ISPAD and IDF, he is a professional member of the American Association of Clinical Endocrinologist (AACE), the Lawson Wilkins Pediatric Endocrine Society (LWPES) and the Endocrine Society and is ISPAD representative on the Steering Committee of GPED, Global Pediatric Endocrine and Diabetes consortium. He has been awarded a Doctor Honoris Causa from the University of Medicine and Pharmacy of Timisoara, Romania as well as the ADA's Outstanding Contribution to Diabetes in Youth award and the JDF's Anne Woolf award.

Dr. Warren Lee did his undergraduate and postgraduate pediatric degrees at the National University of Singapore, and trained in pediatric endocrinology at the Royal Children's Hospital in Melbourne. He was founding head of the KK Children's Hospital Endocrinology Service (2001–2006), and the Adolescent Medicine Service (2006–2008). He was a member of the International Diabetes Federation Executive Board from 1996–2006, is a former IDF Western Pacific Regional Chair and served on the ISPAD Advisory Council. He was a Member of Parliament in Singapore from 2001–2006 and chaired the Ministry of Health Advisory Committee on Adolescent Health from 2006-8. Dr Lee is currently in private practice as a pediatric endocrinologist, and is a part time Senior Consultant in the KK Children's Hospital, while continuing diabetes educational activities within South East Asia, Africa and India.

Dr. Kubendran Pillay did his undergraduate training at the University of KwaZulu-Natal (Durban) and post-graduate training at the University of Cape Town. He was a visiting fellow at the London Centre for Paediatric Endocrinology (1999–2000). He was a founder member and Chairperson of the Paediatric & Adolescent Endocrine and Diabetes Society of South Africa (PAEDS-SA) and of the Sugarbabe Foundation. He has served as a member of the Advisory Council of ISPAD and as Vice-President of the African Society for Paediatric and Adolescent Endocrinology (ASPAE). Dr Pillay is currently in private practice as a pediatric endocrinologist and is a part-time consultant to the Paediatric Endocrinology Clinic at Inkosi Albert Luthuli Central Hospital. He is currently involved in diabetes educational activities in Africa.

Professor John Gregory is joint lead of specialist pediatric endocrine services in Wales, where he is active in providing clinical care for children with endocrine disorders living in south and mid Wales whilst also leading an active research programme into health services for children with diabetes and late-effects of the treatment of childhood malignancy. As a former tutor in residence at the Paediatric Endocrine Training Centre for Africa (PETCA), The European Society for Paediatric Endocrinology (ESPE) Officer-elect for PETCA and a tutor on the ESPE Winter School, he is actively involved in training the next generation of pediatric endocrinologists and has a passion to support the world-wide development of pediatric endocrine services for children. He has published widely in the field of Pediatric Endocrinology including joint authorship of *Practical Endocrinology and Diabetes in Children* now in its third edition.

Associate Professor Christa E. Flück is a Swiss pediatric endocrinologist who was trained in general pediatrics and pediatric endocrinology and diabetology at the University Children's Hospital in Bern, Switzerland. From 2000–2004 she did a postdoctoral fellowship at the University of California in San Francisco (CA, USA) in the steroid laboratory of Walter L. Miller. In 2004 she returned to Switzerland, starting her own steroid research group at the Children's Hospital in Bern with the support of Swiss National Science Foundation grants. She is an associate professor for pediatric endocrinology and diabetology of the University of Bern, with a half clinical, half research and teaching appointment. Her research interests are steroid disorders (including disorders of sexual development) and molecular regulation of androgen biosynthesis. For her achievements in research she received the Young Investigator Award of the European Society of Pediatric Endocrinology 2005 and the Theodor Kocher Prize of the University of Bern in 2007. She is currently a member of the teachers' team for ESPE winter school.

Dr. Chantal Cripe-Mamie born 1966, is a Swiss neonatologist, who trained in general pediatrics and neonatology in various Swiss hospitals. She did a clinical fellowship in neonatology in Cleveland, Ohio, USA from 2001-2004. She then returned to Switzerland to pursue her career in clinical work first in Lausanne then as of 2006 in Bern, Switzerland. Her main interests are nutrition and metabolism of the extreme premature infant and the growth restricted newborn. She is currently training at the University of Bern for a diploma in clinical nutrition.

Professor Angela Huebner is a Pediatric Endocrinologist at the Children's Hospital of the Technical University Dresden where she has been Head of the Division of Paediatric Endocrinology and Diabetes since 1998 and Vice-Director of the Department of Paediatrics since 2005. She graduated from Medical School in Dresden, Germany, with residency in pediatrics at the University Children's Hospital Dresden and the Department of Paediatrics at the University of Hamburg, Germany. She performed

a research fellowship granted by the Deutsche Forschungsgemeinschaft and the Wellcome Trust, UK in molecular endocrinology working with Prof. Adrian Clark and Prof. Martin Savage at St. Bartholomew's Hospital London, UK. Her research has always been focused on the adrenal gland, in particular on monogenic causes of adrenal hypofunction including ACTH resistance syndromes. Angela Huebner was appointed as Professor of Pediatrics in 2004 and twice received the Henning Andersen Prize of the ESPE society. For eight years she acted as the coordinator of the ESPE Winter School and is currently a member of the Website Editorial Board of ESPE.

Dr. Barbara Kind is a PostDoc. at the research laboratory of the Children's Hospital of the Technical University Dresden. From 1999 to 2005 she studied Biology, Molecular Biology, Cell Biology and Genetics at the Technical University of Dresden, Germany, then spent time at University College of Dublin, Ireland, finishing her diploma on telomerase at Technical University Dresden. She gained her PhD thesis in 2010, on the adrenal gland, working in the group of Prof. Angela Huebner at the Children's Hospital of the TU Dresden and now works as a PostDoc. in the group of PD Dr. Min Ae Lee-Kirsch. Her current research is focussed on defects in the innate immune system in autoinflammatory and autoimmunologic diseases.

Dr. Katrin Koehler is a Senior Scientist at the research laboratory of the Children's Hospital of the Technical University Dresden. From 1987 to 1992 she studied biochemistry at the University of Halle-Wittenberg, Germany. Here she performed her PhD thesis at the Institute of Human Genetics and Medical Biology concerning genetic risk factors of cardiovascular disease granted by the "Bundesministerium für Bildung und Forschung". In 1998 she changed as a postdoc. to the group of Prof. Angela Huebner in Dresden. Since then her research has focussed on the adrenal gland, in particular on the pathogenesis of the triple A syndrome. Her research is currently funded by the "Deutsche Forschungsgemeinschaft".

Dr. Michele O'Connell is a pediatrician from Ireland who is now based in Melbourne, Australia. Having completed her general pediatric training in

Ireland, Michele undertook subspecialty fellowship training in Paediatric Endocrinology and Diabetes at The Royal Children's Hospital, Melbourne and has been working as a Staff Specialist in this Department since 2009. Michele's principal clinical and research interests relate to the management of diabetes in youth and more specifically to the optimal use and application of diabetes-technologies in children and adolescents. She is also very involved in medical education and plays an active role in the under-graduate and postgraduate teaching programs at RCH and the University of Melbourne.

Foreword

Existing pediatric endocrinology textbooks and resources primarily serve the needs of health professionals working in developed countries, where sophisticated laboratory testing and imaging equipment, as well as optimal therapeutic approaches, are often readily available. They are ill-designed for the use of health professionals in low-income countries, where many health professionals often only have a vague idea of what "endocrinology" means.

Dr Zacharin should be congratulated for putting together this first edition of *Practical Paediatric Endocrinology*, a textbook that is designed to cater to the needs of health professionals working in a low-income setting. Together with 29 experts in pediatric endocrinology from developed and developing countries, she has put together a reference tool that covers all aspects of pediatric endocrinology through 16 comprehensive, in-depth sections. There is a special emphasis on the diagnosis and treatment of pediatric endocrine conditions when resources are limited.

Do we need a textbook of pediatric endocrinology aimed at low-income settings? Is it appropriate to direct scarce resources from developing countries toward pediatric endocrinology, a subspecialty that addresses medical conditions much less common than infectious diseases or malnutrition? Prevalence data for these conditions are often not available, but it is clear from local initiatives that diabetes and disorders of growth and puberty, sexual development, thyroid function, adrenals, calcium

and bone metabolism—as well as obesity and its complications—affect all populations around the world. Disorders of sexual development have dire consequences for affected children in countries where social and cultural beliefs require a clear-cut definition of being a boy or a girl. Fortunately, education of health professionals can go a long way toward alleviating discrimination against these patients. Pediatric endocrine conditions such as hypothyroidism, adrenal insufficiency or diabetes, if left untreated, are a significant cause of morbidity and mortality. Fortunately, they can be diagnosed accurately with good clinical skills and basic laboratory tests and appropriately treated with affordable drugs. There is an urgent need to deliver expert pediatric endocrine care to children and adolescents living in low-income countries. The importance of addressing the morbidity and mortality of non-communicable diseases in the developing world was recognized at a recent United Nations Summit in September 2011. This textbook is a first step towards providing children and adolescents suffering from pediatric endocrine conditions with the appropriate medical care they are entitled to, irrespective of where they live.

The influence of Dr Zacharin's textbook goes well beyond the diagnosis and treatment of pediatric endocrine diseases in developing countries. It will support existing initiatives that aim at building capacity in pediatric endocrinology in settings where these conditions go largely unrecognized. It will serve as a resource for the training of nurses, dieticians, health officers and other allied health professionals by newly trained pediatric endocrinologists. It will provide them with a tool to advocate for children and adolescents with pediatric endocrine conditions. It will also help them sensitize lawmakers and local public health authorities to the importance of providing patients with simple and relatively affordable drugs that are on the World Health Organization (WHO) Model List of Essential Medicines for Children (such as insulin, hydrocortisone and levothyroxine), but are often not available locally.

Jean-Pierre Chanoine
Clinical Professor,
British Columbia Children's Hospital
and University of British Columbia,
Vancouver

Preface

Although pediatric endocrinology is a relatively new speciality, the pace of change has been rapid over the past 10 − 20 years. Technological advances and electronic communications have totally changed not only the face of medicine in westernized countries but also the ability to reach, recognise, diagnose and treat health problems in the developing world. Along with medical advances, major changes in education and travel have enabled patients to seek advice from major centres and medical staff to access information and specialist training. Formation of new special interest groups and societies with international exchanges provide new options for the future.

Visiting and teaching in several developing countries over recent years, my colleagues and I have been enormously and consistently impressed by the level of knowledge, and dedication achieved under very often difficult circumstances, in resource constrained environments. An outstanding need appeared to be provision of practical guidelines for assessment and treatment of pediatric endocrine conditions for those working in these areas.

This book was conceived as an accessible and useful resource for pediatricians and other health care workers, aiming to provide clear diagnostic outlines and management strategies. Many experienced endocrinologists around the world have contributed to this book, several of whom have travelled and taught widely in the developing world. The resulting book was not intended to take the place of standard texts. It is intended to provide brief, up to date background information for endocrine conditions with an emphasis on diagnostic possibilities, practical low cost investigations and treatment where indicated. A guide as to how to access more sophisticated technologies where needed, is also provided.

Development of a broader knowledge base in medicine requires an ability to access and interpret medical literature. For this reason we have included a short chapter to serve as an introduction to basic molecular biology, so that the reader may better understand, interpret and assimilate an increasingly vast amount of complex information.

We have also included a chapter concerning research. Particularly in the developing world there has been a relative lack of knowledge concerning prevalence and incidence of many endocrine conditions, limited in part by distance, financial constraint and patient education to seek advice. We emphasise the importance of simple research protocols to help recognise these vital issues. Such research will inform local practice and in turn will provide a basis for accessing government support for future funding and preventative care. We hope that undertaking research and providing innovative care will also sustain practitioner interest.

In many places newly trained Pediatric Endocrinologists are returning to their own countries, as perhaps one of the first to practice in the speciality. Although knowledge may be thorough, clinical judgment takes time and experience. For this reason, we have provided a section with typical endocrine scenarios, worked through by different authors, to complement the clinical chapters and to extend and assist with development of this important aspect of medicine, whilst being mindful of possible burdens imposed upon families by possibly excessive expenditure on non- essential investigations.

Two of the most important emerging world-wide endocrine issues are obesity and both type 1 and type 2 diabetes mellitus. Particularly in the developing world with better living conditions and access to improved nutrition, both problems are increasing at a rate similar to that in westernized countries. I am grateful to Professor Stuart Brink for providing a brief version of his recently published book *"Basic Training for Healthcare Professionals in Developing Countries"*. My thanks also go to Drs Justin Brown, Michele O'Connell and Professor Garry

Warne for providing scenarios and helpful suggestions to improve chapters.

Other resources available complement this volume include an e-learning program accessible through the European Society of Paediatric Endocrinology at http://www.sb-elearning. org, and a *Colour Atlas of Paediatric Endocrinology and Growth* by Wales J, Rogol A, and Witt J, that can be accessed through Amazon.com.

We hope we have succeeded in filling a gap, to provide working knowledge and practical application towards pediatric endocrinological diagnosis and management, for pediatricians in circumstances where material resources may be limited and where the need to provide accurate and acceptable care to families is paramount.

Margaret Zacharin
Melbourne, December 2012

CHAPTER

1

Growth: Importance and Implications of Variations

Jaya Sujatha Gopal-Kothandapani, Indraneel Banerjee, Leena Patel

OUTLINE

PART 1: NORMAL GROWTH AND PUBERTY

Introduction

Growth is a complex dynamic process by which the body and various structures within the body increase in size. Normal growth results from the careful co-ordination of three cellular processes: (1) an increase in the number of cells or cell hyperplasia, (2) increase in the size of cells or cell hypertrophy and (3) programmed cell death or apoptosis. It involves tissues, organs, body parts and the whole body, and any or all of these can be affected when growth is disrupted. Although the term 'growth' has a wide definition, we have restricted its use to growth in height or linear growth for the purpose of this chapter. The growth pattern of a child and adolescent is a good indicator of:

- health and general well-being
- nutritional status
- disease activity and response to treatment of any underlying illness.

Commonly Used Terms

Interpreting growth measurements for any individual child requires comparing with reference values. The reference can be the child's previous measurements and/or those derived from measurements of a sample of healthy children in a population. For example, a child's height at a particular age can be compared with the child's height measurements at previous time points, if available, as well as with a height reference such as the WHO Child Growth Standards. The height reference may be available as a table or as a growth chart.

A histogram of height measurements from a reference sample shows a **bell-shaped** or **Gaussian distribution**, also conventionally described as a **'normal' distribution** (Figure 1.1). This is because a greater proportion of the measurements will cluster around the average and the number of measurements that are further away from the average are fewer. The **mean** is the average value for a bell-shaped distribution and **standard deviation** describes the spread of values. **Percentiles**, or **centiles**, represent the percentage of the population that falls below that point. Thus in a bell-shaped distribution the mean represents the 50th centile and this simply indicates that 50% of the values will fall below while 50% will be above the mean. The 3rd, 15th, 50th, 85th and 97th centiles are shown in the WHO growth charts (Figure 1.2).

A 'normal' curve with a mean of 0 and a standard deviation of 1 is called a **standard normal curve** (Figure 1.2; Table 1.1). The **Empirical Rule** can be applied to this, such that approximately:

- 68% of the values will fall within 1 standard deviation of the mean in either direction
- 95% of the values will fall within 2 standard deviations of the mean in either direction
- 99.7% of the values fall within 3 standard deviations of the mean in either direction.

Since only 5% of measurements from healthy children fall outside the range between −2 and +2 standard deviations, a height below or above this range is more likely to be abnormal than normal. In the absence of a defined cut-off for abnormal growth measurements, the probability of whether a measurement is likely to be normal or abnormal is useful in clinical practice.

Any 'normal' distribution can be standardised by converting the mean to zero and the standard deviation to one. For a measured value (e.g. height), the **standard deviation score (SDS)** or **z-score** can be calculated (measured value minus mean value/standard deviation), and then the corresponding percentile can be obtained from probability tables (found in textbooks on statistics). Converting observed growth measurements into SDS is useful in clinical research and allows comparisons to be made irrespective of age, gender and ethnic background.

Types of Growth Charts

Gender specific height, weight and head circumference centile charts are widely used in clinical practice. They represent age on the horizontal axis and include selected centiles for reference populations from different countries (Figure 1.2 shows the WHO length/height-for-age chart for girls). These are described as **distance charts**. The centile lines on a distance chart show the normal pattern of growth through childhood and adolescence. Charts for other growth measurements (such as sitting height and subischial leg length) and disease-specific growth charts (e.g. Turner syndrome, Down syndrome) are also available. **Growth velocity charts** illustrate the rate of change in measurements per year on the vertical axis

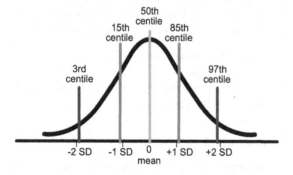

FIGURE 1.1 'Normal', bell-shaped or Gaussian distribution from smoothed out histogram of height measurements from a reference population sample.

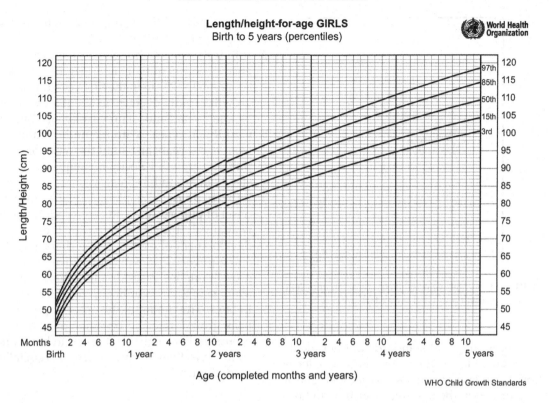

Length/height-for-age GIRLS
Birth to 5 years (percentiles)

World Health Organization

WHO Child Growth Standards

FIGURE 1.2 Length/height distance chart showing 3rd, 15th, 50th, 85th and 97th centile lines for the reference population.

TABLE 1.1 Approximate Relationships Between Percentiles and Standard Deviations for a Standard Normal Distribution

Standard deviation	Percentile
+3	99.9
+2.5	99
+2	97.7
+1	84.1
0	50
−1	15.9
−2	2.3
−2.5	1
−3	0.1

and age on the horizontal axis (Figure 1.3). However, they may not be available for different populations worldwide.

Problems can arise with use of a growth chart derived from different population data. Previously, WHO data were derived from the National Centre for Health Statistics (NCHS) standards from North America. The most recent WHO growth charts are derived from longitudinal growth data in optimally nourished children from six different countries, including those that are relatively underdeveloped. While these charts are not necessarily representative of undernourished children in developing countries, they aim to provide a common international reference standard, which may be adopted for use in countries

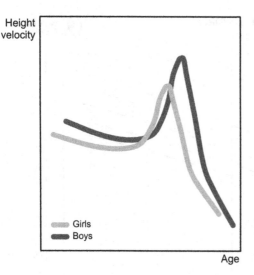

FIGURE 1.3 Height velocity chart showing the 50th centile for girls (light grey) and boys (dark grey).

where recent national standards are not available. If possible, the development of a local national standard should be encouraged. These standards should be updated over time to take into account secular trends and shifting economic and nutritional status in those countries.

Phases of Linear Growth

Normal growth is a continuous process with a predictable pattern. It starts prenatally and continues until the epiphyses at the ends of long bones are fused. The latter occurs when full pubertal maturation is achieved. Deviations from the normal pattern of growth provide clues to the state of health of a child and possible underlying pathology.

The period of growth can be subdivided into a phase before birth and three phases after birth:

1 **Fetal phase:** During this phase a single fertilised egg grows and develops over 9 months into an infant with an average length of about 50 cm. Thus the growth rate or height velocity during this phase is the fastest (approximately 70 cm/year).

2 **Infancy phase:** Although considerable growth occurs initially and length increases by about 23—25 cm in the first year, the rate of growth rapidly declines to about 9 cm/year by age 2 years and 7 cm/year by age 4 years.

3 **Childhood phase:** Through mid-childhood from age 4 years and until the onset of puberty, growth velocity remains relatively steady at around 5—7 cm/year.

4 **Puberty phase:** This phase begins with the onset of puberty and ends when adult height is attained. It is characterised by the development of secondary sex characteristics and a pubertal growth spurt when the peak growth rate increases dramatically to an average of 8 cm/year in girls and 10 cm/year in boys. The timing of the onset of puberty, peak growth rate and cessation of growth occurs earlier in girls compared to boys, and contributes to men being nearly 12.5 cm taller than women.

Key Factors which Regulate Growth and Basic Requirements for Normal Growth

Genes, nutrition and hormones have important effects on fetal and postnatal growth. Fetal growth is determined by the availability of glucose *in utero* and influenced by the IGF system. Nutrition, insulin and IGF-I regulate growth in early infancy and growth hormone begins to have an effect from the second 6 months of life. During puberty, growth is regulated by both growth hormone and sex steroids. Other hormones necessary for normal growth but which do not directly control growth are:

- thyroid hormones
- vitamin D
- insulin
- leptin
- glucocorticoids.

TABLE 1.2 Basic Requirements for Normal Growth and Examples of Conditions When these are not Available and Growth is Adversely Affected

Basic requirements	Conditions when basic requirements are not available
Happiness	Emotional neglect and psychosocial deprivation
Health	Any chronic illness
Nutrients	Malnutrition from any cause
Normal cells and bones	Genetic conditions including skeletal dysplasia, i.e. conditions in which bones are incapable of normal growth
Hormones	Hormone deficiencies or excess such as hypothyroidism or glucocorticoid excess

In addition to these factors, there are some basic requirements for normal growth and without them growth is adversely affected (Table 1.2).

Clinical Assessment of Growth

Clinical assessment of growth requires thorough:

- history
- growth measurements
- pubertal staging
- clinical examination.

History

A history from the child who is able to communicate and carers provides valuable information about their specific concerns, beliefs and expectations. The key components are presented in Table 1.3.

Growth Measurements: Anthropometry

For any growth measurement, repeated measurements over time are more informative

TABLE 1.3 Key Components of the History for the Assessment of Growth

- **Presenting complaint:** short or tall; early, delayed or arrested puberty; associated symptoms such as weight loss or weight gain.

- **Duration** of the problem and progress.

- **Past history:** symptoms associated with specific syndromes, hypothalamic-pituitary lesions, systemic illness.

- **Dietetic history:** estimated food energy and protein intake, history suggestive of vitamin or mineral deficiency, missed meals, lean periods, diarrhoea, vomiting, skin changes suggestive of malnutrition.

- **Medications:** prolonged corticosteroid treatment.

- **Antenatal details:** maternal health, illness, medications, alcohol, recreational drugs.

- **Fetal monitoring history:** ultrasound scan, fetal movements.

- **Birth details:** gestation at birth, mode of delivery, need for resuscitation, birth weight, length, head circumference.

- **Postnatal period:** hypoglycaemia, jaundice, feeding difficulties, floppiness, surgery in the neonatal period, unusual features such as puffy feet, hands and neck.

- **Neurodevelopment:** problems with speech, hearing, learning, vision, behaviour.

- **Family history:** consanguinity, mother's and father's height, mother's and sister's age at menarche, father's and brother's age at pubertal growth spurt and starting to shave, family members with growth disorders, known inherited or auto-immune conditions.

- **Social background:** parents' education, employment, income, stress in family.

- **School and social activities:** academic performance, behaviour, friends; physical and/or psychological impact such as bullying and emotional problems.

than single measurements as they show the pattern of growth and growth velocity.

WEIGHT

Infants should be weighed naked and children with minimal clothing using accurately calibrated scales. Weight should be recorded in kilograms and to the nearest 100 grams.

A number of formulae are available for estimating average weight for a healthy child by age (Table 1.4). The weight derived from these formulae is only a rough guide to the estimated weight. It is advisable to weigh accurately and to plot on reference standards, such as the WHO centiles.

SUPINE LENGTH AND STANDING HEIGHT

Supine length should be measured from birth to 2 years and older children who are unable to stand independently. Standing height is measured in children older than age 2 years who can stand independently. The instruments available for measuring length range from simple, relatively cheap boards, light portable measuring mats which can be rolled up to more sophisticated equipment such as the Harpenden neonatometer. For standing height, fixed wall-mounted stadiometers as well as portable equipment can be used (such as Minimetre and the Leicester Height Metre). The range of error is greater with wall charts compared to a stadiometer. It must be appreciated that even stadiometers may be susceptible to error. Error can arise from:

- inappropriate installation of equipment, positioned incorrectly
- incorrect use, such as faulty setting of the digital counter of a stadiometer owing to rough handling
- incorrect technique of positioning the child
- unco-operative child.

TABLE 1.4   Formulae for Estimating Average Weight and Standing Height

	Age	Formula
Weight in kg	Birth	3.5 kg
	1–12 months	0.5 × Age in months + 4
	1–5 years	2 × Age in years + 8
	6–12 years	3 × Age in years + 7
Standing height in cm	2–12 years	(Age in years × 6) + 77

A solid rod of known length should be used to calibrate the equipment. The most important aspect of measuring length and height is the technique of positioning the child. This remains uniform irrespective of the equipment used (Figure 1.4). Although height can be measured by one person, length requires two people.

The measurements should be recorded in centimetres and to the nearest millimetre. Whenever possible, serial measurements should be made with the interval between measurements at least 3 months or more.

INTERPRETING LENGTH AND HEIGHT MEASUREMENTS

A child's growth measurements should be plotted on centile charts so that comparisons can be made with the reference population. In addition, the child's height needs to be interpreted in the context of parents' heights (Figure 1.5). When possible, parents' heights should be obtained by direct measurement rather than relying on reported values, which are likely to be error prone. Midparental height is an indicator of the child's growth potential based on the genetic background. Midparental height is calculated as:

$$[(\text{fathers height in cm} + \text{mothers height in cm}) \div 2] - 7 \text{ for a girl}$$

$$[(\text{fathers height in cm} + \text{mothers height in cm}) \div 2] + 7 \text{ for a boy}$$

This formula is derived from children in the UK but is also applicable for children in other parts of the world. The target centile range is the standard error on either side of the midparental height. This is approximately 10 cm in boys and 8.5 cm in girls. The midparental height formula is applicable in those where parental heights are not wide apart. In those where maternal and paternal heights are widely discrepant, a midparental height may not be reliable as a marker of genetic growth potential. In

(A) Supine length – if child under 2 years or not able to stand

1. Infant measuring board placed on a firm flat surface and accurately calibrated
2. One person positions head correctly in contact with headboard
3. Another person ensures back and legs are straight and feet are flat against the moving footboard
4. Read length to nearest millimetre

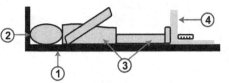

(B) Standing height

1. Height metre accurately calibrated
2. Flat surface, no shoes and socks; heels together, flat and against the wall
3. Shoulders relaxed, back and bottoms against the wall, legs straight
4. Eyes looking straight ahead and in the same plane as the external auditory meati
5. Ensure headboard is on top of the head
6. Ask child to breathe in; exert gentle but firm pressure under the mastoid processes as the child breathes out; arms by the side
7. Read height to the nearest millimetre

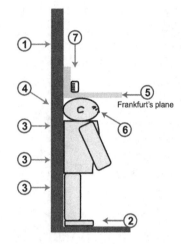

Frankfurt's plane

FIGURE 1.4 Techniques for measuring (A) supine length and (B) standing height.

such cases, the child's height usually tends to follow the centile line for either of the parents' heights.

Parents' heights are plotted on the right-hand side on growth charts as illustrated in Figure 1.5. As the charts are gender specific, subtract 14 cm from father's height to plot it on a girl's chart and add 14 cm to mother's height to plot it on a boy's chart.

Height measurements can also usefully be expressed as standard deviation scores (SDS), where a child's height is compared with the mean of other children of matched age and sex. It can be then used to compare children of different ages and sex. Height SDS is derived by the formula:

$$\frac{\text{Child's height measurement} - \text{mean height for age from a reference chart}}{1 \text{ SD of height for age on a reference chart}}$$

HEIGHT VELOCITY

The increment in height between two time points can be used to estimate the rate of change or height velocity:

$$\text{Height velocity in cm/year} = \frac{\begin{array}{c}(\text{Height at time point 2 [cm]} \\ -\text{Height at time point 1 [cm]})\end{array}}{(\text{Age at time 2 [years]} - \text{Age at time 1 [years]})}$$

The reliability of an estimated height velocity depends on:

- the time interval between the two height measurements
- the reliability with which the two height measurements are made.

The error in measuring height can be about 0.15 cm even with an experienced observer. Since an estimate of height velocity from

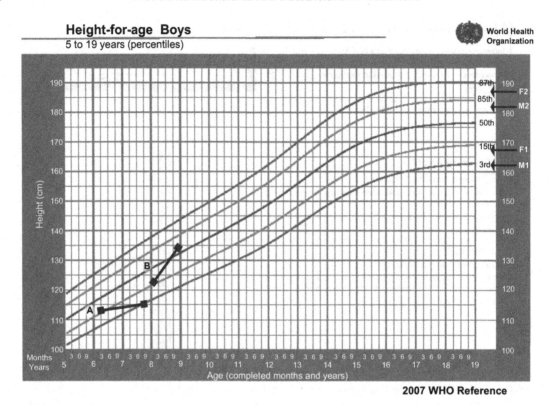

FIGURE 1.5 Height distance chart for boys.
Note: The reference centile lines as well as parents' heights are useful for interpreting the growth of a child. A growth trajectory that is parallel to the reference centiles indicates normal height velocity. Deviation downwards suggests poor linear growth (A), and upwards suggests rapid growth (B). The initial height of child A and child B would be considered appropriate for father 1 (F1) and mother 1 (M1) but short for parents F2 and M2.

intervals less than 12 months requires extrapolating, the error will be magnified. Thus the error is lower when height velocity is estimated from measurements taken 12 months apart and greater with shorter intervals between the two height measurements.

A child's rate of growth in height can be interpreted from a height distance chart and without a height velocity chart. Serial height measurements from a child plotted on a distance chart will reveal the child's growth trajectory. For a healthy child, this trajectory will be reasonably parallel to the reference centile lines on the growth chart. An individual's growth trajectory that deviates downwards from the references centile lines suggests poor linear growth. When it deviates upwards, the growth trajectory indicates rapid growth (Figure 1.5).

Obtaining records of past height measurements from additional sources can be valuable. These include maternal and child health records and records retained by the family from serial measurements at home. Parental observations of increasing divergence in growth patterns between children in the same family may also be useful for growth assessment.

SITTING HEIGHT (CROWN RUMP LENGTH) AND SUBISCHIAL LEG LENGTH

Sitting height should be measured when there appears to be disproportion between the trunk and limbs or if there are any features to suggest a skeletal dysplasia. An alternative to the expensive Harpenden sitting height table is a narrow table positioned against the standing height measuring equipment. The child sits on the table with the back straight and flat against the wall, shoulders relaxed and legs hanging loosely from the edge of the table. The head should be positioned as for standing height. Gentle upward pressure is applied behind the mastoids and a headboard lowered to obtain the reading. Subtracting the height of the table from this value gives the sitting height. Subischial leg length is calculated by subtracting sitting height from the standing height. The values for sitting height and subischial leg length can be interpreted by plotting them on corresponding centile charts.

HEAD CIRCUMFERENCE

Head circumference is measured as the maximal occipito-frontal circumference. A non-stretch tape measure should be used. It should encircle the head above the ears, midway between the eyebrows and the hairline, and over the occipital prominence at the back of the head. The value should be recorded in centimetres and to the nearest millimetre.

BODY MASS INDEX

Body mass index (BMI) provides a crude estimate of adiposity and should be calculated if a child appears overweight or weight is on a higher centile compared to height on a growth chart. It is calculated from weight and height:

$$\text{BMI in kg/m}^2 = \text{weight in kg} \div \text{height in m}^2$$

BMI should be plotted on age specific reference ranges, if locally available.

Pubertal Staging

Assessment of pubertal development is important when there are concerns about puberty and is also essential when there are any concerns about growth. There is considerable normal variation in the timing and pace with which physical changes and the growth spurt occur during puberty. However, the sequence of events remains fixed (Figure 1.6). Assessing pubertal status entails obtaining a history as well as physical examination using Tanner's stages (Figure 1.7). Enquire about the timing of events such as start of breast development, voice breaking, growth spurt and starting to shave facial hair. However, the history may not correspond with examination findings. Early breast development in girls and the changes in testicular volumes in boys are subtle and may go unnoticed.

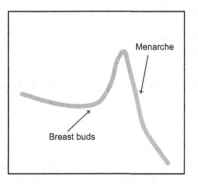

FIGURE 1.6 The sequence of physical changes during puberty in relation to the growth spurt.

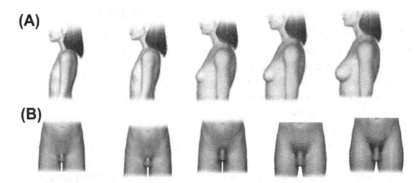

FIGURE 1.7 Tanner stages of pubertal development in (A) girls and (B) boys. *Reprinted with permission from Carel J-C, Léger J. Precocious Puberty. New Engl J Med 2008;358:2366—77.*

Onset of and rate of change of some features of puberty differs markedly between different ethnic groups. For example, pubic hair development in children of Chinese or Vietnamese origin can be minimal until an otherwise late stage of puberty, in comparison with a child of Mediterranean or Middle Eastern origin, where onset of pubic hair is an early feature of puberty.

Peak height velocity occurs relatively early in girls, usually before age 12 years and before menarche. Following menarche, height velocity slows down and the child reaches a near-final adult height in another 2 years. The average age of menarche in girls in the UK and in most Western countries is around 13 years. There is a trend to earlier menarche in most populations, the reasons for which are not fully clear. It is possible that an improved nutritional status may be partly responsible for this trend. In boys, peak height velocity occurs on average between 13 and 14 years. At this time, testicular volumes are between 10 and 12 mL. The later pubertal growth spurt translates to taller stature in boys compared to girls.

Clinical Examination

Specific growth concerns and potential explanations or differential diagnoses for these determine the focus of the clinical examination. Both general and systemic examination can provide valuable clues. For example, in a child with concerns about short stature, general examination needs to focus on:

- head, face and neck for dysmorphic features (as in Turner or Noonan syndrome)
- limbs, hands and feet for unusual appearances (e.g. Madelung deformity in SHOX haploinsufficiency or dyschondrosteosis; abnormal thumbs in Fanconi anaemia)
- disproportional length measurements between the limbs and trunk, other skeletal abnormalities suggestive of skeletal dysplasias
- weight centile and subcutaneous fat in relation to height centile (e.g. truncal adiposity in growth hormone deficiency)
- features to suggest deficiencies of growth hormone, thyroxine, cortisol or sex steroids.

In addition, systemic examination will include identifying any systemic illness, cardiac defects and neurodevelopment problems.

BONE AGE

Bone age is used to assess skeletal maturity and growth potential. Bone age is assessed from the appearances of epiphyses, usually from a radiograph of the non-dominant hand and wrist. Since epiphyses determine linear growth, bone age reflects bone maturation and correlates better with linear growth than chronological age. A number of methods are available for determining bone age. In the Greulich and Pyle method, using photographic reproductions of hand X-rays, the individual ossification centres are compared with published age-matched standards derived from healthy children. In the Tanner—Whitehouse 2 or 3 (TW2 or TW3) method, the maturity of each epiphyses is scored and a bone age is derived from the total score.

Bone age is an important component of growth assessment as many growth disorders are accompanied by a delay in bone maturation, particularly hypothyroidism, growth hormone deficiency and pubertal delay. However, the bone age results can be subjective and may not be accurate, particularly in those under 5 years of age. Nonetheless, bone age X-rays are readily available and serve as a useful additional tool in growth assessment.

PART 2: VARIATIONS IN LINEAR GROWTH

Short Stature and Growth Failure: Definition and Implications

Short stature can be a normal variant in some children and a symptom of underlying pathology in others. Although a height less than two standard deviations below the mean for age and gender at a single point, irrespective of a child's growth rate and/or ethnic origin, is frequently used as an arbitrary cut-off, this is not an absolute definition of short stature.

For an individual, the definition of short stature requires taking into consideration the stage of pubertal development, parents' heights, ethnic background and the growth performance of the reference population. For example, a child with height on the 2nd centile would be considered to be short if the midparental height were on the 50th centile. However, if the midparental height were on the 9th centile, this child would be relatively short for the reference population but not short for parents' heights. Conversely, a child with height on the 50th centile would not be considered short for the reference population but would be short for parents if midparental height were on the 98th centile.

Growth failure or faltering growth implies that a child fails to grow at a normal height velocity. This is independent of initial height and is not restricted to children who are short. By this definition, a boy whose height was on the 85th centile at 6.5 years and 50th centile at 8 years would have faltering growth despite both height measurements being within the 'normal' range. This pattern of growth is usually pathological and warrants careful evaluation. It would not be appropriate to make any sensible assessment of a child's height without plotting the midparental height on the growth chart and thus placing the child in the context of the family. Whenever possible, parental heights should be included in assessment.

School age children and adolescents who are short may have a negative perception about their physical appearance and may suffer more psychosocial limitations than physical disabilities. They can experience feelings of depression, anxiety, bullying at school and social isolation leading to behavioural problems, poor interpersonal skills, low academic performance and a poor quality of life. The physical impact of short stature depends on the aetiology and may include interference with independent activities of daily living such as opening doors, reaching objects, gaining access to public transport or even problems with walking if lower limb deformity is present. Some conditions may be associated with chronic pain which may further limit activity and increase distress. These problems need to be recognised and appropriate support provided.

Clinical Classification of Short Stature

Short stature can be broadly classified according to the dominant clinical feature (Table 1.5).

Epidemiology of Short Stature

A height measurement more than two standard deviations below the mean is only expected in 2.5% of healthy children according to the Empirical Rule. Thus, the shorter the child the greater the likelihood of organic disease (Table 1.6).

Clinical Assessment of a Child with Short Stature

It is important to consider common conditions in the population that may be associated with short stature. These include chronic malnutrition and energy deficiency in many developing countries. Chronic illnesses such as recurrent malaria, haemolytic anaemia, giardiasis and intestinal worm infestations should be excluded first before considering rarer conditions such as coeliac disease, cystic fibrosis and inflammatory bowel disease. Endocrine causes of short stature are relatively rare, but not impossible. These include examples presented in Table 1.6, such as growth hormone deficiency, Turner syndrome and glucocorticoid excess.

Therefore, specific history and examination in children with short stature should be focused on likely causes, as follows:

- Maternal nutrition, birth size and history of poor growth *in utero* (small for gestational age).
- Postnatal events: prolonged jaundice (congenital hypothyroidism, congenital hypopituitarism), neonatal hypoglycaemia (congenital hypopituitarism), floppiness with feeding difficulties (Prader–Willi syndrome), puffy hands and feet (Turner syndrome).
- A detailed medical history for features of chronic energy deficiency and chronic systemic illness, recurrent infections

(malaria, respiratory tract infections, urinary tract infections, gastroenteritis), blood transfusions (haemolytic anaemia), problems with hearing, vision, speech and learning; treatments such as corticosteroids.
- Family history of consanguinity, similar condition in a family member, parents and siblings' height and puberty.
- General examination: head size, body proportions, evidence of malnutrition, signs of chronic systemic illness, hepatosplenomegaly (chronic haemolytic anaemia), dysmorphic features, midline defects, visual defects.

SPECIFIC CONDITIONS PRESENTING WITH SHORT STATURE AND GROWTH FAILURE

Familial short stature and constitutional delay in puberty are the most common physiologic causes of short stature when nutrition is adequate and general health is satisfactory. They must be considered in the context of any short child presenting for assessment and may indeed be part contributors where a pathologic cause also exists.

Undernutrition

Undernutrition, usually secondary to protein calorie malnutrition, is the most important cause of short stature worldwide, is usually accompanied by mineral and vitamin deficiencies and is associated with pubertal delay, aggravating the problem of short stature. Its presence can be assessed as a low weight for height as well as low weight for age and sex-matched peers. Short stature due to undernutrition is complicated by zinc deficiency which alone can cause short stature and delayed puberty. It results in low IGF1 and has been considered as an adaptive mechanism for an energy-restricted environment.

TABLE 1.5 Clinical Classification of Short Stature According to Dominant Clinical Feature

Growth failure Endocrine disorder	Small for gestational age	Dysmorphic features in face and/or limbs	Disproportion between trunk and limbs	Chronic systemic disease	Apparently healthy, normal looking and growth rate normal for stage of puberty
Hypothyroidism	Normal or apparently large head (preserved head size)	Girls	Short limbs	Overt features	Bone age not delayed and parents short
• Growth hormone deficiency	• Intrauterine growth retardation (Russell–Silver syndrome)	• Turner syndrome	• Skeletal dysplasia: hypochondroplasia, achondroplasia	• Malnutrition	• Familial short stature
• Corticosteroid excess	• 3-M syndrome	• SHOX deficiency (Leri–Weill dyschondrosteosis or Langer mesomelia)	• Rickets	• Chronic infection	• Bone age delayed
• Primary IGF-I deficiency	Small head	Girls or boys	Short limbs/back	• Chronic renal failure	• Constitutional delay in growth and puberty
	• Fetal alcohol spectrum disorder	• Noonan syndrome	• Muco-polysaccharidosis	• Cyanotic congenital heart disease	
	• Fanconi syndrome	• Down syndrome		• Juvenile chronic arthritis	
		• Prader–Willi syndrome		Silent or asymptomatic	
		Boys		Coeliac disease	
		• Aarskog syndrome		Chronic inflammatory bowel disease	
				Renal tubular defects	

TABLE 1.6   Estimated Frequency of Short Stature and Organic Cause to Indicate the Scale of these Problems in Western Settings

Criteria	Frequency	Population
Height below 3rd centile	1 in 80	14,346 Prepubertal children at school entry in the UK [Voss. BMJ 1992]
Height below 3rd centile and height velocity less than 5 cm/year	1 in 20	114,881 Elementary school age children in USA [Lindsay. J Pediatr 1994]
• Endocrine disorder	5%	
• Systemic illness	10%	
• CDGP and FSS	75%	
GHD	10%	49 Prepubertal short children with height more
CDGP	8%	than −2.5 SD below the mean and referred for
FSS	0	evaluation of short stature [Moore. J. Pediatr. 1993]
Turner syndrome	4%	
Primordial short stature	2%	

Notes: CDGP − constitutional delay in growth and puberty; GHD − growth hormone deficiency; FSS −familial short stature.

Chronic Disease

Many disorders of chronic illness result in short stature and frequent but not inevitable pubertal delay. Those disorders associated with malabsorption in the upper gastrointestinal tract are more likely to cause slow growth, due to a combination of poor nutrition, necessary medications such as corticosteroids and to active inflammation with high inflammatory cytokines.

In countries where access to healthcare may be limited by distance, financial constraint or lack of knowledge concerning normal growth, other conditions commonly interfere with normal growth. These include cardiac disease, chronic anaemia and vitamin deficiency, chronic asthma, liver and renal disease.

Type 1 diabetes mellitus with chronic poor control, due to lack of access to or use of adequate insulin, results in Mauriac syndrome, characterised by severe growth failure, thickened skin and hepatosplenomegaly.

Coeliac disease may be a hidden cause of growth failure, with very few or no symptoms after infancy, other than growth and pubertal failure.

Intrauterine Growth Retardation and Small for Gestational Age

Most intrauterine growth retardation (IUGR) worldwide is due to problems of maternal nutrition, particularly in the first trimester of pregnancy. There are multiple factors operative, including protein calorie malnutrition, vitamin deficiencies, smoking and intrauterine infections. Epigenetic programming is now well established to occur as a result of maternal and feto-placental factors, with long-term and sometime transgenerational adverse effects on the fetus and child. Some of these effects can be delayed in expression to the second and third decade of life. A strong association is seen between past IUGR, metabolic syndrome and early ischaemic heart disease, diabetes mellitus, and hyperlipidaemia. Reduced fertility due to multiple hormone resistance may also occur.

The major challenge to be met is to reduce maternal factors predisposing to this condition.

Education and service availability need to focus on access to better antenatal care and improved peri-conceptual maternal nutrition and support.

Russell–Silver Syndrome

Characteristic Features

The Russell–Silver syndrome (RSS) is a particular condition within the IUGR range. The estimated incidence is 1 in 3000 to 100,000.

RSS is a heterogeneous condition characterised by some or all of the following features:

- severe prenatal and postnatal growth failure
- feeding difficulties from birth
- short stature and no disproportion between trunk and limbs
- poor weight gain
- hemi-atrophy resulting in limb length asymmetry
- normal head circumference and large forehead; head appears relatively large in comparison to face and body
- small triangular lower face, narrow chin, small jaw, downturned corners of the mouth
- clinodactyly
- pubertal onset at normal age which contributes to compromised adult height
- café-au-lait patches.

Diagnosis is usually clinical and can be confirmed by gene testing.

Genetics of Russell–Silver Syndrome

About 40% of cases are sporadic. Abnormalities in the imprinted genes on chromosomes 7 and 11 have been identified in some cases and include:

- loss of paternal methylation of the central telomeric imprinting centre region I (ICR1) on chromosome 11p15 which disrupts the regulation of H19 and IGF-II (up to 60% reported)

- maternal uniparental disomy of chromosome 7 and therefore absence of the genes that are normally active on the paternal copy of chromosome 7 (7%).

Management

Untreated average adult height is 140 cm for females and 150 cm for males. Growth hormone treatment is beneficial in improving childhood linear growth, where available.

Endocrine Disorders: Hypothyroidism

Causes

- Undiagnosed congenital hypothyroidism in countries where there is no neonatal screening programme: untreated severe congenital hypothyroidism is likely to have a significant impact on neurodevelopment and is unlikely to present with short stature in the absence of other features. However, in those with mild and previously compensated congenital hypothyroidism, short stature may be a presenting feature. Intellectual development may be normal if the underlying problem is of a lingual thyroid, where sufficient thyroxine has been produced to protect the brain in the first 2 years of life. In later childhood, thyroid function may become decompensated to cause significant short stature.
- Acquired hypothyroidism:
  - autoimmune due to Hashimoto's thyroiditis
  - iodine deficiency

Characteristic Features of Hypothyroidism

These include:

- growth failure
- relatively overweight for height

- lack of concentration and poor school performance may be present but the child may apparently be seen as a diligent student, conforming to rules but being methodically slow.

Classical features of lethargy, tiredness, sleepiness, cold intolerance, mottled skin, constipation, coarse features, hoarse voice, slow pulse, goitre and delayed relaxation of deep tendon reflexes are seen less commonly as is delayed bone age which may be severe if the hypothyroidism is congenital.

Investigations When Hypothyroidism is Suspected and Management

These include:

- blood samples for thyroid function (TSH, free thyroxine) and thyroid antibodies
- replacement with levothyroxine and dose adjusted according to clinical response and regular monitoring of thyroid function.

(See Chapter 3, Thyroid Disorders, for details.)

Endocrine Disorders: Growth Hormone Deficiency

Growth hormone (GH) is secreted from the anterior pituitary gland in a pulsatile manner. Its secretion is controlled by the hypothalamus through an interaction between its releasing hormones, GHRH and ghrelin, and the inhibitory hormone somatostatin. GH secretion is also regulated by insulin-like growth factor (IGF-1).

Causes of Growth Hormone Deficiency

Growth hormone deficiency (GHD) can be broadly classified into congenital or genetic conditions and acquired defects (Table 1.7). Although the aetiology remains obscure in many cases of isolated GHD, abnormal pituitary morphology may be seen on MRI (Figure 1.8).

Clues from the History that Suggest Growth Hormone Deficiency

- **Neonatal history:** hypoglycaemia, prolonged jaundice, microphallus.

TABLE 1.7 Organic Causes of Growth Hormone Deficiency

1. Congenital — associated with developmental abnormalities of the hypothalamus/pituitary, characterised by presentation in infancy or early childhood
Eye features such as nystagmus, squint, impaired vision: septo-optic dysplasia and optic nerve hypoplasia
Other midline brain and facial abnormalities: holoprosencephaly, single central incisor, cleft lip/palate

2. Defects in genes necessary for pituitary development and function
Isolated familial GHD

   - Severe short stature and autosomal recessive: GH1 defects
   - Moderate short stature and autosomal recessive or dominant: GH1 or GHRHR defects
   - Short stature with agammaglobulinaemia and X-linked recessive
   - Combined pituitary hormone deficiency
   - PIT1/POU1F1, PROP1, LHX3, LHX4, HESX1, SOX3, SOX2, GLI2, GLI3

3. Acquired
Tumours within the hypothalamic-pituitary axis— craniopharyngioma, germinoma, teratoma
Cranial irradiation — leukaemia, medulloblastoma, astrocytoma/glioma, ependymoma, nasal rhabdomyosarcoma
Trauma to the hypothalamus/pituitary — perinatal or postnatal
Infiltration — Langerhans cell histiocytosis
Central nervous systems infections

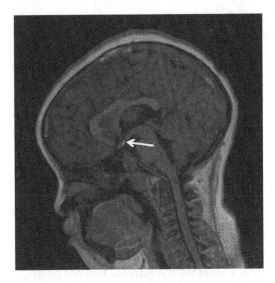

FIGURE 1.8 MRI scan showing small anterior pituitary, absent stalk and ectopic posterior pituitary.

- **Breech delivery:** a high incidence reported in retrospective studies, up to 65%.
- **Childhood history:** head injury, infection, cranial irradiation.
- **Family history:** consanguinity, severe short stature.
- **Symptoms suggesting intracranial lesion:** headache, vomiting, visual loss — up to 25%.
- **Craniofacial and midline abnormalities:** nystagmus, squint, visual impairment, optic nerve hypoplasia, cleft lip/palate, single central incisor.
- Other causes of short stature and growth failure excluded (e.g. small for gestational age, hypothyroidism, chronic systemic disease, Turner syndrome, skeletal dysplasia).

Clinical Features of Growth Hormone Deficiency

These include:

- short stature, frequently below -3 SD for reference population, but no disproportion between the trunk and limbs
- growth failure and progressive decline in height velocity
- high-pitched voice
- cherubic face with crowding of mid-facial structures
- normal head circumference and frontal bossing
- delayed dentition
- chubbiness with more subcutaneous fat compared to muscle bulk
- anterior abdominal adiposity with dimpling of fat
- small phallus (where gonadotrophin deficiency is co-existent)
- delayed bone age
- delayed puberty
- any associated features to suggest an acquired cause, e.g. visual loss, diabetes insipidus.

Investigations When Growth Hormone Deficiency is Suspected

These tests may not be available but an attempt to make a definite diagnosis of GH deficiency should be undertaken for the following reasons:

- to investigate for a possible brain tumour as a cause for pituitary dysfunction
- if there is any consideration for use of GH treatment.

Investigation with dynamic growth hormone testing should be considered when a child is short, below the 3rd centile, growing slowly, falling away from the growth curve, with a growth velocity less than the 25th centile for bone age, with associated risk factors as above and without any features to suggest a chronic disease.

If the growth velocity is normal and an IGF1 is normal for age-matched peers, dynamic testing may not be required. However, on its own, neither a normal growth velocity nor an IGF-I in the normal range would sufficiently exclude the diagnosis of growth hormone deficiency.

To diagnose GHD:

- **Single random plasma IGF-1 and IGFBP3 levels:** In the absence of undernutrition, low levels (below -2 SD) for gender, age and stage of puberty strongly support GHD but normal levels do not exclude it.
- **GH stimulation tests:** As GH is secreted in a pulsatile manner, GH measured from single random blood samples cannot be interpreted. GH secretion can be stimulated by exogenous agents such as arginine, which reduces endogenous inhibitory somatostatin tone. Glucagon injections may lower blood glucose levels and also have a direct stimulatory effect on GH release. Insulin is a powerful stimulant of GH secretion and acts by inducing hypoglycaemia. However, hypoglycaemia may be dangerous and hence the insulin tolerance test should only be considered if adequate medical supervision is available. Other agents that are less commonly used to test GH secretion include pyridostigmine, clonidine, levodopa and propranolol. Although useful, GH stimulation tests are never a 'gold standard test' and can be biased by false positive and false negative results. Peak GH levels can be falsely low in children who are peripubertal and those who are overweight. Children older than 8 years who are prepubertal or in early puberty should have GH stimulation tests after sex steroid priming (testosterone 100 mg intramuscular 3–9 days before the test in boys; ethinyl oestradiol 10 mg daily for 3 days is sometimes used in girls). Two pharmacological stimulation tests are recommended in patients suspected to have isolated GHD and one test in those with acquired pathology, multiple pituitary hormone deficiencies or genetic defects.

To identify whether GHD is isolated or associated with other pituitary hormone deficiencies, the following tests are recommended in order of usefulness to the patient:

- **Thyroid function tests including both free T4 and TSH.**
- A **TRH test** (measurement of TSH following injection of TRH) might help if available but is not essential for diagnosis. A low fT4 without rise in TSH will usually provide sufficient information.
- **8 am cortisol levels.** Similarly, a low cortisol without rise in ACTH may be helpful. The ACTH level is less likely to be available and is of less value. The standard dose synacthen test (measurement of cortisol following an injection of synthetic ACTH) can be used to detect whether the adrenal has not been stimulated for a prolonged time and is therefore unable to respond. It does not differentiate between primary and secondary hypo-adrenalism in the absence of an ACTH level.
- **Plasma urea and electrolytes; plasma and urine osmolality** in the morning after overnight fast (food and water) will define many cases of diabetes insipidus of central aetiology. The presence of diabetes insipidus may indicate a space-occupying lesion in the hypothalamic-pituitary area.
- **Basal FSH and LH** levels; and a GnRH test may be of some use in an adolescent or in early infancy but are of no value at all in mid-childhood as the gonadal axis is quiescent and stimulated gonadotrophin levels will be normally low. Time of onset into puberty and normality of pubertal progress as physical features are far more useful for evaluating the hypothalamic-pituitary-gonadal axis.
- **Prolactin** level might be of minor interest if there has been a tumour or radiation to the hypothalamus but is unlikely to be diagnostic except if a prolactinoma is suspected as the cause for growth failure. In rare cases, children with Pit1 gene defects may have very low prolactin levels.

To define the cause of GHD the following are needed:

- Neuroradiological evaluation with magnetic resonance imaging (MRI) of the hypothalamic-pituitary region: hypoplastic anterior pituitary, interrupted or hypoplastic stalk, ectopically placed posterior lobe (Figure 1.8).
- Where MRI is not available, CT with a request to focus on the hypothalamic-pituitary area may help but definition is less satisfactory. A lateral skull X-ray will demonstrate sellar erosion or enlargement, if that is the only available test.
- Other MRI findings may help define midline lesions. These include midline abnormalities such as: optic nerve/chiasm hypoplasia, which can be detected by a good ophthalmologic assessment. An MRI is required to demonstrate absent septum pellucidum and abnormalities in the corpus callosum, often present in the septo-optic dysplasia spectrum.
- Genetic studies in patients with isolated familial GHD, if facilities exist.

Management of Growth Hormone Deficiency where Available

Children with GHD need replacement doses of recombinant human GH (rhGH) (25–50 mg/kg/day or 0.7–1 mg/m^2/day). Doses should be adjusted according to the growth response and IGF-I levels maintained in the normal range. Final height outcome is better with younger age at start of treatment, longer duration of treatment, smaller height deficit at start of treatment and greater catch-up in height in the first year of treatment. rhGH is continued until near-final height (HV less than 2 cm/year) when GH secretory status should be reassessed to identify patients likely to benefit from continuing rhGH replacement into adulthood.

Hypopituitarism (Combined Pituitary Hormone Deficiencies)

Hypopituitarism or combined pituitary hormone deficiencies is defined as a deficiency of two or more pituitary hormones. Deficiency of all anterior and posterior pituitary hormones is referred to as panhypopituitarism.

Causes of Hypopituitarism

The congenital and acquired causes of growth hormone deficiency (Table 1.7) can also cause hypopituitarism. Genetic defects that affect pituitary development and differentiation include mutations in the transcription factors PROP1 (deficiency of all anterior pituitary hormones) and PIT1 (deficiency of GH, TSH and prolactin).

Clinical Features of Hypopituitarism

The age at presentation and the spectrum of clinical features are determined by the underlying cause and hormone deficiencies. Somatotrophs appear to be most vulnerable and are followed by gonadotrophs, thyrotrophs and corticotrophs. Thus GH deficiency is most common and is followed by deficiency of LH and FSH, TSH and finally ACTH. The number of hormone deficiencies can evolve as the child gets older. This means that children with hypopituitarism can develop additional hormone deficiencies at any age and therefore require regular follow-up and re-evaluation of pituitary function.

Congenital hypopituitarism presents in the neonatal period often with non-specific (lethargy, poor feeding, poor weight gain) features. These include:

- symptoms of hypoglycaemia (jitteriness, apnoea, convulsions)
- jaundice which may be prolonged (unconjugated due to TSH deficiency and conjugated due to ACTH deficiency)

- undescended testes, underdeveloped scrotum and micropenis.

Congenital hypopituitarism can be associated with a history of breech or traumatic delivery. Some cases are secondary to deficiencies in embryonic pituitary transcription factors, as outlined in Table 1.8.

A particular form of hypopituitarism in early life is septo-optic dysplasia. Unlike congenital hypopituitarism, children with septo-optic dysplasia may develop central diabetes insipidus and are therefore prone to dehydration and hypernatraemia. The spectrum and severity of clinical features is wide and includes the following.

- Optic nerve hypoplasia — this is identified by ophthalmoscopy. The eye manifestations range from normal vision to total blindness and can be associated with nystagmus and squint. The intracranial part of the optic nerve is best visualised on MRI scanning.
- Pituitary hormone deficiencies — these are more likely in children with anatomical abnormalities of the pituitary gland and other structures in the brain including the corpus callosum and septum pellucidum.
- Other midline brain abnormalities (thin corpus callosum and absent septum pellucidum).

- Epilepsy — due to a more global brain abnormality in severe septo-optic dysplasia.

During childhood, hypopituitarism should be suspected in any child with poor linear growth and clinical features suggestive of hypothyroidism with or without adrenal insufficiency. An additional clue during adolescence is delayed puberty. Craniopharyngiomas are the commonest hypothalamic tumours of childhood that cause hypopituitarism. They are developmental tumours which arise from remnants of the Rathke's pouch and are characteristically slow growing. They usually present in school-age children and teenagers but can present at any age. The clinical features of craniopharyngiomas and other tumours close to the pituitary and hypothalamus are due to:

- compression of the pituitary gland and thus pituitary hormone deficiencies
- compression of the hypothalamus — disturbance of appetite and excessive weight gain; hypothalamic dysfunction can also contribute to pituitary hormone deficiencies
- compression of optic chiasm with defects in visual fields and visual acuity
- raised intracranial pressure — morning headaches, vomiting and cranial nerve palsy (6th nerve).

TABLE 1.8   Clinical Classification of GH Insensitivity

1. Congenital GH insensitivity		2. Acquired GH insensitivity
Normal birth weight and normal head circumference	Small for gestational age, small head	- Malnutrition
GH receptor defects		- Chronic inflammation
- Low GHBP: mutation in extracellular domain	- Low IGF-I and learning difficulties: IGF-I gene defects	- Liver disease and other chronic systemic diseases
- Normal or high GHBP: mutation in intracellular domain	- High IGF-I: IGF-I receptor defects	- Severe infections
GH signalling defects		
- STAT5B		
- Noonan syndrome: PTPN11		

Investigations for Suspected Hypopituitarism

Depending on the availability of laboratory and radiological facilities, investigations should be directed to:

- assess the spectrum of anterior and posterior pituitary hormone deficiencies (see section on growth hormone deficiency)
- identify intracranial pathology and anatomical abnormalities of the pituitary and brain.

Management of Hypopituitarism

The principles of management of hypopituitarism are to:

- replace the hormones that are deficient and
- treat the underlying cause (such as a tumour) when possible.

When there are multiple pituitary hormone deficiencies, glucocorticoid replacement must be prioritised before replacing thyroxine and growth hormone. For guidance on hormone replacement, see the sections on GH deficiency, gonadotrophin deficiency, hypothyroidism, adrenal insufficiency and central diabetes insipidus.

Growth Hormone Insensitivity

Definition

Children with congenital GH insensitivity are exceptionally short and have clinical features similar to GHD. However, they differ from GHD in that they have high GH levels to stimulation tests. They do not respond to GH treatment and the availability of recombinant human IGF-I makes this the treatment of choice.

Classification of GH Insensitivity Based on Clinical and Biochemical Features

GH insensitivity can be either congenital or acquired (Table 1.8).

Cushing Syndrome

The mechanisms by which excess exogenous or endogenous corticosteroids lead to growth impairment are complex and include disruption of the GH–IGF axis at various levels, direct effects on the epiphyseal growth plate, and inhibitory effects on gonadotrophin secretion and adrenal steroid production.

Causes

- **Exogenous:** iatrogenic secondary to long-term treatment with pharmacological doses of corticosteroids as immunosuppressive and anti-inflammatory agents, for example for asthma and nephrotic syndrome.
- **Endogenous:** adrenal pathology, excess pituitary ACTH secretion (Cushing's disease) and non-pituitary ectopic ACTH syndrome – all rare in childhood.

Characteristic Features of Cushing Syndrome

These include growth failure, excessive weight gain and obesity, tiredness, lack of energy, behaviour and sleep problems, truncal obesity and nuchal fat pad, rounded plethoric face, thin skin, striae, easy bruising, hirsutism, hypertension, proximal muscle weakness and delayed motor milestones, delayed bone age, osteopaenia.

The diagnosis of Cushing syndrome is reliant on the demonstration of excess cortisol secretion due to altered circadian rhythmicity. In addition, in children with Cushing's disease, where the lesion is due to a pituitary adenoma, ACTH levels are high, but suppressible with high-dose dexamethasone. The specific investigations for Cushing syndrome are outlined elsewhere in this book. (*See Chapter 4, Adrenal Disorders.*)

Management of Cushing Syndrome

Management depends on the cause of Cushing syndrome and includes both medical and surgical options. Specialist advice is recommended.

Turner Syndrome

All girls with Turner syndrome do not have the classical textbook features. Therefore Turner syndrome should be considered in any girl presenting with short stature as well as in any adolescent girl presenting with delayed or arrested puberty. The diagnosis of Turner syndrome is confirmed by peripheral blood lymphocyte karyotyping. The estimated incidence is 1 in 2500 live female births and therefore relatively common.

Treatment with growth hormone is beneficial in improving adult height. A woman with Turner syndrome is on average 20 cm shorter than other adult women and untreated final adult height is 136−147 cm.

(See Chapter 2, Puberty, for details.)

Noonan Syndrome

Characteristic Clinical Features

Some of the characteristic clinical features of Noonan syndrome resemble Turner syndrome. However, Noonan syndrome affects boys as well as girls. The estimated incidence is 1 in 1000 to 2500 live births.

Features include:

- short stature and growth failure
- delayed puberty
- facial dysmorphism with ptosis, hypertelorism, downward-slanting eyes, low-set abnormal ears, grooved philtrum, broad nasal tip
- neck webbing
- pectus carinatum often with combined pectus excavatum
- cardiac abnormalities: pulmonary valve stenosis (PS), atrial septal defect (ASD), ventricular septal defect (VSD), patent ductus arteriosus (PDA), hypertrophic cardiomyopathy
- undescended testes
- mild learning difficulties which are sometimes due to or compounded by unrecognised hearing or visual problems
- bleeding tendency due to one or more defects of the coagulation cascade important.

The genetics of Noonan Syndrome

Mutations in a number of genes on different chromosomes have been identified in children with Noonan syndrome. The most common defect is found in the PTPN11 gene on chromosome 12q and is inherited as autosomal dominant. Other genes involved include:

- KRAS − more severe form of the disease
- RAF1 − dilated cardiomyopathy
- SOS1 − heart defects
- NFNS − neurofibromatosis-like features.

Management

The diagnosis is essentially clinical. Genetic testing, where available, can provide confirmation. Growth hormone treatment can be used to improve linear growth in childhood but has little effect on adult height achieved. Some studies suggest modest increments in height in the short term. However, long-term studies do not show convincing evidence to justify growth hormone treatment in children with Noonan syndrome. Moreover, some forms of the Noonan syndrome spectrum, such as Costello syndrome, are prone to malignancy. In such cases, growth hormone treatment may not be advisable.

Recognition and identification of a bleeding disorder is important particularly in girls with Noonan syndrome. The problems are of oozing blood loss in an exposed area of tissue such as after tooth extraction or birth. Postpartum haemorrhage is common and may result in the need for an emergency hysterectomy. These problems may be avoided if prior diagnosis of a bleeding disorder has been established.

Prader—Willi Syndrome

Characteristic Clinical Features

The estimated incidence is 1 in 15,000 and 1 in 25,000 live births. Features include:

- short stature
- floppiness and feeding difficulties from birth and necessitating nasogastric tube feeding in infancy
- failure to thrive infancy
- voracious appetite emerges in childhood between age 2 and 8 years. This is due to an abnormality in the secretion of ghrelin from the stomach. Ghrelin stimulates appetite and GH secretion.
- progressive obesity with greater fat mass compared to lean mass
- sleep disorders
- characteristic facial appearance with almond-shaped eyes and fair hair
- small hands and feet
- mild learning difficulties
- speech delay
- behavioural problems including skin self-mutilation
- scoliosis
- small penis and undescended testes
- delayed puberty.

The Genetics of Prader-Willi Syndrome

A number of genes in the region 15q11-q13 are affected in Prader—Willi syndrome. Normally, the paternal inherited genes in this region are functioning and maternal genes are switched off (this is called genomic imprinting). The paternally derived genes can be affected in a number of ways:

- deletion of the critical part of the paternally derived chromosome — 70% of cases

- maternal uniparental disomy when both copies of chromosome 15 are inherited from the mother — 25% of cases
- imprinting defect inherited from the father which affects functioning of the paternal genes — 5% of cases.

Management

The diagnosis is essentially clinical. Genetic testing, where available, can provide confirmation. Without treatment, average final adult height is about 154 cm in men and 145—159 cm in women. Growth hormone treatment can be used to improve linear growth and adult height as well as to normalise body composition.

3-M Syndrome

Characteristic Features

3-M syndrome is an autosomal recessive primordial growth disorder characterised by prenatal and post growth restriction, significant short stature, facial dysmorphism and prominent heels.

Genetics of 3-M Syndrome

A significant proportion of children with 3-M syndrome have a genetic aetiology — genes such as CUL7 and OBSL1, in growth hormone signalling pathways, have been implicated.

Management

Children with 3-M syndrome have relative GH insensitivity with normal GH levels to stimulation tests and relatively low IGF-I levels. There is no significant improvement in linear growth with growth hormone treatment.

Skeletal Dysplasias

A skeletal dysplasia should be suspected in patients who have disproportionate short stature with unusually short limbs or short trunk and a positive family history. The skeletal dysplasias are broadly classified based on the region of bone involved such as epiphysis, metaphysis and diaphysis.

Hypochondroplasia and **achondroplasia** are most common. These children grow normally but fail to have a normal pubertal growth spurt despite appropriate pubertal development. A sitting and standing height along with full skeletal survey should be undertaken to confirm diagnosis. There is no significant improvement in linear growth with growth hormone treatment.

TALL STATURE

Definition and Implications

As for short stature, the definition of tall stature is relative. Children who are above 99.6th centile and/or above their parental target centile range are considered exceptionally tall for the reference population. Tall stature can have significant psychosocial impact leading to low self-esteem, depression, social isolation and bullying. However, social perceptions around tall stature are not as negative as for short stature and in general it appears to arouse considerably less anxiety among individuals and their families.

Some children who are very tall in early childhood may have advanced bone age with a normal adult height outcome.

Assessment of any child who is unusually tall for his or her family must consider pathologic causes of excessive growth rate.

Clinical Classification of Tall Stature

Tall stature can be classified according to the dominant clinical features as shown in Table 1.9.

Clinical Assessment of a Child with Tall Stature

In addition to the history and examination detailed in Part 1, specific features useful in the assessment of a child with tall stature include arm span, sitting and standing height, height velocity and pubertal staging.

Management of Tall Stature

Investigations and treatment should be tailored according to the clinical diagnosis. Although high-dose oestrogen for girls and high-dose testosterone for boys has been used to attenuate final height in pubertal age

TABLE 1.9 Clinical Classification of Tall Stature

Tall and normal height velocity	Tall and increased height velocity	Dysmorphic features and no disproportion between trunk and limbs	Characteristic features and relatively long limbs
• Familial tall stature if parents tall • Obesity	• Precocious puberty if prepubertal age group and signs of puberty present • Hyperthyroidism • Familial glucocorticoid deficiency • GH excess (very rare)	• Asymmetrical overgrowth: Beckwith–Wiedemann syndrome • Symmetrical overgrowth: Sotos syndrome	Autosomal dominant, characteristic features and normal intelligence • Marfan syndrome Learning and behaviour problems • Klinefelter syndrome • XYY boys • Homocystinuria Anosmia • Gonadotrophin deficiency

children, the side effects and possible adverse late effects of therapy should be borne in mind as these may outweigh the benefits. Many centres no longer offer treatment for tall stature, solely to hasten epiphyseal closure, although there may be individual exceptions.

SPECIFIC CONDITIONS PRESENTING WITH TALL STATURE

Idiopathic or Familial Tall Stature

Characteristics include:

- commonest cause of tall stature
- one or both parents are tall
- the child's height is within the parental target centile
- bone age corresponds to the chronological age
- concordant pubertal growth.

Exogenous Obesity

In general, a child with exogenous obesity will be tall compared to the midparental expectation but will have an advanced bone age, with relatively early puberty resulting in normalisation of adult height. Judicious weight reduction usually slows growth rate.

Endocrine Conditions

Precocious Puberty

Sudden onset of abnormal growth acceleration in comparison with siblings and peers, combined with pubertal changes, provides a diagnosis. Advanced bone age will variably reduce final height.

Growth Hormone Excess

This is very rare in childhood, perhaps less so when associated with the McCune–Albright syndrome. If an affected child has significant facial changes due to sphenoid wing fibrous dysplasia and/or when gonadotrophin independent precocious puberty is also present, onset of GH excess can be extremely difficult to detect clinically. A high index of suspicion together with IGF1 levels and a glucose tolerance test to measure growth hormone levels are required, for diagnosis.

Klinefelter Syndrome

This may be suspected in a child who has learning problems, social isolation, testicular maldescent or in an adolescent with pubertal failure or arrest gynaecomastia or behavioural problems. Unusually tall stature within the family may be seen.

(See Chapter 2, Puberty, for details.)

Marfan Syndrome

This should be suspected when there is an unusually tall child in a family, with some of the following features:

- A family history of early death or lens dislocation should be sought.
- Clinical assessment of arm span greater than 5 cm more than the height, lower segment greater than the upper segment, long slender fingers, upward and outwards dislocated lens, high arched palate and pectus excavatum or carinatum, among others.
- An important component of Marfan syndrome is aortic root widening, which has a high risk for aortic dissection with progressive dilatation.

Marfan syndrome is an autosomal dominant condition due to a mutation in the fibrillin gene (FBN1) on chromosome 15q, but genetic confirmation is rarely required. It is important to consider the diagnosis of Marfan syndrome in children with tall stature, as progressive aortic root dilatation may be prevented with cardiac medication, such as β-blockers. It is prudent to seek a cardiac opinion if Marfan syndrome is suspected but not all physical signs are present.

A diagnostic tool based on the revised Ghent criteria is available on the web site: www.marfan.org

Management

Management includes:

- annual echocardiographs irrespective of the cardiac involvement at the time of diagnosis
- β-blockers should be started for children to prevent aortic complications
- advice given not to take part in contact sports
- annual eye assessment is recommended for lens dislocation and or myopia
- orthopaedic monitoring and management are indicated for kyphoscoliosis.

Beckwith—Wiedemann Syndrome

Cardinal features include fetal macrosomia, neonatal hypoglycaemia secondary to hyperinsulinism, which varies from mild and short-lived to extremely severe, hemihypertrophy and omphalocoele.

Early diagnosis is important for hypoglycaemia management and for surveillance for increased risk for Wilm's tumour and adrenal carcinoma.

Soto Syndrome or Cerebral Gigantism

This is an autosomal dominant condition from a mutation in the NSD I gene on chromosome 5q. Clinical features include intrauterine excessive growth, large birth weight and growth from infancy, large head and prominent forehead, downward-slanting palpebral fissures, high arched palate, a long pointed chin, large hands and feet, scoliosis, developmental delay, and behavioural problems including attention deficit hyperactivity disorder (ADHD).

Advanced bone age is present. Children with this condition may not be exceptionally tall as adults. No specific treatment is indicated.

References and Further Reading

Gluckman PD, Hanson MA, Cooper C, Thornburg KL. Effect of in utero and early-life conditions on adult health and disease. *N Engl J Med* 2008;**359**:61—73. Review.

Lindsay R, Feldkamp M, Harris D, Robertson J, Rallison M. Utah Growth Study: growth standards and the prevalence of growth hormone deficiency. *J Pediatr* 1994;**125**:29—35.

Moore KC, Donaldson DL, Ideus PL, Gifford RA, Moore WV. Clinical diagnoses of children with extremely short stature and their response to growth hormone. *J Pediatr* 1993;**122**:687—92.

Voss LD, Mulligan J, Betts PR, Wilkin TJ. Poor growth in school entrants as an index of organic disease: the Wessex growth study. *BMJ* 1992;**305**:1400—02.

Wit JM, Ranke MB, Kelnar CJH. ESPE Classification of paediatric endocrine diagnoses. *Horm Res* 2007;**68** (Suppl 2): S1-120.

Wit JM, Kiess W, Mullis P. Genetic evaluation of short stature. *Best Pract Res Clin Endocrinol Metab* 2011;**25**: 1—17.

Resources

The WHO Child Growth Standards. Available at URL: www.who.int/growthref/en/ (Growth reference charts and tables for length/height, weight and BMI for children under age 5 years and age 5—19 years.)

Puberty: Normal and Abnormal

Margaret Zacharin, Indraneel Banerjee, Leena Patel

NORMAL PUBERTY

Background

Physiology of Puberty

It is now recognised that there is a complex cascade of hormonal signals that trigger puberty and regulate its progress. These include input from central signalling through complex brain pathways, involving excitatory glutamate and inhibitory gamma aminobutyric acid (GABA)

neurotransmitter changes and modulated by nutritional signals such as leptin and ghrelin. At the onset of puberty, kisspeptin, a hypothalamic neuronal peptide, is secreted, which in turn stimulates gonadotrophin stimulating hormone (GNRH) from GnRH neurons in the hypothalamus. GNRH is secreted into the blood vessels of the infundibulum of the hypothalamus, to commence the cascade of pituitary secretion of the gonadotrophins, follicle stimulating hormone (FSH) and luteinising hormone

(LH). Gonadotrophins activate production of sex steroids, testosterone and oestradiol from the testes and ovaries respectively, and these in turn are responsible for the secondary sex characteristics of puberty. Although the HPG axis is active in early infancy, there is a resistance to sex steroid action. Therefore in normal infants there is no development of secondary sex characteristics. At 6–12 months of age, the HPG axis enters a period of quiescence and this lasts until adolescence. Anytime after age 8 years in girls and 9 years in boys, the HPG axis becomes reactivated to bring about normal pubertal development.

Although the precise trigger for pubertal onset remains elusive, our current understanding of peptide and hormonal signals is sufficient to provide a basis to understand aberrations in the onset and progress of puberty.

Timing of Puberty

The age of normal pubertal onset in boys or girls varies considerably, determined in part by genetic factors and influenced by many external factors, such as adequacy of nutrition, occurrence and severity of chronic disease processes and tempered by exercise levels.[1,2,3]

Over the last hundred years there has been a slow but marked transgenerational decrease in the age of onset of puberty in both boys and girls, and with onset of menarche in girls. This has been contributed to in a large part by improved conditions of childhood nutrition and general health around the world.

Consequences of Altered Physical Health

In addition to secular changes in health, medical management and outcome of many disease processes have radically improved over the last 20 years.

Longevity has improved for children and adolescents who have diseases involving chronic inflammation such as inflammatory bowel disease and vasculitis, and chronic infections such as hepatitis B, C and HIV. New managements and improved survival after childhood cancer and organ transplantation have all had a major impact on life expectancy, although mainly in countries where infrastructure and funding for medical management provide better opportunities for care.

Now that the immediate consequences of many diseases have been satisfactorily addressed, a more long-term focus has emerged, with the need for progression through puberty, maintenance of adult sex hormone levels and improvement in consequent bone health for this large group of adolescents and young adults. As peak bone mass accumulation is achieved by the end of adolescence, many conditions of ill health at this time are likely to have an adverse impact on the status of bone mineralisation. Therefore, puberty becomes a crucial point in optimising bone mass accrual for future adult life.

Bone Mass Accrual

Puberty has a major effect on bone size and mass. Just under 50% of total bone mass for life is accumulated during puberty in females and slightly less in males, making puberty a crucially important event for functional future strength and bone health. The presence of oestrogen inhibits periosteal apposition of bone, while increasing endosteal bone formation. This results in narrowing of the medullary cavity. Testosterone, by contrast, increases bone size by increasing bone apposition on the periosteal surface while simultaneously increasing the distance of the cortex from the neutral axis, by bone removal from the inner table.

The net result is, for a male, a larger, stronger bone than for a female with thicker trabeculae, to withstand any future impact, either physiological or pathological. These physical differences in bone size are the reason for the difference in strength in the adult male bone from that of a female and the reason for women sustaining fractures more often than men during ill health, although the rate of bone loss is similar for both sexes during ill health. The difference is further exacerbated in women through successive pregnancies, lactation and menopause.

Psychosocial Issues

Whether the time of onset and rate of progress through puberty is due to physiological delay compared to one's peers or whether a pathological process has caused the problem, disordered puberty can have a major impact on psychological and social health of the affected child and his or her family.

Concerns about altered body image or short stature in the context of delayed puberty can generate fears for ultimate height outcome and adult physical appearance, in both parent and child. This can cause much unnecessary anxiety, which has implications for emotional and social disharmony within families and for behavioural disorders in the child. In turn, these problems can spread to behaviour issues within the classroom, with a lack of understanding with school staff, contributing to poor learning and increasing social isolation.

CLINICAL SETTING

Physiology of Normal Puberty

Normal Puberty for Girls

Pubertal onset in a girl tends to occur at an age of just over 10 years, with a normal range 8–13 years. Onset of puberty is tempered by variation in ethnicity as well as general community health and nutritional status. For example, pubertal onset in African nations tends to be somewhat earlier than the same process in the Indian subcontinent. This difference occurs despite the fact that apparent levels of health and nutrition in both communities may be similar. Relatively poor nutritional status for some communities may delay the normal age of puberty to around age 14–16 years.

At about the same time that the HPG axis is activated in puberty, the adrenal glands start secreting adrenal androgens. This is called adrenarche and is responsible, in part, for androgen dependent signs of puberty, such as pubic and axillary hair, body odour and facial acne. Usually, adrenarche is synchronous with true puberty. However, the timing of adrenarche may occur earlier and ahead of breast development or testicular enlargement. This is called early or exaggerated adrenarche.

The first sign of true puberty in a girl is of breast budding. The onset of and progress of pubic hair varies markedly between genetically different communities with, for example, a much later onset of pubic hair in those of Chinese or Vietnamese extraction than in either African, Indian or Caucasian.

Although progress through puberty takes place in an ordered fashion, with menarche usually 2–2.5 years after onset, it is not infrequent to have minor vaginal bleeding at intervals just after the onset of thelarche. This is usually minimal and disappears after 2–3 months, as baseline oestrogen levels rise. It is reflection of fluctuations in oestrogen at the onset of puberty with erratic endometrial response.

Although this physiologic phenomenon is benign, persistent or regular vaginal bleeding prior to the physical changes appropriate for menarche should lead to a thorough evaluation for other causes of oestrogen excess, vaginal foreign body or sexual interference. Onset of oestrogenic activity is accompanied by increased vaginal mucus production, often a cause for parental concern and confused with infection.

Growth of the uterus and elongation of the vagina are accompanied by the appearance of multiple follicles in the ovaries, identifiable on ultrasound as a multicystic ovary. This is a perfectly normal appearance in an adolescent ovary and is not to be confused with a polycystic ovary, where follicles are peripherally located, greater than 20 in number in a large-volume ovary.

Normal Puberty for Boys

For boys the normal age of onset of puberty is just over 11 years, with a normal range of 9—14 years. Secular variations in the onset of puberty occur in boys as for girls, but the association with nutritional status seems less tight than in girls.

The first changes of puberty in a boy are signalled by an increase in testicular volume to 4 mL (measured with a Prader orchidometer) with rugosity of the scrotal skin and onset of pubic hair following rapidly, along with commencement of penile growth.

A growth spurt occurs in the later stages of puberty, compared with girls, where the growth spurt occurs in the first 12—18 months after pubertal onset. Spermarche, that is the beginning of sperm development in the testes, occurs during the later stages of puberty, achieved in many boys by age 14.

The normal variation in linear growth patterns between children of different sexes often causes major concern for parents, who may be unaware of such differences and who may thus erroneously believe that the short pubertal boy who is older than his pubertal younger sister has some form of disordered growth.

DELAYED PUBERTY

Definition and Implications

Puberty is delayed if the early signs of puberty are absent at an age when most other children are relatively advanced in puberty, i.e. the age of onset of puberty exceeds two standard deviations (SD) from the mean. Figure 2.1 shows the variation in timing of puberty in a population. The age at onset of puberty follows a 'normal' distribution with age greater

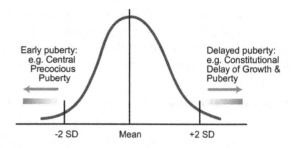

FIGURE 2.1 The timing of normal puberty in humans is normally distributed.
Note: The tails of the curve on either side represent +2 and −2 standard deviations (SD) from the mean as the limits of normality. Those entering early puberty at an age less than −2 SD are considered to be in early puberty, while those greater than +2 SD have delayed puberty.

than +2 SD at the right-hand tail of the curve representing children with delayed puberty. The specific age at which puberty is delayed is likely to vary because of the variability in the onset of normal puberty in different parts of the world. If we accept that most girls are in normal puberty (breast budding) at age 10—11 years, and most boys enter normal puberty (testicular volume greater than 4 mL) at age 11—12 years, then an additional 2 years for girls and boys would represent the age at which puberty is delayed. In children in North America and in the United Kingdom, lack of breast development by the age of 13 years in girls and lack of testicular enlargement by the age of 14 years in boys suggests delayed puberty (Table 2.1).

General Considerations Regarding Assessment

Constitutional delay of growth and puberty is the most common diagnosis in boys referred for delayed puberty. Girls are less commonly referred, partly because they have a growth spurt at an earlier stage of puberty than boys and perhaps because normal physical growth and maturation is more eagerly sought after

TABLE 2.1   Age Definitions for Normal and Abnormal Puberty

Onset of puberty	Girls	Boys
First sign of normal puberty	Breast bud development (not pubic hair)	Enlargement of testes $\geq$ 4 mL (not pubic hair)
Average (range) age for normal children	11 years (8–13)	12 years (9–14)
Age definition for precocious puberty	Before 8 years	Before 9 years
Age definition for delayed or absent puberty:		
1 SD	> 12 years	> 13 years
2 SD	> 13 years	> 14 years

by boys in most societies. Girls who are referred with delayed puberty often present at a much later age. Therefore in girls who present with delayed puberty, it would be prudent to investigate for an underlying medical reason for their problem, more so than in boys with delayed puberty.

The questions for a physician confronted with a child with delayed puberty are therefore to determine the following.

- Is puberty delayed or possibly arrested?
- What is the cause?
- Is intervention required?

Secondary considerations will involve the duration of intervention of treatment and the optimal method for management in any given case.

Assessment

Assessment of a child with delayed puberty must be put in the context of:

- parents' and family height measurements
- timing of puberty of parents, siblings and other relatives
- examination of the child for signs of puberty and evidence of progress through puberty.

It seems curious that the simple relationship between midparental height expectation and a child's potential height outcome is consistently underestimated by a majority of healthcare providers. Perhaps the most commonly omitted event in the assessment of a child with short stature and delayed puberty is the addition of the midparental height expectation to a growth chart. The height of the parent of the same sex as the child (i.e. mother of a girl who is under investigation) can be plotted directly onto the growth chart. The height of the parent of the opposite sex can be plotted by either adding 12.5 cm to a female parent height for a male child or subtracting 12.5 cm from a male parent for a female child. The target centile range is the range of height measurements, which represents the variability or error around the midparental height. In girls, the variation is around 8 cm on either side, while in boys the variation is greater at around 10 cm on either side of the midparental height. Unfortunately, where the heights of biological parents are unavailable, this important contributor to assessment is missing. Therefore, where possible, parental heights should be measured and if parents are not present at the consultation, reported values should be plotted, at least. In some cases, however, midparental heights are not meaningful, particularly when one parent is significantly taller or shorter than the other. Nonetheless, recording the parents' height on the growth chart is useful as the child of parents with significant height divergence usually tracks the centile line of one of the parents, which can be confirmed by visual inspection of the growth chart.

A predicted height outcome can be made when growth is plotted on a centile chart with the midparental height expectation carefully documented on the chart. If available, a maternal and child health record may help to assess the previous rate of growth and a bone age measurement may provide extra evidence for biological growth rate and thus of growth potential. A point on a chart is very difficult to interpret if midparental height is unknown.

The contributors to normal growth are intrinsic to any assessment:

- adequate nutrition
- growth factors: growth hormone IGF1
- insulin and thyroid hormones
- presence of sex hormones
- bones which are capable of a growth response.

GROWTH MONITORING

Monitoring a child's growth pattern with plotting growth on a growth chart must be part of routine assessment for all children. This provides rapidly accessible and important information about the impact of any illness or its treatment on the child.

Any deviation from a normal growth pattern seen on a growth chart may provide corroborative evidence of ill health. Often, growth may appear to improve with improving health, commonly seen in the context of malnutrition. Sometimes, the growth trajectory may have alternating phases coincident with waxing and waning in health or nutrition or both. The growth chart is a useful tool to visualise the impact of treatment of a child's underlying condition. It is useful to predict the likelihood of a child entering puberty at a normal age.

Patterns of growth failure differ, depending on the nature of the underlying condition. Likewise, the extent to which puberty impacts on linear growth also depends on the underlying condition. The timing of onset of any disease process and its severity is very likely to have a significant impact on the growth trajectory.

Failure to attend to pubertal disturbance in the context of chronic illness can result in a potential loss varying between 5 and 15 cm of final height outcome. This loss of height potential is often very distressing to the child and the family. Regular monitoring of growth and puberty may provide information on which to act, so that treatment choices such as induction of puberty may be introduced to alter the growth trajectory more favourably. Hence, assessment of growth and puberty at regular intervals is important in all children with chronic illnesses.

In all children presenting with short stature and delayed puberty, the foremost consideration should be whether nutrition is adequate. The total energy intake and in particular dietary protein content should be assessed for deviation from what is perceived as normal and adequate for the population. If nutritional intake is felt to be normal, the possibility of bowel malabsorption, such as that occurring with coeliac disease and inflammatory bowel disease, should be considered. Type 2 diabetes that is poorly controlled can also cause delay in growth and puberty. Therefore, physical examination of a child should be thorough and include signs of autoimmune disorders, vasculitis and other chronic disorders.

A number of hormones are related to the pubertal growth spurt. Abnormalities in such hormones have an adverse influence on the pubertal process. In puberty, the gonadotrophins and sex steroids potentiate the action of growth hormone. If growth hormone deficiency is present, growth may appear to slow down. However, isolated growth hormone deficiency is relatively uncommon at this age, and certainly so for a congenital cause. However, new onset of growth failure may present due to a midline space-occupying lesion in the brain, affecting the hypothalamus-pituitary axis. Therefore, in adolescents in good health and with adequate nutrition but with evidence of growth hormone deficiency, the possibility of a brain tumour should be seriously considered.

Although not directly related to growth, the thyroid hormones also have an impact on growth and puberty. While prolonged and severe hypothyroidism can cause precocious puberty, milder forms can be associated with short stature, but not usually with delayed puberty. It is therefore useful to assess for signs of hypothyroidism and the presence of goitre in children in the pubertal age range. Insulin like growth factor 1 (IGF-I) is a marker of the adequacy of growth hormone secretion. IGF-I is influenced by puberty and may appear to be low in states of delayed puberty. However, in any chronic illness IGF-I is often low, switched off by poor health and inadequate nutrition. While it is unnecessary to measure IGF-I as a marker of poor health, it is useful to understand the mechanism of growth failure under these conditions.

HYPOTHALAMIC PITUITARY DISORDERS (SECONDARY HYPOGONADISM)

Constitutional Delay in Growth and Puberty (CDGP)

Clinical Setting

Constitutional delay in growth and puberty (CDGP) is the commonest cause of delayed puberty.[4] Children with CDGP are delayed in the onset of puberty and are short. CDGP is not a permanent condition; a spontaneous growth spurt occurs later than usual with final height in the target centile range and genitalia achieving adult dimensions. Often there is a family history of delayed puberty or short stature in childhood in one or both parents, but not invariably so. CDGP is apparently more common in boys than in girls, but the gender disproportion may be due to the fact that boys seek medical attention earlier than girls for short stature.

Characteristic Features of CDGP

- Short stature during childhood and adolescence but with growth potential to reach a final adult height in keeping with parental heights.
- Height velocity normal for stage of puberty.
- Lack of signs of puberty in the absence of underlying pathology or chronic ill health.
- Family history of delayed puberty in the one or both parents or siblings is often elicited, although not necessary. It is often difficult to elicit an accurate history of pubertal delay in the parents. Late shaving is not a reliable marker of delayed puberty in men. Similarly, age at menarche in mothers is often open to recall bias. A history of being short as a child with late catch-up growth compared to peers may be more helpful, but by no means confirmatory.
- Delayed bone age.

Clinical Assessment

A family history of pubertal delay is helpful and a bone age markedly less than chronological age is useful as a diagnostic guide; however, these signs are not specific to CDGP. The parental complaint is usually of short stature, although the adolescent, most commonly a boy, is usually more concerned about lack of pubertal progress. Although not strictly a disease, CDGP can be a cause of significant distress to the child. Refusal to use a public urinal at school is often a sign of distress in a boy with CDGP. In girls, lack of breast development may cause similar anxiety. As a result, some girls may choose to wear clothes that conceal the lack of breast development.

Functional disorders of the hypothalamic-pituitary-ovarian axis are particularly common in adolescent girls and may be related to deliberate dietary restriction, with subclinical anorexia nervosa now affecting up to one in 10 adolescent girls in Western society. Intensive and prolonged exercise schedules, such as training for long distance running, gymnastics or ballet on several days every week, are all common culprits for pubertal delay.

Nutritional deficiency in conditions such as Crohn's disease and severe neurologic disorders such as cerebral palsy with consequent low body weight may also delay puberty, by switching off the hypothalamic-pituitary-gonadal axis, with cumulative reductions in linear growth rate, pubertal progress and bone health. Such associated features are usually absent in constitutional delay of growth and puberty.

Diagnostic Approach

Clinical Evaluation: Constitutional Delay in Growth and Puberty (CDGP)

CDGP remains a condition where the diagnosis is made by exclusion of other serious illnesses. It is important that a thorough history is obtained to assess the impact of chronic illness and long-term medication. Evaluation of dietary intake may be helpful, particularly in children with a low body weight and low body mass index. Puberty may be delayed in children in deprived areas with inadequate dietary intake. The possibility of food avoidance, such as in anorexia nervosa, also needs to be considered, mainly in girls. A history of anosmia may help to differentiate CDGP from Kallmann syndrome. Most importantly, a history of headaches, visual disturbances and/or polyuria needs to be elicited, as these are often features of hypothalamic-pituitary tumours, such as a craniopharyngioma.

The clinical assessment of children with delayed puberty should involve a detailed general history, followed by a thorough examination (Table 2.2).

Although CDGP is common, the diagnosis of secondary hypogonadotrophic hypogonadism due to brain tumour should be actively considered in every child. In girls with delayed puberty, Turner syndrome should be excluded. Likewise, in boys with delayed puberty, the possibility of Klinefelter syndrome must be considered. General examination should include observation of signs that may suggest underlying illnesses as well as those that indicate specific disorders. Examination of children with CDGP is usually normal, except for lack of signs of puberty. Sometimes, early signs of puberty are present, but progress is slow and effectively 'arrested'. In all children, accurate anthropometric measurement with growth plotting on a growth chart and careful pubertal staging are essential (Table 2.2). Pubertal assessment by verbal report is often erroneous and therefore not reliable. Nonetheless, in some cases, self-reporting of puberty may have to be accepted if the child refuses to be examined.

It is important to look out for signs of:

- chronic or recurrent infections
- cardiovascular or respiratory illness
- malnutrition
- malabsorption including coeliac disease and inflammatory bowel disease
- renal abnormalities including distal renal tubular acidosis, which may masquerade as short stature and pubertal delay without obvious bony changes of rickets
- visual fields and fundal examination are essential to consider the possibility of a hypothalamic tumour.

Pubertal assessment may occasionally be misleading, in the situation of a unilateral testis,

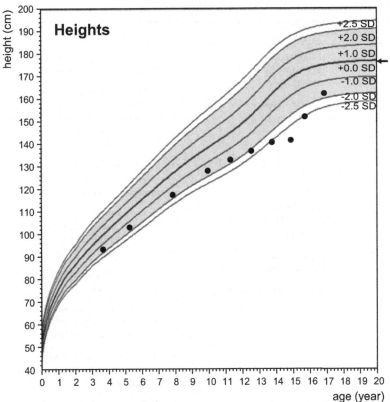

FIGURE 2.2 Growth trajectory in a boy with Constitutional Delay of Growth and puberty.

where previous absence or surgical failure to find a testis has occurred. In this case the remaining testis undergoes compensatory hypertrophy and may appear large and out of proportion to other signs of pubertal progress.

Investigations that will Yield Results Useful to the Patient, in Order of Priority

- Bone age − provides corroborative evidence of delay in puberty and reassurance of future growth potential; however, results are not always reliable and are subject to variation in reporting.
- Exclusion of underlying medical problems as above.
- Blood tests for basal or stimulated gonadotrophins and sex hormone levels in a prepubertal child are usually unhelpful except where primary gonadal dysfunction is suspected (e.g. with Turner or Klinefelter syndrome, where gonadotrophins are elevated).

- Karyotype, particularly when Turner or Klinefelter syndromes are suspected. In many countries this expensive test is now being replaced by a molecular karyotype using polymerase chain reaction (PCR). This will give an accurate diagnosis in most cases but will currently only detect mosaicism down to a level of at least 10%. Y mosaicism at low levels around 5% may not be detected by this method. If a clinical phenotype of Turner syndrome is suspected, a formal karyotype, counting 60−100 cells, may be required.

TABLE 2.2 Clinical Assessment of Delayed Puberty

History	Examination	Investigations
• Short stature	• Pubertal staging (Tanner staging, testicular volume by orchidometer)	• Karyotype (Turner syndrome, Klinefelter syndrome)
• Feels 'different' from peers	• Serial accurate height and weight measurements	• Pubertal response to a short course of low-dose sex steroids (response if CDGP, poor response in hypogonadotrophic hypogonadism)
• Poor self-esteem		
• Behaviour problems, learning difficulties	• Signs of malnutrition	
• Parental history of pubertal delay	• Evidence for underlying chronic systemic disorders	• Baseline pituitary function testing (thyroid function, IGF-I, cortisol, prolactin, electrolytes)
• Anosmia	• Visual field examination by confrontation perimetry (peripheral constriction in sellar/ suprasellar tumours)	• Dynamic anterior pituitary function testing (indicated if multiple pituitary hormone deficiency likely)
• Headaches		
• Visual disturbances		
• Cranial or gonadal radiation	• Fundoscopy for signs of papilloedema (brain tumours)	• Basal gonadotrophins (high in gonadal failure)
• History of chronic illness, prolonged medication	• Anosmia (Kallmann syndrome)	• Gonadotrophin releasing hormone (GnRH) test (low gonadotrophins in HH)
• Dietary intake — evidence of malnutrition, malabsorption or food avoidance		• Human chorionic gonadotrophin (hCG) test (abnormal in gonadal dysfunction)
		• Anti-ovarian antibodies (autoimmune ovarian dysfunction)
		• MRI hypothalamus-pituitary (sellar/suprasellar tumours)

Rationale for Management

The impact of treatment for CDGP is primarily for psychosocial and emotional benefit because final height, normal adult physical parameters and fertility are all likely to be normal. One should not underestimate the benefits of short-term intervention where indicated. The decision for treatment depends on the level of concern expressed by the child and the family (Figure 2.3). Sex steroids (testosterone in boys, ethinyl oestradiol in girls) prime the pituitary to release gonadotrophins, resulting in spontaneous progression of puberty. At low doses and in short courses, this treatment may be useful to augment growth, hasten puberty and improve psychological well-being. At low doses, there should be no concern regarding early epiphyseal fusion or retardation of growth potential.

Boys

ACUTE TREATMENT

Testosterone may be administered by various routes, preferably by the intramuscular route. One regimen is as follows:

Intramuscular Testosterone esters injection: 125 mg followed by two injections each of

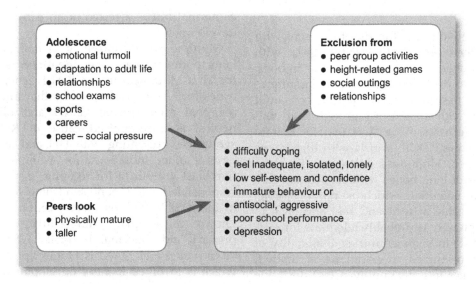

Adolescence
- emotional turmoil
- adaptation to adult life
- relationships
- school exams
- sports
- careers
- peer – social pressure

Exclusion from
- peer group activities
- height-related games
- social outings
- relationships

- difficulty coping
- feel inadequate, isolated, lonely
- low self-esteem and confidence
- immature behaviour or
- antisocial, aggressive
- poor school performance
- depression

Peers look
- physically mature
- taller

FIGURE 2.3   Psychological problems associated with delayed puberty.

250 mg, 3 weeks apart. This should suffice to stimulate the hypothalamic-pituitary axis, particularly when puberty is imminent, i.e. when testicular volume is at least 4 mL at the time of treatment commencing. However, if testicular volumes are less than 4 mL at first examination, suggesting that pubertal onset is not imminent, a second short course of testosterone may be required.

Other options include a slower introduction of testosterone, at 50 mg intramuscular injection (IMI) monthly for 6 months.

FOLLOW-UP PLAN

Treatment should be followed by review at the end of 6 months, for pubertal progress. Evidence should be sought for increasing testicular size, indicating stimulation of the hypothalamic-pituitary-gonadal axis. Further increments in testicular volume confirm spontaneous endogenous pubertal progress. Virilisation after treatment, without increase in testicular volume, is a reflection of exogenous administration of testosterone. Once testis volume has reached 8–10 mL, puberty is likely to progress spontaneously without the need for further treatment. In some boys, particularly if those in whom testicular volumes are much less than 4 mL, a second course will probably be required 6 months later, even if the diagnosis of CDGP is very likely.

EXPECTED OUTCOMES

Testosterone treatment for boys with CDGP is best given as short courses and continuous treatment is not appropriate for this condition. Continuous treatment, particularly with high doses of testosterone, will cause virilisation and bone age advance but will not have a desirable magnitude of growth spurt.

Reassessment should be made regularly for evidence of pubertal progress.

If virilisation occurs but testicular size does not increase in spite of two or more courses of testosterone treatment, the possibility of hypogonadotrophic hypogonadism should be suspected. In contrast, if there is absence of virilisation, no increase in testicular size but continuing acceleration of linear growth rate, primary hypogonadism, i.e. testicular damage, is likely.

Girls

It is relatively rare for girls to present with CDGP; therefore treatment for girls with delayed puberty is not as common as in boys. Explanation of the condition and reassurance that a growth spurt is due sometime soon could be helped with the aid of a growth chart and a bone age assessment. It is usually best to avoid treating CDGP in girls with high doses of oestrogen. High-dose oestrogen fuses the epiphyses of long bones with consequent loss of height potential, which is not desirable. Where possible a 'wait and see' approach to delayed puberty is probably adequate for girls with CDGP. In some countries availability of low-dose oestrogen preparations is limited, which makes intervention even less desirable (see section on HRT).

Isolated Hypogonadotrophic Hypogonadism

Hypogonadotrophic hypogonadism (HH) is characterised by delayed or arrested puberty due to impaired gonadotrophin secretion from the pituitary gland. HH can be either isolated or associated with other pituitary hormonal deficiencies (Table 2.3).

In the newborn period, HH may be suspected in baby boys with significant undervirilisation, i.e. those with a small penis and undescended testes. In girls, the diagnosis of HH is usually delayed until adolescence with absent or slow breast development and delayed menarche.

Isolated HH is relatively rare in children, and the diagnosis is often delayed until late childhood and young adult life. The possibility of CDGP needs to be considered first before arriving at a possible diagnosis of isolated HH. In boys with presumed CDGP who have received two short courses of sex steroids (each for 3 months' duration) but have persistently small testicular volumes (less than 4 mL), HH is likely.

Clinical Setting

Isolated HH results in failure to enter puberty in most cases. Occasionally, puberty may begin as normal but is arrested at an early stage of development.

Multiple genes controlling several hypothalamic pathways have been identified as causes for HH. Mutations in the KAL1 gene, which codes for a transcription factor that influences neuronal migration of GnRH and olfactory nerves, is a recognised cause of Kallmann syndrome, presenting with HH and anosmia. Several other mutations, for example in the fibroblast growth factor receptor, may also be responsible for Kallmann syndrome. Mutations in the KISS gene, G-protein receptor 54 (now known as KISS1R), intracellular adhesion proteins and abnormalities of the GNRH axis all can cause HH. DAX1 is a transcription factor which is involved in early development of the adrenal cortex and GnRH neurons; mutations in DAX1 can be a cause of HH in association with adrenal insufficiency.

Diagnostic Approach

Organic causes of hypothalamic dysfunction such as structural lesions in the region must be excluded. A relatively recent history of headaches, visual disturbances, fluid imbalance and arrest of puberty may be pointers to a space-occupying lesion causing HH.

An abnormal sense of smell should raise the possibility of Kallmann syndrome. Anosmia may occur associated with failure to enter or progress through puberty, or may be found in other relatives who have otherwise normal gonadal function. Anosmia is a typical feature of Kallman syndrome, although a few children with FGFR1 mutations may not have anosmia. In the absence of anosmia, the diagnosis of Kallmann syndrome is not very likely. In such cases, other abnormalities in hypothalamic gene networks controlling puberty should be considered as causing HH.

The diagnosis of Kallmann syndrome can be confirmed genetically, but gene mutation testing for this condition is not routinely available. In the absence of genetic mutation testing, it is

TABLE 2.3   Causes of Hypogonadotrophic Hypogonadism

1. GENETIC

Kallmann syndrome

Isolated gonadotrophin deficiency

Gonadotrophin deficiency in association with other disorders
- Adrenal insufficiency
- Genetic defects [NR5A1 (SF1), NR0B1 (DAX1)]

Pituitary hormone deficiency
- Septo-optic dysplasia
- Genetic defects (PROP1, LHX3, HESX1)

Other abnormalities
- Genetic obesity (Lep, LepR)
- Hypoglycaemia (PC1)

2. ACQUIRED

Brain tumours
- Craniopharyngioma
- Hypothalamic glioma/astrocytoma
- Pituitary adenoma

Central nervous system irradiation

Infiltration
- Histiocytosis

Traumatic brain injury

Post central nervous system infections: meningitis, encephalitis

3. SYNDROMES

Prader–Willi
Bardet–Biedl
CHARGE
Noonan
Down

4. FUNCTIONAL

Systemic disease
- Malnutrition
- Malabsorption
- Chronic lung disease
- Chronic haemolytic disorders (e.g. thalassaemia, sickle cell anaemia)
- Chronic renal failure
- Arthritis, inflammatory disorders

Anorexia nervosa
Intensive exercise
Hypothyroidism
Hyperprolactinaemia

reasonable to assign a diagnosis of Kallmann syndrome on clinical grounds. MRI scan evidence of absent olfactory bulbs is not a requisite for the diagnosis (Figure 2.4). MRI is usually performed for exclusion of tumour.

Assessment of HH

Testing for sense of smell is needed. It is not possible to rely on a patient report, because most who cannot smell think they can. A testing kit is a simple and effective tool to examine for sense of smell and may be prepared locally. This must utilise simple and easily identifiable substances such as orange, chocolate and coffee. Peppermint and pepper are not suitable as testing substances as they can be detected by irritation of the nasal mucosa.

Investigations that will Yield Results Useful to the Patient, in Order of Priority

- Basal FSH, LH and sex steroid levels — gonadotrophins and sex steroids are expected to be low, but are not diagnostic. However, unstimulated gonadotrophins do not reliably rise to detectable or elevated levels under the age of 10 years. Reliance on this test may therefore be misleading in children and a diagnosis of *primary* gonadal failure could thus be missed.
- MRI of the pituitary and hypothalamus with specific views to visualise olfactory bulbs, if suspecting Kallmann syndrome. The principal value of the MRI is to exclude secondary organic pathology.
- GNRH test, expecting to see no increase in gonadotrophins after stimulation. However, for some genetic disorders this may provide false reassurance because exogenously administered GNRH may be able to stimulate production of gonadotrophins while endogenous GNRH is entirely lacking.
- Basal levels of testosterone and oestradiol are not helpful in a prepubertal child.

FIGURE 2.4 Magnetic resonance imaging (MRI) of the brain (coronal views, T2-weighted images) showing (a) presence of olfactory bulbs marked by the arrow; and (b) absence of the olfactory bulbs, consistent with the diagnosis of Kallmann syndrome in a 17-year-old young person with anosmia and delayed puberty.

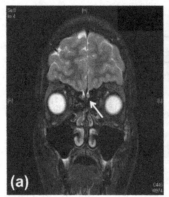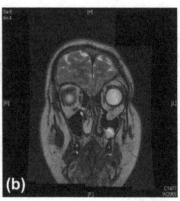

- Karyotype is usually of less value in the older child or adolescent who has low gonadotrophins. With the advent of the cheaper, accurate and rapidly performed molecular karyotype, this test is likely to be performed more frequently for specific diagnosis of many conditions.

Rationale for Management

The aims of treatment are to complete puberty, to reach adult height potential, to relieve anxiety and to optimise achievement of fertility where possible.

Boys

Where established gonadotrophin deficiency exists, it has now been shown that optimal outcome, in terms of spermatogenesis and future fertility, can be obtained, using gonadotrophin replacement rather than testosterone.[5] Prolonged use of testosterone in this condition may not promote spermatogenesis in adulthood.

It is well recognised that a small proportion of young adults with HH appear to have a reversible form where gonadotrophin secretion is established at a later age, after stopping sex steroid replacement.

Gonadotrophin treatment may not be available in all countries or to all patients, given its high costs. However, as fertility is so important in most communities an outline of both types of treatment is suggested here.

HCG and FSH

Human chorionic gonadotrophin (HCG) 500 IU twice weekly is used as a subcutaneous starting dose, administered twice per week, increasing slowly to 1000 and then to 1500 IU x 2/week, over around 18—24 months.

If the boy is at least 16 years of age, addition of FSH is commenced 4 months after the HCG reaches 1500 IU dose, and is given three times per week, as a subcutaneous administration, while HCG is continued.

Evidence for spermatogenesis should be sought with semen analysis, after 6 months of combined treatment. Once sperm are seen, treatment can be changed to maintenance testosterone until the man wishes for fertility, at which time HCG and FSH are recommenced.

Expected Outcomes

Gonadotrophin treatment has been shown to be effective in adolescent males, with evidence of sperm production by 6—9 months of treatment. Current evidence indicates that second and subsequent rounds of induction of spermatogenesis can be achieved in 5–6 months, thus permitting improved adult fertility outcomes for these men.

Sex Hormone Replacement

Boys

Where HCG and FSH is not an option, the alternative is to commence testosterone, using intramuscular testosterone esters if the boy is of reasonable height and of an age where he desires and needs rapid pubertal progress.

A commencing dose of 125 mg, increasing to 250 mg at 3-weekly intervals, can be used.

Once linear growth is complete, transfer to a longer acting, flat-profile testosterone preparation such as intramuscular testosterone undecanoate is preferred. This is only available in some countries but its use is likely to become more widespread. It is not painful even though a large volume (4 mL) is administered slowly. It provides more even release of androgen over 3 months, reducing mood swings and assisting with adjustment to the need for long-term treatment.

(See treatment of primary hypogonadism for more detail.)

Girls

As spontaneous pubertal progress is not expected, oestrogen can be commenced at diagnosis, assuming the girl to be at least 12 years at that time.

If other conditions such as growth hormone deficiency co-exist, some delay in onset of hormone replacement therapy (HRT) may be needed, to allow for growth hormone action and hence to optimise growth potential. However, contrary to expectation, prolonged delay in commencement of treatment may not be beneficial to final height outcome.

A similar regime is used for all types of hypogonadism and is detailed below (see treatment of primary hypogonadism for more detail).

Oestrogen should be commenced in a small dose (ethinyl oestradiol 2 or 2.5 µg day or oestradiol valerate 0.5 mg second daily) and the dose increased slowly, over 2.5 to 3 years. It is essential to avoid over-rapid increases in oestrogen dosing, in order to optimise breast development. Premarin® is very difficult to manage in sufficiently small doses, due to limitations on available tablet sizes.

Secondary Causes of Hypogonadotrophic Hypogonadism

Cranial Radiation

Clinical Setting

Cranial radiation at high doses of 40–55 Gy, used for management of malignant brain tumours in childhood, and occasionally lower doses (18–24 Gy) used in whole brain radiation, as part of previous leukaemia chemotherapy protocols, may result in evolving hypothalamic pituitary deficits.

Childhood cranial radiation between 25 and 40 Gy often causes disinhibition of the normal childhood hypothalamic restraint of puberty, with consequent early pubertal onset, usually about 2 years earlier than other family members. These children may progress through a stage of normal pubertal progress, to later gonadotrophin failure with pubertal arrest.

It is important for parents to be aware of the evolving nature of such deficits so that repeated evaluation on a regular basis is undertaken and pubertal failure is not missed.

Diagnostic Approach

- Assessment of height in the context of familial growth patterns.
- Careful plotting of growth velocity so that a combination of evolving growth hormone deficiency (slowing growth rate) with onset of early or precocious puberty (increasing growth rate) is not missed.

- Understanding that spinal radiation causes loss of vertebral growth capacity. Radiation in the prepubertal years can result in a significant loss of height potential.

Investigations

- Full assessment of the hypothalamic-pituitary axes, including growth hormone status.
- Primary or secondary hypothyroidism can both occur so fT4 and TSH are required.
- Bone age for growth potential.

Rationale for Management

The aims of treatment in this situation are:

- to optimise final height
- to reduce psychosocial, emotional and physical impact of hormonal deficiencies
- to improve bone health.

ACUTE MANAGEMENT

- To treat hypothyroidism if present.
- If growth hormone deficiency is present, this should be addressed if circumstances permit use of GH.
- Pubertal induction and long-term management follow guidelines as for primary hypogonadism (see treatment of primary hypogonadism for more detail).

FOLLOW-UP PLAN AND EXPECTED OUTCOMES

As radiation exposure is also associated with other hypothalamic pituitary deficits, ongoing regular pituitary function should be assessed, including growth and thyroid function. Clinical evaluation should take place every 4—6 months during time of growth and annually in long-term follow-up. Biochemical tests such as thyroid function should be performed when indicated. Once established, the need for HRT is likely to be permanent.

Chronic Disease

Clinical Setting and Diagnostic Approach

The course of chronic diseases tends to fluctuate, with periods of better health during which normalisation of linear growth and onset of puberty or progress through puberty can take place. However, with the relapsing nature of many of those disorders, pubertal progress can halt, particularly when nutritional status is poor. In addition, the elevated cytokines associated with inflammatory conditions, together with treatment regimes involving corticosteroid or immunosuppressive agent use, even on an intermittent basis, can cause deficits in bone mass accrual.

In the setting of chronic disease, onset of and progress through puberty becomes particularly important, in terms of optimising bone mass by the end of adolescence, to decrease cumulative lifetime fracture risk. A particular example is thalassaemia major, which requires frequent blood transfusion, resulting in deposition of iron in the hypothalamic pituitary area, with consequent pubertal failure and hypogonadism. In this scenario, long-term HRT is vitally important in order to maintain secondary sexual characteristics and to preserve adequate bone mineralisation for later life.

It is important to judge whether or not a child with a chronic disorder and delayed puberty will need induction of puberty.

Assessment of growth rate using a growth chart against midparental height expectation is useful to understand the extent of growth slowdown. The stage of puberty is helpful to assess if the child is completely prepubertal or if some advance in puberty has already occurred. The disease severity has to be judged to appreciate the depth and extent of likely influence on growth and puberty. Further, treatment with growth-restricting medication, such as corticosteroids, has to be factored into a composite assessment to judge the timing of pubertal induction, if required.

Investigations that will Yield Results Useful to the Patient, in Order of Priority

Follow-up repeated review of general health and evaluation of growth and puberty are key elements to assess the need for treatment of delayed puberty.

Rationale for Management

The rationale for sex steroid treatment is different from that for children with constitutional delay of growth and puberty. However, treatment regimens are similar in dose and duration.

Boys

ACUTE

Intramuscular testosterone can be used in a similar regime to that of constitutional delay, with 125 mg followed by 2 injections, each of 250 mg of testosterone ester, 3 weeks apart. This should only be administered in a window of opportunity when health is relatively good and growth-restricting treatment such as corticosteroid is low. If used during a period of ill health, it will cause virilisation without stimulation of growth or of puberty. On the contrary, if used appropriately, a significant pubertal growth spurt can be obtained.

Along with induction and management of pubertal progress in chronic disease processes, attention to intake of vitamin D, calcium, magnesium and phosphate balance may also contribute to the improvement in bone health, particularly while linear growth is taking place.

LONG-TERM AND FOLLOW-UP PLAN

As chronic disease processes usually have a relapsing and remitting course, it may well be necessary to utilise further short courses of testosterone, 6 months apart. Ultimately, it may be necessary to take a boy completely through puberty, using exogenous testosterone, administered at regular intervals, in order to achieve adequate virilisation and associated psychosocial and emotional well-being.

This action will also improve bone health and thus reduce lifetime fracture risk, in a condition where ill health, immobilisation and corticosteroid use all mitigate against good-quality bone.

EXPECTED OUTCOMES

Careful discussion with the boy and his family is required prior to instituting longer term testosterone treatment, because ultimately the affected boy will probably not reach his midparental expectation. Unfortunately, this is likely to happen whether or not testosterone is given. The adolescent should be aware of the relative benefits of intervention, in terms of psychosocial and emotional benefit and virilisation, versus the possible loss of 3–5 cm of final height.

Girls

In the situation of chronic inflammatory conditions which are unlikely to resolve or remit, use of administered oestrogen is appropriate. However, oestrogen has a propensity for epiphyseal closure and therefore the dose of oestrogen should be relatively low at the start of treatment.[6]

ACUTE

If the affected girl is showing little or no sign of pubertal advance, or where physical changes are slow but a growth spurt is failing to take place as expected, it is reasonable to commence oestrogen replacement. Oestrogen can be replaced in a variety of ways. Commonly administered routes are transdermal and oral oestrogen, in slow increments over a period of 2.5–3 years, with the addition of progestogen at the end of that time, for regular endometrial shedding. (See treatment of primary hypogonadism for a more detailed regime of oestrogen.)

LONG-TERM AND FOLLOW-UP PLAN

Treatment with sex steroids has to be reviewed at regular intervals. Growth should be assessed at each review and oestrogen treatment stopped when growth slows and near-final height is achieved, as measured by a bone age, checking for epiphyseal fusion. Biochemical parameters to check adequacy of oestrogen secretion should be performed approximately 8 weeks later, to check if endogenous oestrogen secretion is adequate or whether it needs to be re-instituted.

Should physical progress and growth spurt greatly exceed the expectation of the paediatrician at any time during treatment, it can be withdrawn, with a similar assessment, to identify spontaneous HPA activity.

EXPECTED OUTCOMES

In anorexia nervosa and other states characterised by loss of adipose tissue, oestrogen treatment has not been shown to be beneficial for bone health. However, it may be premature to discount the benefits of oestrogen as most reports have used oral oestrogen, which is disliked and poorly tolerated by many girls with anorexia nervosa. One strategy may be to use oral oestrogen in a low dose (ethinyl oestradiol 2–2.5 µg/day) over a short period (3–4 months) to induce puberty in the context of improving nutrition. Transdermal oestrogen can be helpful, in the author's experience, as a girl fearful of gaining weight seems to have less fear of weight gain if the treatment is not given by mouth. When the transdermal route is acceptable, treatment may improve bone health status. It can be withdrawn once adequate and sustained weight gain has been achieved.

Immobilisation and Disability

Clinical Setting

Severe neurological deficit as a result of congenital or acquired brain injury may be associated with poor nutritional status and consequent severely delayed puberty.

Affected children are also at high risk for long-bone fractures, due to immobilisation osteopaenia, complicated by low muscle mass and poor muscle pull, with consequent narrow, gracile bones. In these states, the potential to achieve bone mineralisation through puberty assumes much significance, to improve bone mass accrual and thus to reduce short and long-term fracture risk.[7]

Assessment and Diagnostic Approach

- Assessment of puberty in the context of parental and sibling history.
- Nutritional assessment as a contributor to pubertal delay.
- Drugs, e.g. anticonvulsants, which may adversely influence bone density.
- Careful questioning as to fracture history, particularly as to whether any fracture occurred in the setting of significant injury or whether it occurred with minimal trauma, as in a no-impact fragility fracture. This will help define the need for HRT, to improve bone quality and reduce future fracture risk.

Investigations that will Yield Results Useful to the Patient, in Order of Priority

- Calcium, magnesium, alkaline phosphatase.
- Vitamin D, parathyroid hormone (PTH) if available.
- Bone density, with volumetric adjustment for body size. (If available, it is a measure for comparison of treatment effectiveness reported using reference standards comparable for the height and size of the population.)

Rationale for Management

Parents may sometimes wish for their severely disabled child to remain small and prepubertal to be able to lift and care for the child. They may be fearful that puberty will cause a deterioration or alteration in their relationship with the child. While this is maybe a reasonable consideration by parents, in fact progress through puberty enhances the parent–child relationship, with significant improvement in brain maturity as well as bodily function.

Some less disabled children may, after treatment of delayed or arrested puberty, subsequently be able to help with lifting and transfer activities, thus reducing the risk of carer injury. An improvement in growth and physical development concomitantly reduces lifetime fracture risk and often also has a rewarding effect on the parent–child interaction in the long term.

ACUTE

- Attention to adequacy of nutrition as growth and pubertal progress will not occur without adequate caloric intake.
- Correction of vitamin D deficiency because bone mineral accrual and consequently bone density will be impaired without adequate mineral substrate.
- Induction of puberty with testosterone or oestrogen as previously described for constitutional delay of growth and puberty.

FOLLOW-UP PLAN

Pubertal status and progress over 6–18 months.

EXPECTED OUTCOMES

Normal maintenance of adult sex hormone levels, once puberty is complete. In exceptional circumstances where the patient is extremely thin, it may not be possible to maintain adult sex hormone levels and long-term treatment may be required. (See treatment of primary hypogonadism for a more detailed regime.)

Menstrual Management with Complex Disorders

(See Chapter 10, Paediatric and Adolescent Gynaecology, for further information.)

For girls who have severe physical disabilities such as bleeding disorders, immobility secondary to deformity, bone fragility or orthopaedic problems or for those with neurologic disabilities, regular menstrual periods may be extremely inconvenient and difficult to manage.

Use of the oral contraceptive pill, in a continuous fashion, without withdrawal bleeds is possible but missed pills cause intercurrent bleeding and accurate administration of medication is dependent upon a regular carer.

Depot progestogen should not be used alone, as it causes switch-off of the hypothalamic-pituitary-ovarian axis, with resultant bone loss, in a situation where the skeleton is already at risk. If used at all, addition of continuous oral or transdermal oestrogen is required in addition to the progestogen.

A progestogen-bearing intrauterine device (IUD) can be considered once the uterus has reached full adult dimensions with a length of at least 7 cm. These IUDs are rarely extruded. In general they cause either complete amenorrhoea or minimal menstrual loss for a period of 5 years after insertion, together with adequate contraception for the same period. This type of device, where available, can prove to be extremely helpful to manage menstrual periods in girls who have a chronic disability such as severe cerebral palsy.[8] As the amount of progestogen is minimal, this has the added advantage of not interfering with normal hormonal secretion. Unlike depot injections of medroxyprogesterone, releasing relatively large doses of progesterone in the circulation, these devices carry a lesser risk of inducing osteopaenia.

Hyperprolactinaemia

Clinical Setting

Prolactin-secreting tumours of the pituitary gland are extremely uncommon in childhood, although they occur with increasing frequency in late adolescence and early adulthood. In late adolescence, hyperprolactinaemia may be due to a microadenoma, where the prolactin levels are relatively high, usually several thousand mU/L. Lesser levels may be associated with a non-functioning pituitary adenoma, although the difference from a microadenoma may not be simple. In adults, prolactinomas are not an uncommon cause for secondary amenorrhoea in girls and hypogonadism in both sexes.

A prolactinoma causing hyperprolactinaemia is rarely a primary cause for pubertal failure. In girls, galactorrhoea is possible but rare, and is more often seen in older patients. In boys, presentation with pubertal failure is also uncommon. However, some large tumours may be associated with pubertal failure and galactorrhoea.

After cranial radiation or with a lesion such as a craniopharyngioma or a hypothalamic glioma, mild hyperprolactinaemia may occur. Similarly, in some individuals with ovarian hyperandrogenism secondary to polycystic ovarian syndrome, prolactin levels may be slightly elevated. This should not be confused with a diagnosis of a prolactinoma.

However, identification of hyperprolactinaemia is useful, as it may inhibit pubertal progress or later menstrual function and it is amenable to effective treatment.

Assessment and Diagnostic Approach

- Presence of medications likely to raise prolactin — particularly antipsychotic agents (e.g. olanzapine), anti-nausea agents (such as domperidone).
- Clinical assessment of growth rate, pubertal onset/progress or arrest.
- Café-au-lait marks as seen in neurofibromatosis type 1 may suggest the presence of an underlying optic nerve glioma. Although rare, McCune—Albright syndrome may be considered in the presence of café-au-lait marks, because acromegaly with co-secretion of prolactin is a complication seen in children and adolescents.
- Mildly elevated prolactin levels can be associated with pubertal arrest, and primary

or secondary amenorrhoea in girls. These conditions include other midline lesions such as craniopharyngioma, glioma or after cranial radiation, in association with other pituitary hormone losses.

Investigations that will Yield Results Useful to the Patient, in Order of Priority

- Prolactin level — a prolactinoma is likely if prolactin levels >2000 mU/L. In non-functioning adenomas, prolactin levels are usually less.
- MR scanning of the pituitary and hypothalamus — helpful to identify tumours such as a pituitary micro or macroadenoma, craniopharyngioma or other hypothalamic tumours.

Rationale for Management

Hyperprolactinaemia reduces sex hormone levels, contributes to poor pubertal progress, increases psychosocial and emotional disorders and adversely affects bone health. Therefore, there are long-term implications of treatment of children with hyperprolactinaemia-induced delayed puberty. Treatment options are outlined as given in the section below.

Treatment

- Cessation of agents causing high prolactin, if possible.
- Treatment of tumour such as a hypothalamic glioma, on its merits.
- Dopamine agonists such as cabergoline which are relatively long acting — these have been shown to reduce prolactin and to reduce tumour size.
- Neurosurgery to debulk a prolactinoma is not indicated except in specific circumstances with a large tumour compressing on the optic nerves. In such cases treatment with dopamine agonists may not cause rapid decompression in order to preserve visual fields.

Follow-up Plan

- Regular prolactin levels, at least every 6 months.
- MRI for lesion size reduction — annually.

Expected Outcomes

- Resolution of problems of growth, puberty, galactorrhoea.
- Possible tumour resolution up to 5–10 years, if isolated prolactinoma.

Other Conditions Causing Pubertal Problems with Incomplete Delayed or Abnormal Progress

If pubertal progress is discordant, or incomplete, consideration should be given to structural abnormalities or hormone resistance.

- **Mullerian agenesis** with failure of uterine development but normal ovarian function results in normal growth, breast and pubic hair but primary amenorrhoea. Surgical vaginal reconstruction may be required. HRT is not needed as oestrogen action is normal.
- **Complete androgen insensitivity (CAIS),** an X-linked disorder of androgen action in a 46XY individual with a female phenotype, results is normal growth and breast development but no pubic or axillary hair and primary amenorrhoea. The risk of gonadoblastoma is low and gonadal removal is not required, but may be preferred due to presence of gonads in the inguinal area in some affected children.
- **Incomplete androgen** insensitivity (PAIS) is associated with partial virilisation at puberty. Gonadoblastoma risk is reported up to 50% particularly if the gonads are intra-abdominal.[9] Gonadectomy is advised, although optimal timing varies depending on the position of gonads. Opinions vary across different centres. Most children with PAIS

will need exogenous testosterone treatment if the child is raised as a male. If the gonads are removed, further testosterone replacement is required in long-term follow-up.

PRIMARY HYPOGONADISM

Hypergonadotrophic hypogonadism is characterised by lack of pubertal signs due to gonadal failure. Unlike CDGP or hypogonadotropic hypogonadism (HH), serum gonadotrophin levels are elevated. However, the hypothalamic-pituitary-gonadal axis is not activated during childhood and thus elevation of gonadotrophins is an unreliable marker of gonadal status in childhood and can give false reassurance.

Primary gonadal problems include gonadal dysgenesis or acquired damage by surgery, radiation or chemotherapy, resistance to action of gonadal hormones or more rarely inflammation as an auto-immune disorder of oophoritis.

Girls

Turner Syndrome

Clinical Setting

PRESENTATION

The most common presentation to an endocrinologist in a girl is for short stature, with or without pubertal delay. Although relatively rare, occurring in 1/2500 live births, Turner syndrome should always be excluded, unless of course another obvious cause such as gross primary hypothyroidism is identified.

EXAMINATION

Short stature is the commonest manifestation of Turner syndrome. Other phenotypic findings of webbed neck, widely spaced nipples with shield chest, increased carrying angles and low posterior hairline are not always easily recognised. It is usual for subtle phenotypic manifestations to be visible to the trained eye but may not be easily identifiable for the majority of physicians whose primary activity is not paediatric endocrinology. Common physical changes are of narrow deep-set nails, very mild epicanthic folds, high arched palate and increased number of moles. These will normally alert the clinician to the condition. Absence of these findings does not preclude the need for karyotype. Failure of puberty can occur in association with growth failure. In some children with Turner syndrome, puberty starts but does not progress as normal.

No matter how mild the phenotypic features or how minimal the karyotypic mosaicism may be, all girls with Turner syndrome have an increased risk for associated features such as bicuspid aortic valve and abnormalities of the renal tract. It is therefore important to examine the cardiovascular system in some detail and measure blood pressure in all children with Turner syndrome.

DIAGNOSIS

Karyotype is required for confirmation of diagnosis. In many countries this expensive test is now being replaced by a molecular karyotype using PCR. This will give an accurate diagnosis in most cases but will currently only detect mosaicism down to a level of at least 10%. Y mosaicism at low levels around 5% may not be detected by this method. If a clinical phenotype of Turner syndrome is suspected, a formal karyotype, counting 60–100 cells, may be required.

INVESTIGATION

Once Turner syndrome has been diagnosed, they should be investigated for a number of autoimmune conditions. There is a lifetime risk of 10% for coeliac disease, with varying risks for autoimmune hypothyroidism, psoriasis, inflammatory bowel disease and diabetes mellitus type 2. Screening surveillance should be undertaken regularly, as any or all of them will impinge upon both growth and pubertal progress and in the long term may cause serious health problems if not detected and managed appropriately.

Some spontaneous pubertal change is noted in 30–40% of girls with Turner syndrome. However, only 4% of these girls proceed to menarche and less than 1% are spontaneously fertile. The common assumption that entry into puberty excludes Turner syndrome is thus incorrect. In girls with short stature and delayed puberty, the diagnosis of Turner syndrome has to be excluded by a karyotype.

When Y mosaicism is found, early bilateral gonadectomy is indicated, due to high risk for gonadoblastoma. This tumour may be found even in very young children, where surgery has been delayed.

MANAGEMENT

The majority of management for this condition is usually undertaken by paediatric endocrinologists. As there are many health issues throughout life, information is therefore provided for associated non-endocrine conditions, to ensure that these are attended as well as specific endocrine problems. These include the following.

CARDIAC Currently, MRI and angiography of the base of heart and great vessels is considered as the gold standard for assessment of cardiovascular status of a girl with Turner syndrome. Cardiac MRI delineates the aortic valve, aortic arch and thoracic aorta more efficiently than ultrasound echocardiography, which may not be able to detect rare congenital abnormalities such as an anomalous pulmonary venous drainage defect or even occasionally miss a bicuspid valve in a girl who has a shield chest.

In places where access to MRI is possible, it is considered appropriate for cardiac MRI heart to be undertaken by the end of puberty and to be repeated every 5 years thereafter, with particular emphasis on a pre-IVF pregnancy assessment.

The risk of aortic dissection during the 2nd and 3rd trimester of pregnancy is significant in the presence of bicuspid aortic valve or short segment coarctation, with cystic medial necrosis being commonly found at autopsy in such patients. However, this type of investigation may not be readily available in all situations and if not available, two-dimensional echocardiography should be performed at roughly the same time intervals. Aortic root diameter must be assessed in relation to body surface area.[10]

RENAL Anomalies of the renal collecting system or the presence of a horseshoe kidney should be identified in all girls with this condition, partly because there is a mild increase in risk for recurrent urinary tract infections where some mechanical alteration of the collecting system exists and partly because an unidentified horseshoe kidney may be accidentally removed if injured during a motor vehicle accident, if its presence is not recognised. The horseshoe kidney, by nature of its position anterior in the abdomen, is significantly more prone to injury during trauma than the usual placement in the retroperitoneal space.

AUTOIMMUNE DISEASES Hashimoto's thyroiditis with hypothyroidism, coeliac disease and inflammatory bowel disease all cause significant ongoing ill health, and where present in childhood and adolescence may contribute to delayed or arrested puberty. Screening should be undertaken every 12–18 months where resources are available.

HEARING Increasing hearing loss due to middle ear effusion and Eustachian tube dysfunction is so common in girls with Turner syndrome that 70% of adult women with this condition are reported to have some hearing loss or to require some form of hearing aid. Regular audiology assessment every 12–18 months from infancy onwards should be undertaken so that accrual

of language and optimisation of learning can take place throughout childhood and adolescence.

LIVER FUNCTION Abnormalities of liver enzymes are frequent in Turner syndrome and relate to intrahepatic small vessel malformations or to autoimmune liver disease. It is important to document changes so that HRT is not blamed for elevated liver transaminases.

Y MOSAICISM If a Y component of the karyotype is found, early bilateral gonadectomy is advised, due to gonadoblastoma risk at any age.

Diagnostic Approach

Pubertal Status and Progress

As 30–40% of girls with Turner syndrome enter puberty spontaneously, intervention for pubertal failure may not be required for some time. Provided a normal growth rate is taking place, and puberty appears to be progressing, a wait and watch policy is sensible. Intervention with HRT can be delayed until there is evidence for lack of progress of breast development.

Timing of HRT in Turner syndrome depends on the age of the individual. For children who also have concomitant use of growth hormone for short stature, there is no reason to delay commencement of HRT treatment in the hope that a delay in epiphyseal closure may improve final height outcome.

A consistent complaint in adult women with Turner syndrome, relating to past treatment, is that of adverse psychological and emotional effects of a very late puberty, in comparison with peers. Therefore, unless there is sufficiently strong evidence otherwise, HRT should be commenced at around the time of normal puberty.

Spontaneous puberty is more likely with some mosaic karyotypes but can occur with 45,XO individuals. Mosaicism examined in chromosomes from peripheral blood lymphocytes may differ from the karyotype at the tissue level, in particular within the ovary. However, phenotype does not follow genotype consistently. In some mosaics with specific deletion of either arm of the X chromosome or XXX karyotype, puberty and even fertility may be normal. Even with an XO karyotype, spontaneous pregnancy has been reported.

INVESTIGATIONS

- FSH, LH, oestradiol to assess ovarian status. Gonadotrophins are usually but not always elevated after age 8–9 years but are often low prior to that age and are not helpful as a diagnostic aid.
- Thyroid function
- Coeliac screen
- Liver function tests
- Lipid studies
- MRI/echo of heart and great vessels
- Renal ultrasound.

Other Causes of Primary Gonadal Failure in Girls

Clinical Setting

Congenital Disorders

Other forms of gonadal dysgenesis in a phenotypic female are rare and include sex reversal due to various genetic disorders including Denys–Drash syndrome and abnormalities of SRY and other sex determining genes. Abnormalities of the steroidogenic pathway within the adrenal gland associated with primary gonadal dysfunction include abnormalities of the StAR (steroid acute regulatory) protein, 17a hydroxylase and 17,20 lyase deficiencies, which cause hypergonadotrophic hypogonadism.

(See Chapter 4, Adrenal Disorders and Chapter 5, Disorders of Sexual Development in Resource-limited Settings.)

GONADOTROPHIN RESISTANCE

This problem is associated with Albright's hereditary osteodystrophy (AHO) or pseudohypoparathyroidism type 1a. Rarely, genetic abnormalities in the gonadotrophin receptors may also cause gonadal failure. Some children with severe intrauterine growth retardation may present with pubertal delay or more commonly with late pubertal arrest due to apparent resistance to multiple hormones.

Acquired Disorders

INFILTRATIVE DISORDERS

Some disorders, such as galactosaemia, a rare inborn error of metabolism, may affect the ovary and cause ovarian failure. Other infiltrative disorders with deposition of iron can cause ovarian dysfunction, in situations where transfusion requirement is high, such as thalassaemia major or marrow dysplasia such as Diamond–Blackfan syndrome, or in primary iron deposition disorders such as haemochromatosis. It is more common for iron deposition to occur in the hypothalamic area, as outlined previously, but deposition can occur simultaneously in the gonads and hypothalamus.

LOCAL RADIATION

Ovarian failure is the rule after direct abdominal radiation, such as with some regimes for the management of Wilms' tumour or sarcoma of the pelvis. Usually, with this type of problem, radiation is unilateral and the contralateral ovary potentially may be capable of future function. However, despite shielding techniques, the contralateral ovary may also be subject to radiation, from backscatter of radiation from the bones. Further, additional chemotherapy with agents such as cyclophosphamide can also damage the non-irradiated ovary, which is potentially capable of later recovery, even though total ova numbers will be attenuated.

Total body radiation (TBI) used as conditioning treatment prior to bone marrow transplant also ultimately causes ovarian failure, although 50% of girls who have had TBI may have sufficient ovarian function to progress into or through puberty before failure supervenes. The younger the patient at the time of radiation, the more likely it is to have some residual ovarian function, with a decrease in the chance of spontaneous preservation of ovarian function with every year of age at time of treatment.

CHEMOTHERAPY

The use of certain types of chemotherapy may cause some reduction in ovarian function. The use of cyclophosphamide is common in many chemotherapeutic regimes. Recovery from high-dose cyclophosphamide can take place 2–10 years after treatment, with preservation of some ovarian function, although with reduced total numbers of ova. Other alkylating agents including melphalan, busulfan and procarbazine are even more gonadotoxic but similar recovery has been reported.

Girls who have had past gonadotoxic chemotherapy should be advised not to postpone pregnancy until their mid to late thirties because a reduced total ova population may reduce chances of a successful pregnancy.

Rationale for Management

Treatment aims are to achieve optimal linear growth, adequate feminisation, adult bone mass accrual and psychosocial and emotional maturity over a time frame similar to peers.

Management of Female Primary Hypogonadism

ACUTE

Oestrogen causes epiphyseal fusion in boys and girls. In boys, epiphyseal fusion takes place via peripheral aromatisation of androgen to oestrogen and is therefore slower than in girls. For girls one has to be cautious with the dose of oestrogen used, in order to optimise linear growth while allowing pubertal progress. While small doses may be additive to height gain, moderate to high doses will hasten the fusion of epiphyses. The use of oestrogen for induction of puberty is therefore more difficult to manage for girls than for boys.

Female pubertal induction with oestrogen involves the use of oral or transdermal routes. In general, girls do not prefer the application of gel preparations or even transdermal patches. Therefore prescription of topical preparations may not result in suitable compliance, with a desirable effect. There may be a tendency to omit medication, except when coming to visit the doctor. It is important to recognise such lack of compliance and to change to oral oestrogen where required.

Oral oestrogen as a natural, non-ethinyl radical oestrogen is preferred for girls with Turner syndrome, a condition where hypertension is common and the ethinyl radical of ethinyl oestradiol (as in most contraceptive pills) induces renin substrate to a far higher degree than natural preparations of oestrogen. If ethinyl oestradiol is the only preparation available, the risk of inducing hypertension should not preclude treatment with HRT, as long as blood pressure and lipid profiles are checked and healthy lifestyles are maintained. However, effort should be made to provide a natural oestrogen. Oestradiol valerate is inexpensive and available in most countries.

For girls with other conditions such as after radiation or chemotherapy, it is a reasonable option to use ethinyl oestradiol for induction of puberty as it is longer acting than natural estrogens.

A typical treatment regime for gonadal dysfunction is 0.5 mg of natural oestrogen (oestradiol valerate every second day for 3–6 months, then increasing slowly, to 1 mg daily for 12 months, then to 2 mg/day, with the addition of progestogen for regular menstrual cycling).

If Premarin is used, commencing dose should be 0.15 mg second daily, increasing to 0.3 mg/day at around 12 months, then to 0.625 mg/day by 2 years, with addition of progestogen at that time.

If ethinyl oestradiol is the only available oestrogen, it can be commenced at 2 µg/day, if this preparation is available locally. Alternatively, a 10 µg tablet could be quartered to give 2.5 µg every day or halved to give 5 µg every other day. Treatment with ethinyl oestradiol can be increased stepwise over a period of 2 years, simulating the progress from early breast development to regular menstrual cycles to a maximum of 20 µg/day, with the addition of progestogen at this point.

For all girls who have a uterus, progestogen must be used to manage the menstrual cycles, in order to ensure regular endometrial shedding. The addition of 14 days of a progestogen, administered every 1–3 months, is adequate for endometrial shedding. Some girls prefer to have a period each month but others prefer to have only 4 periods per year. The duration of progestogen use is important, to ensure complete endometrial shedding, such that any residual endometrium at the end of a menstrual cycle is less than 1 mm in thickness to prevent against the possibility of endometrial cancer. Whether oral or transdermal oestrogen is used, oral progesterone must be administered in both cases. Available progestogens include medroxyprogesterone acetate 10 mg or norethisterone acetate 5 mg.

LONG TERM

When ovarian failure is permanent, such as with Turner syndrome, a final long-term HRT regime should include continuous oestrogen and intermittent progestogen, as outlined, with a minimal requirement for 14 days every 3 months. More frequent use of a progestogen with an increased frequency of menstrual bleeds may be preferred by the patient; therefore HRT treatment regimens may have to be tailored to suit the individual.

FOLLOW-UP PLAN

For girls who have had unilateral radiation or chemotherapy alone and where resolution of ovarian failure might occur at an unpredictable time, it may be wise to change to long cycles of a contraceptive pill when the girl becomes sexually active, to avoid the possibility of an unwanted pregnancy. The long cycle utilises an oral contraceptive pill for longer periods (simply by omitting the lactose pills for two cycles out of three) and allowing for withdrawal bleeds every 3–4 months. This regimen improves the amount of oestrogen exposure in contrast to the traditional approach of using the pill for 3 weeks followed by a gap of 1 week.

Boys

Primary gonadal abnormality results from structural gonadal dysgenesis, or functional abnormality of androgen production or action, including defects of testosterone pathway production and/or acquired insult to the testes.

Clinical Setting

Anorchia

This rare condition presents in infancy with a normal male phenotype but absent testes. The cause may not be easily identifiable but is assumed to be due to testicular loss occurring after male phenotypic development; that is, after 10–14 weeks' gestation. Identification of possible residual intra-abdominal testicular tissue is required, to enable surgical retrieval to be attempted.

Klinefelter Syndrome 47XXY

This condition affects 1/580 live born males and is the commonest cause for primary gonadal dysfunction in boys. The vast majority of males with this condition are either never diagnosed or are first seen as an adult in an infertility clinic. Most have clearly progressed normally through puberty without need for intervention. However, a significant proportion of children with Klinefelter syndrome are either diagnosed antenatally (through procedures such as amniocentesis) or at the time of puberty. Some children may be diagnosed in infancy at the time of investigation for undescended testes, while in others diagnosis may occur in mid-childhood when investigated for behaviour disorders or social isolation.

Although very rare, Klinefelter syndrome may present at birth with female genitalia. Rarer variants of Klinefelter syndrome include mosaicism with 46,XY/48,XXXY and 49,XXXXY. Some of these are associated with significant developmental delay.

Boys with this condition are usually of at least average size and may often be above average for their midparental expectation. The diagnosis may therefore be very significantly delayed because short stature is absent and more subtle problems may not be recognised by parents or carers. If a boy presents for endocrine assessment due to a failure to enter or progress through puberty, the typical features may not be obvious. These are as follows:

- eunuchoid appearance with body disproportion and a greater lower body to upper body segment ratio, implying longer limbs compared to spinal length.
- gynaecomastia, which may be prepubertal
- 'female' body habitus
- report of relatively lower intelligence particularly when compared to other family members
- small and firm testes, usually less than 4 mL in volume, even if pubertal progress has occurred.
- developmental delay, particularly in those with increasing complement of X chromosomes
- abnormality of radio-ulnar orientation, elbow dislocation and congenital heart

abnormalities, particular in those with more X chromosomes.

However, even these typical findings may not be present in all children and the diagnosis may therefore be somewhat difficult. Even with hyalinised testes, the typical feature of testes in Klinefelter syndrome, some boys with Klinefelter syndrome may appear to have relatively large testes, up to 12 mL by mid-puberty. However, these testes tend to shrink with time, as fibrosis progresses. If in doubt about the possibility of Klinefelter syndrome, a peripheral blood lymphocyte karyotype is a prudent test, particularly in the presence of mild learning difficulties and social and behavioural disorders.

Autoimmune disorders for boys with Klinefelter syndrome are more common than in other members of the community. Evidence for these should be sought on a regular basis, for coeliac disease and hypothyroidism. Teratoma and seminoma of the testes, leukaemia and lymphoma are also seen with increased lifetime frequency in this group. Rarely, children with this condition may present with mediastinal tumours.

Radiation to the Testes

- Direct radiation treatment always causes damage to the testes, principally affecting the germ cells.
- 4 Gy is required to cause permanent azoospermia.
- 20–30 Gy is required to cause Leydig cell damage at any age.
- Chemotherapy causes permanent azoospermia in a postpubertal boy and often causes some damage to spermatogenesis when used prepubertally.

If lower doses of radiation are used, progress into and through puberty may take place. Testicular size is misleading, as testes will be relatively small with poor growth potential after radiation exposure.

Abnormalities of Testosterone Action

- **5α reductase deficiency** results in inability to produce the active testosterone derivative, dihydrotestosterone. It can present in infancy or childhood with sex reversal, genital ambiguity or delayed or arrested puberty.
- **Partial androgen insensitivity**, as an X-linked disorder of the androgen receptor, varies widely in presentation ranging between genital ambiguity at birth to delayed progress through puberty.

Diagnostic Approach

PUBERTAL STATUS AND PROGRESS

Children with testicular damage may enter and progress in puberty, despite raised gonadotrophins and/or small testes. The time for intervention with medical treatment needs to be assessed by following the growth trajectory in an affected individual An absent growth spurt together with lack of progress in puberty suggests the need for treatment with sex steroids. Treatment decision making may be further modulated by the underlying diagnosis, general health, other concurrent treatment and growth potential.

A random testosterone level is not always helpful, although morning testosterone levels are better than those in the afternoon or evening. If a boy is progressing through normal stages of virilisation and linear growth, there is no need to measure testosterone, as it can be misleading.

Investigations in Order of Value to the Patient

- FSH/LH
- Bone age for growth potential
- Karyotype where indicated
- HCG test to evaluate presence of possible functional testicular tissue.
  Infants: 1500 to 2000 Units by subcutaneous injection, with testosterone (and in some

cases, other androgens) measured at 72 hours.
  Older children: 5000 Units as a single dose or 3000 Units/m^2 for 3–5 days with measurement of testosterone on day 6.
- AMH/inhibin may be of value where available to indicate presence of intra-abdominal testicular tissue which needs to be surgically repositioned. However, AMH and inhibin levels can be difficult to interpret, and these tests should be used only if age and sex matched reference standards are available.

Rationale for Management

Treatment aims are to achieve normalisation of growth, optimise final height and attain adequate virilisation and adult genital status with normal bone accrual.

Libido and sexual function in a young adult male is not entirely dependent on testosterone levels and sexual function can appear to be relatively normal in the presence of low levels of serum testosterone. However, chronically raised gonadotrophins are associated with significant testicular damage and therefore with the possibility of inadequate bone accrual. Any condition with hypogonadism should be adequately treated for both physical and bone health.

Management of Boys with Primary Hypogonadism

If testes are intra-abdominal, efforts should be made to investigate for their presence and exact location. If puberty is unable to progress, one option is to attempt to reposition the testes through surgery. While orchidopexy is fairly successful in young children, it is less so in older children. Testes which are significantly high may not be amenable to repositioning in the scrotum without damage to the vascular supply to the cord and epididymis.

If puberty will not occur such as with anorchia or after early testicular irradiation, it is reasonable to commence testosterone replacement at a time appropriate for peers; that is, around age 12–13 years.

If puberty is severely delayed or if growth hormone is being used for growth after cranial radiation, time of pubertal induction may need to be modified to allow for further linear growth. If sex steroid is commenced at an older age, probably greater than 15 years, a higher dose can be used to achieve more rapid changes, in order to allow pubertal progress appropriate for the peer group. Rate of change of dose should be determined based on height and growth potential.

At age 12–13 years it is better to use either an oral or transdermal testosterone preparation initially, for the comfort of a young patient. If that option is not available, the use of low-dose intramuscular testosterone can be utilised, although uncomfortable for the child, with doses increased slowly over 2–3 years to mimic the normal course of puberty.

Testosterone undecanoate (oral) 40 mg every second day as a commencing dose can be increased to 40 mg/day and then to 40 mg twice a day over 12 months. For the second year 40–60 mg three times daily can be used, changing to intramuscular testosterone when the boy is halfway through puberty.

Transdermal testosterone as gel preparations are available but generally are not complied well by adolescents as they are somewhat messy. However, for an adolescent with severe neurologic disability, transdermal testosterone can be an excellent alternative to more conventional methods of testosterone replacement. Further, a number of boys will electively choose a topical preparation, particularly if they wish to avoid monthly intramuscular injections.

If a female parent or member of the family is administering transdermal testosterone, it must be done with the use of plastic gloves. Testosterone gel absorption and plasma concentration is dependent on the area of skin treated, with higher concentration achieved using a small area of administration, around 2–4 cm in diameter. Testosterone gel is usually applied to the anterior abdominal wall or thigh, but may also be applied to the upper arms for adequate absorption.

Intramuscular testosterone: Long-acting intramuscular testosterone preparations are now available in many countries, with a flat profile plasma testosterone attainable, with each injection lasting 10–12 weeks.

In the absence of long-acting preparations, shorter acting conventional preparations of testosterone are a reasonable option. The pharmacokinetics and pharmaco-dynamics demonstrate that each injection achieves a supraphysiological level of testosterone over 7–10 days, decreasing to baseline by 14 days. Therefore, optimal replacement treatment requires administration every 2 weeks, being uncomfortable and time consuming for the patient. Therefore, for older children and young adults, the longer acting preparations are preferable. For boys with Klinefelter syndrome, the use of adequate amounts of testosterone with a flat profile will usually diminish and obliterate the gynaecomastia that is a common problem with this condition, over about 12 months, without the need for surgery.

Use of dihydrotestosterone for management of 5α reductase deficiency is limited by lack of availability and formulation as a powder only, available for local application. As such it is relatively ineffective. High-dose testosterone use at puberty can in part override the enzyme defect and permit virilisation.

PRECOCIOUS PUBERTY

Puberty Variants

Premature Adrenarche

Early or premature adrenarche is due to premature activation of adrenal androgens

TABLE 2.4   General Summary: Assessment of Pubertal Delay

Assessment

- Plot growth: on a growth chart appropriate for the population being assessed.

- Obtain any past growth measurements to construct a growth curve and include observation of weight curve.

- Plot midparental height expectation.

- Estimate mature height: based on calculation of midparental heights (adding 12 cm to mother's height for plotting her centile on a male chart or subtracting 12 cm from father's height when plotting on a female chart).

Observe growth pattern

Girls with Turner syndrome are usually short but have a sharp reduction in growth velocity at age 5–7 years, usually falling below the 1st centile.
Those who have a chronic disease process have an erratic growth pattern, dependent on nutrition and treatment with corticosteroids, both of which inhibit growth rate. Episodes of better health are accompanied by improved growth velocity.

Evaluate pubertal status

- Tanner staging plus testicular size as measured with a Prader orchidometer for boys.

- Assess evidence for progress if possible.

- Bone age evaluation: expecting a bone age delay of 1–4 years, depending on age and severity of the underlying condition.

- Assess bone age for growth potential.

- FSH/LH for evidence of gonadal failure.

- Karyotype where indicated.

- Other tests for coeliac disease, thyroid, growth hormone status etc.

Exclude or treat underlying causes for pubertal delay: nutritional deficit, disorders of thyroid function, organic lesion in the hypothalamic pituitary axis hyperprolactinaemia

(DHEAS) before gonadal activation. Premature pubarche is the appearance of pubic hair as a result. Although usually a benign process, an unusually young age at adrenarche (under 5 years) or significant virilisation, tall stature and accelerating linear growth may be indicative of underlying adrenal pathology such as late onset congenital adrenal hyperplasia or an androgen secreting tumour (Figure 2.5).

Premature adrenarche alone may need no treatment, particularly if not associated with disorders of adrenal enzyme biosynthesis. As it occurs frequently in children who are overweight, judicious instruction regarding weight-loss programmes will usually reduce the rate of pubertal change back closer to population norms.

(Treatment of congenital adrenal hyperplasia is discussed in Chapter 4, Adrenal Disorders.)

Premature Thelarche

In some girls, mild breast development may occur without the presence of other signs of puberty. Typically, a child with premature thelarche is about 2 years of age, but late-onset variants have been recognised. Usually, breast development fluctuates but is not progressive and there are no other features to suggest rapidly progressive puberty. Height velocity is normal and bone age is not advanced. However, thelarche variants occur across a spectrum and, in addition to breast development, other changes such as rapid growth, increased bone age and some uterine changes are also present. This condition may share common ground with slowly evolving central precocious puberty (CPP).

Investigations are not required for isolated premature thelarche but may be necessary if the distinction between progressive puberty and thelarche is not clear. Thelarche and its variants often have FSH dominance in response to GnRH stimulation. High FSH may stimulate aromatase and therefore oestrogen production but oestrogen is not usually measurable. Often a period of observation is helpful to judge the

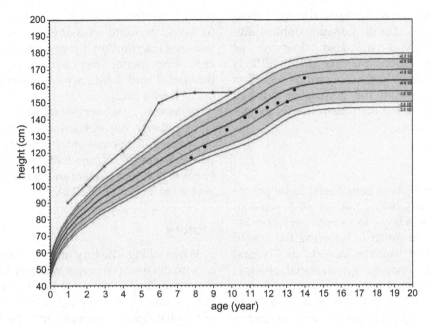

FIGURE 2.5 Height chart in a child with late presenting 21-hydroxylase congenital adrenal hyperplasia. Note: Although initially tall, final height has been compromised by early fusion of the epiphyses.

pace of evolving change and to estimate if true CPP is evolving.

PATHOPHYSIOLOGY OF PRECOCIOUS PUBERTY

Precocious puberty occurs because of early reactivation of GnRH neurons, which are in turn influenced by other hypothalamic factors, such as kisspeptin-1, secreted by hypothalamic kisspeptin neurons and acting through kisspeptin (GPR54) receptors. In addition, there are multiple neuronal pathways that impact directly or indirectly on GnRH neurons. These include inhibitory factors such as γ-amino butyric acid (GABA) and excitatory factors such as glutamate and leptin. It is likely that excitatory factors prevail over inhibitory factors to trigger early onset of puberty.

The intrinsic neuronal trigger for precocious puberty is likely to be modulated by other influences, both intrinsic and extrinsic. While a low body fat mass inhibits the progression of puberty, conversely obesity may facilitate a relative earlier onset of puberty. Children born small for gestational age may have early adrenarche and/or puberty. A radical change in environmental factors, such as in children adopted from impoverished conditions into affluent societies, may also lead to an earlier pubertal timing. Brain injury, such as that sustained by intraventricular haemorrhages in preterm babies, prior meningitis or encephalitis and cranial irradiation may predispose to an earlier activation of puberty. Early puberty may also occur in families with a history of early puberty, suggesting the contribution of familial and hence genetic factors to the process of puberty.

Gonadotrophin dependent precocious puberty is due to central activation of the hypothalamo-pituitary-gonadal (HPG) axis, and therefore is also termed central precocious puberty (CPP). This is the most common mechanism for early puberty. Rarely, precocious puberty is due to gonadotrophin-independent mechanisms, also known as peripheral precocious puberty (PPP). PPP is due to endogenous and autonomous secretion of sex steroids from the gonads or adrenal glands, or due to the administration of exogenous sex steroids.

Clinical Setting

Onset of puberty is considered to be precocious if it occurs below the age of 8 years in girls or 9 years in boys. In recent times, consideration has been given to lowering the age of normal onset of puberty in girls to 7 years, because a tendency to generational change, probably associated with increased nutrition across communities, has resulted in a large number of young girls developing somewhat early pubertal changes under the age of 8 years.

However, when the age of 'normality' is lowered it has to be remembered that not all children presenting at such an early age with pubertal changes will simply have a constitutional problem and a proportion of them may harbour some more sinister cause. A high index of suspicion should therefore be undertaken, for making a diagnosis of constitutionally early puberty, before the age of 8 years in girls and 9 in boys.

It must be remembered that the appearance of pubic or axillary hair does not necessarily constitute true puberty and represents adrenarche. Therefore to diagnose precocious puberty, breast maturation using Tanner staging for girls, and testicular and genital development for boys, are mandatory. In overweight girls, fat over the pectoralis muscles can be difficult to differentiate from pubertal breast bud development. Ultrasound scan of the breast may help to define an echogenic breast bud. Additionally, pelvic ultrasound scan appearances of the size and shape of the uterus and ovaries may

provide evidence for the effects of oestrogen. In boys, accurate measurement of testicular volumes is important, using a Prader orchidometer. Prepubertal testicular volumes range between 1 and 3 mL, while pubertal volumes are at least 4 mL.

In general, girls over the age of 5 who develop early puberty are not usually found to have an organic hypothalamic pituitary disorder, whereas over 70% of boys with a similar presentation will be found to have an organic brain lesion such as a tumour (Table 2.5).

History

When taking a history for precocious puberty, as with delayed puberty, the family history is of significant importance, not just for the parents, but for other older siblings as well. A history of familial central precocity may be reassuring that a space-occupying lesion is unlikely as a cause.

It is best to evaluate a growth pattern over time. For this, any available measurements from maternal and child health data or family records will be helpful. For example, if a child has always been on the 97th centile in height for age, where the midparental expectation is on the 25th centile, it is much more likely that this child will have constitutionally early puberty instead of sinister pathology. This situation should be compared with a child who was growing perfectly normally at the age of 4 years, with a sudden escalation from the 50th to the 97th centile in the next 8 months. The latter situation is highly likely to be pathological.

A markedly advanced bone age may give extra assistance in diagnosis, although all children who have advanced puberty will automatically have an advanced bone age. If, however, the bone age is significantly advanced, for example greater than 4 years ahead of the chronologic age, this will give an indication of a highly active endocrine axis, with a large amount of sex hormone

TABLE 2.5   Causes of Precocious Puberty

Central precocious puberty (CPP) or gonadotrophin dependent precocious puberty (GDPP)	Peripheral precocious puberty (PPP) or gonadotrophin independent precocious puberty (GIPP)

1. Central nervous system abnormalities
Congenital abnormalities
• Septo-optic dysplasia spectrum
• Hydrocephalus
 	
Acquired abnormalities
• Hypothalamic-pituitary tumours
  - Hamartoma
  - Germinoma
  - Optic nerve glioma
 	
• Cranial irradiation
• Hydrocephalus
• Meningitis/encephalitis
• Intraventricular haemorrhage
 	
2. Ectopic source of human chorionic gonadotrophin (HCG)
• Hepatoblastoma
• Choriocarcinoma
 	
3. Prolonged primary hypothyroidism
 	
4. Cause not identified
 	
5. Familial (autosomal dominant) precocious puberty
 	
6. Prolonged exposure to sex steroids
 	
7. Late onset 21-hydroxylase congenital adrenal hyperplasia
	1. Ovarian overstimulation
	• McCune–Albright syndrome
	• Ovarian cysts, tumours
	
	2. Adrenal
	• Congenital adrenal hyperplasia
	• Adrenal tumours
	
	3. Exogenous sex steroids
	
	4. Testicular overactivity
	• Testotoxicosis (activating LH receptor mutation)
	• GSα activation in McCune–Albright syndrome
	• Leydig cell or Sertoli cell tumours

production. This would suggest the presence of precocious puberty, either gonadotrophin dependent or independent, in contrast with minor variants of early puberty. One example is that of a boy with late onset congenital adrenal hyperplasia due to 21-hydroxylase deficiency. Such a child might present with early pubic hair and mild penile enlargement at the age of 6 years but with a bone age of 12–13 years, suggesting an underlying pathological process. In contrast, a boy presenting with tall stature, a few pubic hairs at the age of 7 years with a bone age of 8.5 years and a family history of early puberty is more likely to have constitutional early puberty.

Examination

When assessing a child with precocious puberty, examination is of particular importance, in terms of physical clues to an underlying disorder.

• **Multiple small café-au-lait marks** and axillary freckling are highly suggestive of neurofibromatosis Type 1. If a child with NF1 has precocious puberty at an early age, usually under the age of 5 years, the chance of an optic chiasmal glioma is very high. Rarely, however, precocious puberty can occur in the absence of glioma.[11]

- **Larger café-au-lait marks,** particularly with a coast of Maine appearance and often not crossing the midline, are associated with McCune–Albright syndrome, a G protein mutation with constitutive activation of GTPase activity. This results in affected end organ hormonal excesses, which include precocious puberty in both boys and girls.
- **Associated neurologic changes**, particularly with strabismus or ocular nerve palsies, should be carefully sought. If present, they may suggest a midline tumour.
- **Concomitant onset of diabetes insipidus** would also indicate a structural lesion in this area. However, absence of these findings does not exclude such a problem.
- **Severe hypothyroidism** may be associated with precocity in both sexes due to high TSH levels interacting with the FSH receptor.

Additional Features that Should be Sought

If the history of pubertal onset is extremely rapid and progress significantly rapid over a short time, evidence for a possible peripheral lesion should be sought.

While examining the testes, the presence of asymmetry should be noted. The presence of a unilateral significantly larger testis may be suggestive of possible tumour. However, a Leydig cell tumour may not be very large as the major component of testicular size is composed of Sertoli cells. In the relatively rare cause of testotoxicosis, due to an activating mutation in the LH receptor gene, testes are not enlarged in the presence of significant virilisation.

Blood pressure measurements may help to identify a specific adrenal enzyme block. **Hypertension** may occur with 11-hydroxylase deficiency where excess deoxycorticosterone prior to the enzyme block is responsible for hypertension.

Diagnostic Approach

It is important to establish if a child is in early or precocious puberty and whether puberty is slow or rapid in its progress. Once certain that puberty is progressing rapidly, the physical examination should concentrate on finding signs that may point to a specific cause. Café-au-lait patches may suggest the presence of either NF1 or McCune–Albright syndrome.

Girls

In girls, breast development without pubic hair may suggest an oestrogen-producing ovarian tumour, such as a granulosa cell tumour, which may be palpable in the abdomen.

Primary hypothyroidism may also present with isolated breast development (thelarche), and precocious puberty due to high TSH levels stimulating the gonadotrophin axis, although this is rare. Unlike other causes of precocious puberty, in this condition bone age is delayed.

Isolated pubarche (pubic hair) development suggests androgen excess rather than onset of true puberty. Early pubic hair may occur with late-onset or non-classical congenital adrenal hyperplasia. Rarely, pubic hair may also develop in children with rapidly growing adrenal or ovarian tumours.

Boys

For a boy, the size of the testes is very important in the assessment of puberty. Where testicular size is less than 4 mL, the source of androgen is unlikely to be within the hypothalamic pituitary area and is much more likely to be peripheral, such as an adrenal lesion. Such a lesion could be a congenital adrenal hyperplasia due to 21 hydroxylase or 11 hydroxylase enzyme deficiency. More rarely, a beta HCG-producing tumour may occur, stimulating androgen production from the testes. Lateralising discrepancy in testicular size should therefore be sought for evidence of a testicular tumour. If a single testis only is present or if one testis has been damaged (orchitis or trauma), there is compensatory hypertrophy of the remaining testis, so it may appear larger than expected for the degree of apparent pubertal change.

For males who have primary androgen excess, the high levels of androgen may cause secondary stimulation of the hypothalamic-pituitary axis and subsequent onset of central precocious puberty.

Investigations that will Yield Results Useful to the Patient, in Order of Priority

Investigations should focus on finding a cause for the problem.

BIOCHEMICAL

- Gonadotrophin measurement, where available, will demonstrate whether the problem is central or peripheral. LH is a better indicator of gonadal activity, while FSH is a more sensitive marker of gonadal reserve.
- The level of the secreted sex hormones may give an indication as to origin of puberty. In an oestrogen-secreting ovarian tumour, the level of oestrogen will be extremely high. However, this is not entirely reliable and the level of oestrogen should only be used as an index of suspicion.
- Serum 17-hydroxyprogesterone levels: If suspicious of adrenal hyperplasia, measurement of 17-hydroxyprogesterone levels 60 minutes after administration of synacthen will diagnose congenital adrenal hyperplasia due to 21-hydroxylase deficiency.
- Hypertension with virilisation will usually indicate 11-hydroxylase deficiency; specialised tests including a urinary steroid profile or measurement of deoxycorticosterone (DOC) will confirm the diagnosis. These tests are not commonly available in many places.
- Tumour markers for βHCG, αFP where indicated — these may be elevated in germ cell tumours.

The GNRH test is potentially more useful in precocious puberty compared to delayed puberty. A GnRH test uses intravenous GnRH (100 μg bolus) with gonadotrophin levels in blood samples taken basally and at 30 and 60 minutes helps to differentiate between CPP and PPP. In CPP gonadotrophins are elevated, with peak LH (typically more than 5 IU/L) greater than FSH levels. Conversely, in PPP, gonadotrophin levels are low but sex steroid levels are high.

IMAGING

Imaging will be dependent on history, examination and basic biochemistry.

- Where appropriate, abdominal imaging will demonstrate a lesion within the ovary or adrenal gland.
- Skeletal survey and/or bone scan for fibrous dysplasia.
- Bone age.
- Pelvic ultrasound.
- Where the lesion is considered to be central, MRI is the appropriate investigation for the hypothalamic pituitary area. Lesions in this area such as hypothalamic hamartoma or germinoma are frequently small and commonly missed on CT.

Rationale for Management

Precocious puberty is often distressing to the child and parents. In girls, parents worry about possible menstrual bleeding at an early age. They worry that the child may not 'cope' with rapid body changes while not mature enough to understand the implications of puberty. Psychological support for an affected child and family is of great importance in management of precocious puberty. The affected child may be highly emotional, tearful and occasionally depressed. He or she does not relate well to age-appropriate peers and may wish to play with those considerably older. This in turn can lead to significant difficulties, particularly at school.

Parents can lack empathy if not properly informed as to the effect of pubertal hormones on the child.

The child is often a high achiever in the classroom, due to the maturing effect of sex hormone on brain function. This can lead to overload by school staff, in the mistaken belief that the 'sensible' child will be able to multitask beyond his or her capacity.

Therefore, there may be genuine psychological concerns to consider treatment to stop puberty. Another reason for stopping puberty is to attenuate the pubertal growth spurt and bone maturation with the aim of improving final height prognosis. However, improvement in final height gain is more effective when treatment is started under age 6 years, and rarely effective in those older than 7 years. In some children with significant physical disability, puberty may need to be halted at parental request at an older age, with adequate consideration given to management of personal hygiene for periods and other factors such as epilepsy being triggered by periods.

MANAGEMENT OF PRECOCIOUS PUBERTY

Acute Management

If an organic lesion is found, treatment of the primary disorder is paramount. For hypothalamic hamartomata, disconnection or removal via a transcallosal approach can reduce or cure gelastic and partial seizures but does not cure the CPP. For this condition treatment will be needed.

Disorders of the hypothalamic ovarian gonadal axis need to be treated, depending on the source of the sex hormone. In the relatively rare situation where the cause for precocious puberty is of primary gonadal hormone excess with secondary stimulation of the central axis, as in adrenal hyperplasia or McCune–Albright syndrome, it may be necessary to treat both the underlying condition and to address the

secondary stimulation of the hypothalamic pituitary axis. Once this axis has been activated it often does not switch off despite control of the underlying condition. If the primary condition is tumour, treatment of that problem will usually result in regression of all pubertal activity.

Options for treatment of central precocious puberty may be limited by cost and the availability of preparations.

GnRH Agonist

GnRH analogues, which feed back to inhibit endogenous GnRH secretion, are preferred for the treatment of CPP. However, if unavailable, progestogen may be used as an alternative. Over the age of 7 years in a girl, the use of GnRH analogues will not usually make any difference to final height outcome. Its use in this age group should therefore be limited to the reduction of psychological distress for the child and family.[12]

GnRH agonist can be administered using a long-acting preparation, given once every 12 weeks, if this is available. This will usually control the precocity and will cause reversal of most physical changes of puberty.

For the first month of treatment, stimulation via the LHRH agonist action may occur, with potential exacerbation of the pubertal changes. These may need to be blocked initially with cyproterone acetate, in doses varying between 12.5 to 50 mg or medroxyprogesterone acetate 15–20 mg/day. In girls, vaginal bleeding is possible at the end of this first month of treatment with a GnRH analogue. Parents must be instructed as to the possibility that this phenomenon could occur or they become very anxious and distressed, as does the child.

If the lesion is peripheral, blockade of sex hormone is much more difficult and is currently limited to the use of aromatase inhibitors such as letrozole or anastrozole. In girls, tamoxifen, as a selective oestrogen receptor modulator (SERM), can be added at a dose of 20 mg/day, in an effort to try to reduce the marked bone age advance that occurs in the presence of high levels of sex hormone and thus to try to preserve final height outcome.

Progestogen

In a situation where these very expensive medications are unable to be provided, the use of progestogen can be extremely helpful. Medroxyprogesterone in a dose of 15–20 mg/day, on a regular basis will, in many cases, reverse most of the changes of puberty. The progestogen causes some degree of fluid retention and may make the child somewhat bad tempered, but these changes are usually quite mild and better than the behavioural changes induced by abnormally early puberty.

This treatment is effective in both boys and girls. However, it is not quite as efficacious as a GnRH analogue and tends not to stop bone age advance, thus producing a somewhat truncated final height expectation at the end of treatment. However, for the vast majority of children who have precocious puberty, final height, although lower than the midparental expectation, is not very severely reduced.

Long-term Management

Central precocious puberty treatment needs to be continued until other peers are at an age where puberty is acceptable or for as long as the family wish. A useful guideline for cessation is to treat until the bone age is close to chronological age. As bone age is always advanced in precocious puberty, this may mean that treatment has delayed bone age progression for several years, until bone age and chronologic age converge. A more practical management plan may be to continue GnRH analogues till the child reaches an age which is compatible with puberty occurring in the normal population. This may vary between 10 and 11 years, but is subject to parental and patient choice.

Expected Outcomes After Precocious Puberty

Use of GnRH agonist has not been shown to cause fertility problems in future. However,

after cessation of treatment it may take many months to re-establish normal pubertal progress in some children.

Central precocious puberty occurring in a child who had a history of intrauterine growth retardation can be followed by later adolescent onset of polycystic ovary syndrome.

Both males and females can transmit the tendency to precocious puberty to their own children and should be informed of this possibility.

GYNAECOMASTIA

Clinical Setting

Gynaecomastia is common in both sexes in early infancy, presenting with breast development secondary to maternal oestrogen and occasionally at later stages if a child has been exposed to exogenous oestrogen. Sources of exogenous oestrogen include the excessive ingestion of soy products or, rarely, by access to other sources of oestrogen such as a parent's contraceptive pill.

However, the majority of infantile cases of gynaecomastia, usually presenting in girls and referred to as premature thelarche, do not have an obvious cause. The condition is most often mild and disappears over 1–4 years, without sequelae.

Prepubertal gynaecomastia in males is uncommon and may be associated with serious medical ill health. A cause should also be diligently sought in this age group. In contrast, pubertal gynaecomastia in boys occurs in over 50% of normal adolescent males. Its usual course is to be of minor breast growth, with complete resolution by 2 years after onset.

Gynaecomastia occurs as a response of normal breast tissue to oestrogen. An increasingly common cause in all age groups is via the aromatisation of androgen to oestrogen in peripheral fat. As the degree of obesity increases within populations, a significant rise in the frequency of complaint of gynaecomastia occurs.

Multiple other hormones are responsible for alterations in breast growth.

- Testosterone inhibits breast tissue differentiation.
- Prolactin increases breast tissue via stimulation of lactating cells.
- Thyrotoxicosis can be associated with gynaecomastia, via high levels of sex hormone binding globulin, having a preferential action on testosterone binding, thus providing regularly excessive levels of bioavailable oestrogen.
- Relative oestrogen excess via exogenous oestrogen administration, altered liver function delaying oestrogen excretion or altered oestrogen and testosterone binding should be considered as possible causes.

Klinefelter syndrome can present with gynaecomastia at an early age. Evidence for firm, small testes should be sought. If the affected child is above 8—9 years of age, raised gonadotrophins are likely to be found. Evidence for social isolation or behavioural disorder in childhood should be sought. Their presence increases the likelihood of this possibility. Karyotype should provide a confirmatory diagnosis.

HCG producing tumours of the brain (germinoma), testes, lung or liver are rare but will produce gynaecomastia usually with onset of puberty. Presence of acute onset of diabetes insipidus or lateralising difference in size of the testes should alert the physician to urgent further investigation. A βHCG level is essential for early diagnostic confirmation of these disorders.

Other endocrinopathies associated with gynaecomastia include acromegaly, Cushing syndrome or adrenal hyperplasia with androgen excess.

Disorders of sexual development in an undervirilised male can rarely cause this problem: occasionally ovotesticular disorder of sexual development with oestrogen production.

Partial androgen insensitivity can present as gynaecomastia in late childhood, in a child who was otherwise considered to have normal male genitalia.

Drugs causing gynaecomastia include marijuana, phenothiazine, tricyclic antidepressants and some antipsychotic agents, androgen antagonists such as spironolactone, cimetidine, and ketoconazole. Calcium channel blockers and phenytoin may also cause gynaecomastia.

Diagnostic Approach

The commonest cause of presentation with gynaecomastia is that of pubertal onset in an overweight or normal male. It is rare to find a pathological cause but if breast tissue is significantly large or prepubertal in origin, it is reasonable to consider pathologic causes.

Assessment

This includes a careful history of drug or oestrogen exposure or for systemic disorders including Klinefelter syndrome. Examination should include evidence for testicular masses, liver disease, eunuchoid body habitus, under virilisation or genital ambiguity.

Investigations that will Yield Results Useful to the Patient, in Order of Priority

- FSH, LH, oestradiol, testosterone, prolactin, βHCG, liver function and karyotype are routine.
- Dihydrotestosterone may occasionally be indicated but availability is limited to specialist centres.
- If βHCG is elevated, imaging of abdomen, brain, chest and testes as required.

Management

Acute

The majority of pubertal gynaecomastia is self-limiting and requires no intervention except judicious weight reduction, where indicated. However, in some boys the breast tissue is extremely firm and shows no sign at all of decreasing as puberty progresses. Even if it is likely that some of the breast tissue will disappear with the passage of time, the condition can be so emotionally disabling as to require surgical referral at an early date.

Tamoxifen has been used, as have aromatase inhibitors in adult men with this condition, with some success. However, in children and adolescents these drugs cause failure of appropriate bone mass accrual, particularly in accrual of cortical thickness of bone, an essential part of pubertal bone growth. Therefore, the use of oestrogen-blocking agents should be used with extreme caution in adolescent boys.

Long Term

For boys with Klinefelter syndrome or other undervirilising conditions, testosterone use can completely resolve gynaecomastia over around 12 months' use. Long-acting preparations of intramuscular testosterone or subcutaneous pellets have both been shown to be of more benefit than short-acting preparations, where they are available.

Surgical intervention should utilise sub-areolar mastectomy rather than liposuction, particularly in a boy who has chest wall obesity. Removal of chest wall fat and removal of breast tissue can result in a 'negative breast shape', which is irremediable and severely disfiguring.

Follow-up Plan

Recurrence is rare unless in the context of rapid weight gain or the use of marijuana. Sometimes surgical methods may not provide complete cure and second surgery may need to be undertaken. Occasionally, the child is left with redundant skin either following mastectomy or following a period of significant weight loss.

OTHER DISORDERS OF THE BREAST

These are usually not endocrine conditions but frequently present to the paediatric endocrinologist for first assessment.

Virginal Breast Hypertrophy

Clinical Setting

This is a rare condition, characterised by grossly excessive increase in breast size, which can occur extremely rapidly, with onset even in the early to mid stages of puberty. It usually affects both sides but can be unilateral.

It is occasionally associated with genetic abnormalities, including PTEN mutations and thus may be seen in association with conditions such as Cowden syndrome, where a lifetime increase in risk for multiple malignancies is increased including thyroid, breast and endometrial cancers as well as benign hamartomatous lesions.

Virginal breast hypertrophy is characterised by discomfort, skin stretching, strial formation and when severe by skin breakdown, particularly around the nipple.

Management

This is ultimately surgical, with reduction mammoplasty and sometimes total mastectomy if the problem is recurrent. However, post-operative infection and wound breakdown is common. To reduce these risks, consideration should be given to peri-operative medical management, to reduce the impact of oestrogen effect on breast tissue and thus to stabilise breast growth.

Tamoxifen, as a selective oestrogen modulator (SERM), has been successfully used, at a dose of 20 mg/day, for a period of 6–12 weeks prior to surgery and the dose continued after surgery for 12 weeks, until wound healing is complete and the scars firm and stable.

Unilateral Breast Hypoplasia

Clinical Setting

This is not an endocrine condition, although it frequently presents to the paediatric endocrinologist for assessment and advice.

It is common for breast growth during early stages of puberty to be more prominent on one side with apparently unilateral breast development causing parental concern. This tissue usually either regresses then growth commences on the contralateral side, or the second side catches up over several months.

A diagnosis of breast hypoplasia should therefore not be made until at least Tanner stage IV development has been reached.

Assessment

This should include a careful check for possible associated lesions of the Poland anomalad, with absent pectoralis major, unilateral kidney and abnormalities of radius formation.

However, the condition is usually isolated.

A clue to severity is nipple hypoplasia, which if present usually indicates that breast growth on that side will be absent or minimal.

Management

The treatment is solely surgical. However, surgical referral should never be considered until the affected girl has completed her linear growth and the breast growth has been stable bilaterally for at least 12 months. Referral for surgery made too early will result in potential for an unsatisfactory outcome, possibly with the contralateral side continuing to grow.

The girl herself will need to identify her preferred breast size; that is, whether she wants augmentation on the hypoplastic side or reduction on the 'normal' side.

It is inappropriate to consider that a concerned adolescent girl, worried about her self-image and with fears as to her appearance, can make a rational decision on this subject at the age of 13–14. It is usually advisable to give careful instructions to child and parents as to use of some form of 'filler' for the small side, while waiting for a final outcome. In countries where cosmetic availability of lingerie is accessible, small bra inserts called 'chicken fillets' are easily obtained. Their use can markedly reduce distress for the affected girl. Purchase of these low-cost items via Internet suppliers is possible.

References

1. Banerjee I, Clayton P. The genetic basis for the timing of human puberty. *J Neuroendocrinol* 2007;**19**:831–8.
2. Gajdos ZK, Henderson KD, Hirschhorn JN, Palmert MR. Genetic determinants of pubertal timing in the general population. *Mol Cell Endocrinol* 2010;**324**:21–9.
3. Kaminski BA, Palmert MR. Genetic control of pubertal timing. *Curr Opin Pediatr* 2008;**20**:458–64.
4. Sedlmeyer IL, Palmert MR. Delayed puberty: analysis of a large case series from an academic center. *J Clin Endocrinol Metab* 2002;**87**:1613–20.
5. Liu PY, Baker HW, Jayadev V, et al. Induction of spermatogenesis and fertility during gonadotropin treatment of gonadotropin-deficient infertile men: predictors of fertility outcome. *J Clin Endocrinol Metab* 2009;**94**:801–8.
6. Zacharin M. Disorders of ovarian function in childhood and adolescence: evolving needs of the growing child. An endocrine perspective. *BJOG* 2010;**117**:156–62.
7. Zacharin MR. Puberty, contraception, and hormonal management for young people with disabilities. *Clin Pediatr (Phila)* 2009;**48**:149–55.
8. Zacharin M, Savasi I, Grover S. The impact of menstruation in adolescents with disabilities related to cerebral palsy. *Arch Dis Child* 2010;**95**:526–30.
9. Pleskacova J, Hersmus R, Oosterhuis JW, et al. Tumor risk in disorders of sex development. *Sex Dev* 2010;**4**:259–69.
10. Matura LA, Ho VB, Rosing DR, Bondy CA. Aortic dilatation and dissection in Turner syndrome. *Circulation* 2007;**116**:1663–70.
11. Zacharin M. Precocious puberty in two children with neurofibromatosis type I, in the absence of optic chiasmal glioma. *J Pediatr* 1997;**130**:155–7.
12. Carel JC, Eugster EA, Rogol A, et al. Consensus statement on the use of gonadotropin-releasing hormone analogs in children. *Pediatrics* 2009;**123**:e752–62.

Further Reading

Banerjee I, Clayton P. The genetic basis for the timing of human puberty. *J Neuroendocrinol* 2007;**19**:831-38.

Banerjee I, Clayton PE. Puberty. In: Warrell DA, Cox TM, Firth JD (eds), *Oxford Textbook of Medicine*, 5th ed, Vol. 13.9.2., Oxford: Oxford University Press, 2010. Available at URL: http://otm.oxfordmedicine.com/cgi/content/essentials/med-9780199204854-chapter-130902

Thyroid Disorders

Anna Simon, Margaret Zacharin

OUTLINE

HYPOTHYROIDISM

Hypothyroidism is a common problem encountered by paediatric endocrinologists. In children, the prevalence of hypothyroidism is about 0.15% with a female to male ratio of 2.8:1.[1] Normal thyroid hormone synthesis and its action on target tissues are necessary for normal metabolism throughout life, linear growth after birth and for normal development of the brain until 3 years of age.

Background

A brief review on thyroid gland development, physiology and actions of thyroid hormones will serve to understand the pathology of thyroid disorders, their therapeutic implications and the effect of treatment modalities. For more complete thyroid physiology the reader is referred to standard texts.

Normal Thyroid Gland Development and Function

The thyroid gland develops from an outpouching of the floor of the pharynx — the median anlage which migrates from the base of the tongue to its location in the neck between the fifth and seventh week of embryonic life. As the thyroid gland descends down the neck, it remains attached to the foramen caecum by the thyroglossal duct. The thyroglossal duct later obliterates; failure of

Practical Pediatric Endocrinology in a Limited Resource Setting
http://dx.doi.org/10.1016/B978-0-12-407822-2.00003-7

obliteration of the thyroglossal duct predisposes to the formation of thyroglossal cysts. The median anlage is joined by the two lateral anlages from the fourth branchial pouches. The follicular cells of the thyroid are mainly derived from the medial anlage, while the parafollicular or C cells (calcitonin-producing cells) are derived from the lateral anlages. The thyroid follicle consists of a monolayer of follicular cells surrounding a colloidal centre and the C cells are dispersed between the thyroid follicles. The hypothalamic-pituitary-thyroid (HPT) axis also develops simultaneously with multiple levels of regulatory function. The fetal thyroid is able to concentrate iodine by 12 weeks and the HPT axis is functional by 18 weeks of gestation.

Physiology of the Thyroid Gland

Iodine is the key requirement for thyroid hormone synthesis. Ingested iodine is converted to iodide in the gut then transported via the bloodstream to the thyroid gland with the help of the sodium-iodine symporter (NIS) and transports the iodine to the colloid-cell membrane interface with the help of the iodide transporters pendrin and other proteins. Thyroid peroxidase (TPO) catalyses oxidation of iodide, in the presence of peroxide. Hydrogen peroxide is produced by the thyroid oxidases, THOX2 and THOX1. This is the rate-limiting step in thyroid hormone synthesis. TPO also catalyses the iodination of tyrosine residues (organification) in thyroglobulin and the coupling of the mono-iodotyrosine and diiodotyrosine to form T_3 and T_4. Thyroglobulin is produced by the follicular cells of the thyroid and concentrated in the colloid. Excess iodine is stored in intrathyroidal colloid and released as required. The thyroid hormones are metabolised by the deiodinases to release the iodine which is recycled and absorbed by the thyroid gland. Triiodothyronine, by mono de-iodination of T_4, mainly peripherally, is the active thyroid hormone. Its

production is limited during pregnancy by maturation of hepatic deiodinase which occurs by 30–32 weeks' gestation.

The thyroid gland is under the regulatory control of pituitary thyroid-stimulating hormone (TSH), otherwise called thyrotropin, which is a glycoprotein, acting on the thyroid gland to stimulate iodine uptake, organification and release of thyroid hormones as well as cell growth. TSH in turn is regulated by thyrotropin-releasing hormone (TRH), a tripeptide synthesised in the supraoptic and the supraventricular nuclei of the hypothalamus. The thyroid hormones exert a negative feedback control over TSH and TRH secretion. TSH secretion rises precipitously within 30–60 minutes of birth,

TABLE 3.1   Actions of Thyroid Hormones

Growth and development – essential for normal growth in childhood

- Direct effects

- Stimulates pituitary GH synthesis and secretion

- Stimulates insulin-like growth factor (IGF) synthesis and action

- Increases protein synthesis and facilitates muscle growth

- Enhances IGF-1 action on the bone/cartilage

Central nervous system development and function

- Stimulation of neuronal cell maturation and migration

- Increases myelin formation

- Stimulates dendritic branching and synaptic formation

- Influences other neurotransmitters, enzymes and cell proteins

Metabolic effects

- Increases basal metabolic rate and heat production

- Increases gluconeogenesis, glycogenolysis and stimulates insulin-mediated glucose uptake

- Increases lipolysis and fatty acid oxidation

- Stimulation of adrenergic receptor binding

with resultant increase in thyroid hormone secretion, then decreases to a stable range by 72 hours after birth.

Important Physiologic Considerations for Management of Thyroid Disorders

- Placental transfer of T_4 takes place throughout gestation, permitting relative protection of brain development in the hypothyroid infant, provided the mother is euthyroid.
- Placental transfer of maternal antithyroid drugs also occurs whereas exogenously administered thyroxine does not cross the placenta efficiently.
- Thyroglobulin as a storage pool for iodine and thyroid hormones acts as a marker for the presence of thyroid tissue. It is raised during conditions of thyroid damage and disappears in the absence of thyroid tissue. It is therefore a useful diagnostic tool.
- As a consequence of immaturity of the hypothalamo-pituitary-thyroid axis, the TSH surge after birth is less marked and the decline in T_4 levels after birth more profound, resulting in 'hypothyroxinaemia of prematurity' most marked in infants born prior to 30 weeks' gestation.
- Pre-term infants have very low levels of T_3 due to immaturity of hepatic deiodinase.
- Screening for neonatal hypothyroidism should either be performed at 72 hours after birth or on cord blood for accurate estimation.

Actions of Thyroid Hormones

The major effects of thyroid hormones are mediated via the thyroid hormone nuclear receptors and function as DNA transcription factors.

Serum concentration of T_4 is 80–100 times that of T_3, with most of its activity occurring via conversion to T_3 as the active hormone which has a 10-fold higher affinity than T_4 for the nuclear receptors.

Hypothyroidism can result from defective secretion at any level of the hypothalamic-pituitary-thyroid axis, from tissue resistance through to thyroxine or accelerated hormone degradation. Hypothyroidism can therefore be classified in the following categories.

Primary Hypothyroidism

Primary hypothyroidism refers to decreased production of T_4 and T_3 and increased TSH as a result of loss of inhibitory feedback on the pituitary. Primary hypothyroidism is again classified into:

- overt hypothyroidism, when the serum TSH is high and fT_4 concentration is low.
- subclinical hypothyroidism when the serum TSH is high, but fT_4 concentration is normal.

Central Hypothyroidism

This is characterised by low TSH and low fT_4 which can be caused by:

- deficiency of TSH — secondary or pituitary hypothyroidism
- deficiency of TRH — tertiary or hypothalamic hypothyroidism.

Acquired forms of central hypothyroidism can occur with infiltrative, vascular, neoplastic conditions. It also may occur as a long-term effect after irradiation of the CNS.

Congenital forms of central hypothyroidism are rare and are often a result of gene mutations of the TRH receptor, β-TSH or PIT1.

1. Resistance to Thyroid Hormones

Resistance to thyroxine is a rare condition which is dominantly inherited. Affected patients have high serum levels of free T_4 and T_3 with mild elevation or normal TSH. Goitre is a usual finding, but clinical manifestations vary widely depending on the T_3 receptor isoforms which are predominantly involved.

2. *Consumptive Hypothyroidism*

Consumptive hypothyroidism is caused by increased release and activity of Type 3 deiodinase from vascular tumours, particularly hepatic haemangiomata. Other tumours like astrocytomas and glioblastomas can cause rapid degradation of T_4 and T_3 resulting in hypothyroidism.[2] The requirement of thyroxine in these patients far exceeds the normal replacement doses.

CLINICAL SETTING

Primary Hypothyroidism

Primary hypothyroidism is the most common thyroid disease encountered in a paediatric endocrinology clinic. Primary hypothyroidism can be further classified as congenital hypothyroidism or acquired hypothyroidism.

Congenital Hypothyroidism

Based on newborn screening programmes, the incidence of primary congenital hypothyroidism (CH) ranges from 1/2500 to 1/4000 newborns.[3] A higher prevalence has been reported from the Middle East and Asian countries[4] and is likely in regions with severe iodine deficiency. The importance of early diagnosis of congenital hypothyroidism and appropriate replacement with thyroxine stems from the fact that the brain damage incurred in congenital hypothyroidism is irreversible and results in permanent neurocognitive sequelae.

In countries where comprehensive and universal neonatal screening programmes are not available, this outcome remains a major cause for serious long-term morbidity in many communities. The reader is referred to more extensive discussion of options regarding development of neonatal screening programmes.[5,6]

Paediatricians should be well aware of the symptoms of CH and have a high index of suspicion to make an early diagnosis. Though newborn screening for hypothyroidism has been an effective tool for early detection of CH, the delayed manifestation of some cases of dyshormonogenesis and ectopia can result in the condition being missed. Paediatricians must continue to be alert to the possibility of CH even if the newborn screening test has been negative.

In many countries, the majority of births do not take place in a hospital setting or the mother and infant are discharged from hospital within 24 hours of the birth. Screening programmes therefore must consider the value of cord blood TSH rather than the more usual use of TSH on day 3, at 72 hours after birth.

The symptoms and signs of congenital hypothyroidism are listed below in Table 3.2 and the aetiology in Table 3.3.

The clinical diagnosis of congenital hypothyroidism is difficult and often delayed, as the early symptoms and signs are subtle. The underlying pathology and the duration of thyroid deprivation will influence the severity of the clinical manifestations (see below for diagnosis).

TABLE 3.2 Symptoms and Signs of Congenital Hypothyroidism

At birth	During early infancy
Postmaturity	Prolonged physiological jaundice
Macrosomia	
Large head, open posterior fontanelle	Poor feeding and lethargy
	Somnolence
Delayed skeletal maturation	Hypothermia
	Constipation
	Macroglossia
	Hoarse cry
	Umbilical hernia
	Dry, mottled skin
	Goitre

TABLE 3.3 Aetiology of Primary Congenital Hypothyroidism

Aetiology	Mutations known and associated features
Thyroid dysgenesis (80%) Ectopy Agenesis Hypoplasia Hemiagenesis	TTF1 — Hypotonia, choreoathetosis, respiratory distress TTF2 — cleft palate, kinky hair PAX8 — thyroid hypoplasia or apparent athyreosis TSH receptor — family history
Thyroid dyshormonogenesis (15%)	NIS, PDS,THOX2,TPO, Tg Goitre common, + deafness in Pendred syndrome
Resistance to thyroxine	Mutations in T_3 receptor isoforms Goitre, variable neurological and cardiac effect
Endemic cretinism	Iodine deficient regions
Transient congenital hypothyroidism	Transplacental transfer of TSH-receptor blocking antibodies Maternal antithyroid drugs Acute iodine overload

Aetiology of Primary Congenital Hypothyroidism

Thyroid Dysgenesis

Developmental defects of the thyroid are referred to as thyroid dysgenesis. About 80% of primary congenital hypothyroidism is secondary to thyroid dysgenesis. Thyroid dysgenesis includes athyreosis, hypoplasia, hemiagenesis and ectopic thyroid. Though initially considered sporadic, recent evidence point towards a genetic basis with mutations involving the transcription factors (TTF1, TTF2, PAX8) and thyroid growth (TSHR). Thyroid dysgenesis, especially ectopia thyroid, has a female predominance.[7]

Although it is unlikely that a precise genetic diagnosis can be reached in countries where resources are limited, it is worth considering recognised associated features, as outlined in Table 3.3. It may then be possible to locate a laboratory in any country that has a current interest or that offers a research programme to undertake testing of DNA from an affected infant. Pendred syndrome, in particular, is an example of a condition that should be recognised as early as possible, to avoid potentially catastrophic and complete later hearing loss.

True athyreosis has to be differentiated from 'apparent athyreosis' due to transplacentally transferred TSH-receptor antibodies or Na/I symporter defect. Apparent athyreosis can be confirmed by ultrasound study demonstrating the presence of the thyroid gland, and clinical examination may reveal a goitre.

Ectopic thyroid develops from a migrational defect and can be placed anywhere along the path of migration, but is most often sublingual. A lingual thyroid may present as a mass at the base of the tongue.

Apparent athyreosis or hypoplastic thyroid gland results from mutations involving the TSH-receptor.

An ectopic or hypoplastic gland may produce sufficient hormones for a variable time, from weeks to many months and may present with later hypothyroidism, in infancy or early childhood.

Thyroid Dyshormonogenesis

A defect in any one of the steps involved in the biosynthesis of thyroid hormone results in thyroid dyshormonogenesis. These defects are inherited as autosomal recessive traits and therefore are more prevalent in communities with consanguineous parentage. These inborn biosynthetic defects include defects in iodide trapping, organification, coupling, deiodinase activity and abnormalities in thyroglobulin synthesis, storage and release.[8]

Due to variable times of presentation and detection of hypothyroidism, these conditions are easily missed and can result in major problems of late postpartum onset of intellectual disability, growth failure and sometimes deafness, with consequent speech delay.

Goitre is a common occurrence with thyroid dysgenesis; goitre may be present at birth or appear later.

Gene mutations affecting the following defective thyroid biosynthesis steps have been identified.

- **Thyroid peroxidase (TPO)** in the presence of H_2O_2 catalyses the oxidation of iodide and coupling of iodotyrosine. This is the most common cause for dyshormonogenesis and can present with a complete or partial defect.
- **Transport of iodide from the cell into the colloid lumen through pendrin**, a protein complex functioning as iodide transporters. Pendred syndrome may present at any time from the neonatal period to the second decade of life and is associated with sensorineural deafness. Untreated thyroid disease presents as multinodular or diffuse goitre with variable severity of hypothyroidism. Deafness may be initially mild. The evolution of a Mondini malformation of the cochlea, in the second year of life, can result in precipitous and severe further loss of hearing, with consequent serious implications for speech development.
- **Thyroid oxidase 2 (THOX2)** generates hydrogen peroxide (H_2O_2) which is required for the oxidation of iodide. This is the rate-limiting step for thyroid hormonogenesis and is dependent on Ca^{++} and NADPH.
- **Transport of iodide across the follicular cell membrane against a concentration gradient by the sodium-iodide symporter (NIS).** Defective NIS may present as apparent athyreosis on a pertechnetate scan. Ultrasonography will demonstrate a normally placed thyroid gland with normal or increased size.
- **Defects in the synthesis, storage and release of thyroglobulin** can present with varying severity of hypothyroidism and low levels of thyroglobulin. Thyroglobulin is synthesised

in the follicular cells and then stored in colloid. The tyrosine residues of thyroglobulin undergo iodination to form mono and diiodotyrosine. These molecules couple, to form T_4 and T_3.

Iodine Deficiency

Iodine deficiency is a widely prevalent nutritional disorder in many regions of the world, especially the developing nations. National programmes of iodine supplementation, usually using salt as a vehicle, are making inroads on reducing the burden of this condition.

However, implementation of these programmes continues to be complicated by issues of distribution, dissemination of information, education, understanding of need for change, relative financial consideration where iodised salt may cost more, distrust of packaging and sometimes concerns regarding discolouration of the iodised product. For uniformity of success, each country must address issues particular to its own region, in order for successful permanent eradication of iodine deficiency.

The major source of iodine is as a trace element in food, its presence determined in any area by availability in soil and complicated in some places by ingestion of goitrogens.

Goitre is the most common manifestation of iodine deficiency, consequent upon inadequate substrate availability increasing the feedback loop for TSH production with consequent thyroid gland hyperplasia. A goitre prevalence of 5% or more in a population classifies the area as endemic for iodine deficiency. Around 10% of infants born in areas of profound iodine deficiency are estimated to be at risk for hypothyroidism and its consequences in terms of neurologic deficit.

The endemic form of severe iodine deficiency hypothyroidism is termed as cretinism. Two forms of cretinism have been identified — the neurological form and the myxedematous form.

- Neurological cretinism is frequent in South America and the South Pacific region. Neurological manifestations predominate with mild to profound degrees of intellectual disability, deaf-mutism, spastic diplegia and growth retardation.
- Myxedematous cretinism is more prevalent in endemic areas in Africa and presents mainly with myxedematous features such as coarse face, dry skin, hoarse voice, constipation and severe growth retardation.
- A mixed form with both neurological and myxedematous forms is also seen in certain regions, e.g. Himalayan areas.

Milder forms of iodine deficiency are recognised as causing varying degrees of impairment of intellect, learning difficulty and hearing impairment, as well as goitre.

Diagnosis of Congenital Hypothyroidism

Congenital hypothyroidism is detected on screening tests or otherwise on clinical grounds. A good clinical history and physical examination provide clues to the diagnosis. A high index of suspicion should exist where the infant comes from an area of known iodine deficiency.

The only distinguishing clinical findings at birth which should prompt immediate testing of thyroid function are:

- large fontanelle, macrosomia and postmaturity[9]
- prolonged physiological jaundice.

A history of somnolence, poor feeding and constipation are usually elicited after a positive test result. Family history for other cases of CH and history of maternal thyroid disorders are important for diagnostic evaluation.[10]

Physical examination should include careful palpation for a goitre with the neck hyperextended. Care should be taken to examine for dysmorphic features and other organ anomalies.[11]

Transient congenital hypothyroidism can be considered if there is a family history of autoimmune thyroid illness, use of antithyroid drugs in the mother, or excessive exposure to iodine. Dyshormonogenesis should be considered when siblings are affected.

Hypothyroidism occurs with or without goitre.

Biochemical Confirmation of Hypothyroidism

Locating the Patient

Due to the frequency of minimal hospital stays or home births in many countries, every attempt should be made to document as effectively as possible the whereabouts of the family, so that appropriate location and effective tracing may be undertaken, for follow-up of abnormal screening results. As named streets, villages and specific homes may be lacking, it becomes a matter of serious importance that such information is elicited by a designated staff member employed specifically for that purpose. Loss to follow-up and lack of early treatment of hypothyroidism becomes a major financial and public health burden to a community, with potential loss of long-term functional value within the workforce.

Confirmation of Diagnosis

Once detected on newborn screening or clinically suspected, hypothyroidism can be biochemically confirmed by elevated TSH and a low fT_4. The severity of hypothyroidism is usually judged on the basis of the level of T_4 and the degree of delay in skeletal maturation.

An elevated TSH with normal fT_4 suggests subclinical hypothyroidism and requires close follow-up clinically and also by repeat biochemical assays of TSH and fT_4 every 2–3 weeks till a definite diagnosis can be reached.

Caution should be exercised in the situation where a marginally elevated TSH is present with an inappropriately low T_4. In this situation central hypothyroidism may be present and should prompt further investigation for other aspects of pituitary dysfunction.

Care should be taken to use age-appropriate values while interpreting the biochemical results.

Absence or stippled appearance of the lower femoral epiphysis on an anteroposterior X-ray of the knee in a term newborn along with clinical features can also be considered as a diagnostic test for hypothyroidism when thyroid hormone assays are not available.

Aetiological Diagnosis of Hypothyroidism

Aetiological diagnosis of congenital hypothyroidism is important for establishing the permanence of CH and also determining recurrence risk in the family. These investigations should be considered if available but treatment should never be delayed beyond a maximum of 7–10 days from birth, in order to complete such investigations.

Technetium-99 Nuclear Scan

This assists in the aetiological work-up of CH. Anatomical anomalies of absent, hypoplastic, ectopic positioning of the gland or hemiagenesis can be demonstrated on the Tc99 thyroid nuclear scan.

Many forms of dyshormonogenesis may be suspected, with the finding of a normally located, large gland, with 15–25% uptake on scan (compared to a normal 2–5%). This test, however, cannot clearly distinguish dyshormonogenesis from iodine deficiency, where uptake is also high.

Ultrasonography

Ultrasonography of the thyroid gland can also be used to assess the size and location of the thyroid gland and in skilled hands may replace nuclear scans in the aetiological diagnosis of CH.

For example, estimation of maternal TSH-receptor blocking antibodies can help to diagnose

transient CH, whereas undetectable thyroglobulin levels may confirm the diagnosis of agenesis thyroid. Although these tests are likely not to be available, ultrasound (US) examination of the thyroid helps to distinguish apparent athyreosis from true athyreosis. Apparent athyreosis due to transplacental transfer of maternal TSH receptor-blocking antibodies is not common.[12]

Perchlorate Discharge Test

This test is occasionally used, less so now that genetic diagnosis has become more available. A perchlorate challenge test shows excessive release of iodine that accumulates due to defective hormonogenesis. Normally, less than 10% of the infused iodine is discharged 2 hours after the administration of perchlorate, whereas almost 15–80% iodine release occurs in dyshormonogenesis.

Rationale for Management of Congenital Hypothyroidism

Early treatment of congenital hypothyroidism of any cause, instituted within the first 10–14 days of life, has been shown to result in a neurocognitive outcome indistinguishable from that of a normal population. Delay after that time results in continuing loss of IQ points.

Practical Management of Congenital Hypothyroidism

In a situation where access to scintigraphy is limited, thyroxine treatment should be instituted

TABLE 3.4   Inverse Relationship of IQ to Age of Commencement of Thyroid Replacement[13]

Age in Months	IQ mean	IQ range
0–3	89	64–107
3–6	71	35–96
> 6	54	25–80

without delay. Ultrasonography can be performed at a later stage, and scintigraphy can be performed after withdrawal of thyroxine treatment at an older age (see re-evaluation of thyroid status below).

Replacement with L-thyroxine (LT_4) to achieve normalisation of free T_4 and TSH is the primary aim of therapy. The dosing has to be individualised, based on clinical and biochemical monitoring. LT_4 should be replaced in doses sufficient to normalise TSH and correct fT_4 to the upper half of the normal range.

In situations where free T_4 assays are not available, total T_4 assays may be substituted. T_4 bound to thyroglobulin is measured and is susceptible to errors when thyroglobulin levels are abnormal or abnormal protein binding is present.

LT_4 tablets should be used which should be crushed and immediately administered with a small amount of water or milk formula. This should be given at the beginning of a feed, preferably in a 1 mL syringe inserted towards the back of the mouth, to maximise effective dosing. Thyroxine should not be given with substances that interfere with absorption such as iron, soya or fibre. Liquid preparations are unstable and should not be used.

Counselling parents on the aetiology, thyroid physiology, outcome with treatment and the devastating effect on neurocognitive development if left untreated is crucial for successful long-term management.

In the newborn period, early replacement, at the latest by 10–14 days of life, with thyroxine, 10–15 µg/kg/day and normalising TSH within the first month has been advocated, to achieve near normal neurocognitive function.[14] Regular clinical monitoring with growth and development and biochemical assessment every 2–3 months should be undertaken during the first two years of life and thereafter every 6 months. Non-compliance is associated with poor developmental outcome.

Re-evaluation of the thyroid status after ceasing treatment for 6–8 weeks should be undertaken after the age of 3 years if the initial diagnosis was suspect or if there was an unusually low requirement of LT_4 to maintain a euthyroid state. Special attention must be given to any neurodevelopmental needs as required.

In countries where newborn screening is not available, screening of all siblings of patients with CH should be undertaken for early diagnosis and intervention.

Long-term Outcome

Early adequate treatment (within the first 2 weeks of life) with high-dose thyroxine replacement usually results in normal to near-normal neurocognitive outcome and normal growth. Skeletal maturation also proceeds in a normal pattern. Delayed or inadequate treatment is associated with adverse outcome with permanent and significant neurological and cognitive defects.

Genetic Counselling

With recent recognition of a range of genes being responsible for thyroid dysgenesis and with AR inheritance of dyshormonogenesis, genetic counselling is important and screening of siblings and offspring offers a new potential level of care for affected families.

CLINICAL SETTING

Acquired Hypothyroidism in Childhood

Aetiologies of acquired hypothyroidism are listed.

- Autoimmune
  Goitrous Hashimoto's thyroiditis
  Atrophic (primary myxoedema)
  Polyglandular autoimmune syndrome (Type I, II and III)
- Systemic disease
  Cystinosis
  Histiocytosis X

- Others
  Radiation exposure
  Thyroidectomy
  Antithyroid drugs, amiodarone, lithium
  Radioiodine
  Haemangiomas of the liver
- Central hypothyroidism

Chronic Autoimmune Thyroiditis

The most common cause for childhood acquired hypothyroidism is autoimmune, chronic lymphocytic thyroiditis,[15,16] known as Hashimoto's disease. Hashimoto's thyroiditis is characterised by lymphocytic infiltration, thyroid cell destruction and elevated antibodies to thyroid peroxidase (TPO) and thyroglobulin. One to two percent of children have evidence of autoimmune thyroid disease, with or without goitre. If present, the goitre is usually non-tender. It may be soft early in the course of the disease, later becoming firm and gritty in texture. There is a female preponderance with a 2:1 female to male ratio and a familial clustering.

Chronic lymphocytic thyroiditis has a variable course necessitating prolonged follow-up. Children may be euthyroid, or may have overt or compensated hypothyroidism. Initially, they may have a thyrotoxic phase due to the discharge of preformed T_4 and T_3 from the damaged gland. Most children who are hypothyroid remain hypothyroid; however, spontaneous recovery of thyroid function may occur and some initially euthyroid will become hypothyroid over time.

Chronic autoimmune thyroiditis may be the initial presentation of an autoimmune polyglandular syndrome and therefore the possibility of co-existing or evolving T1DM, pernicious anaemia and Addison's disease should be considered.

Autoimmune thyroid disease also has a higher prevalence in Down syndrome and Turner syndrome.

Radiation Exposure

Childhood exposure to radiation as part of cancer treatment protocols is common, either directly to the gland with older mantle radiation treatments for lymphoma, spinal radiation for brain tumours or by indirect exposure at the time of cranial radiation. Other radiation exposure from both external beam and radionucleotides such as occurred at Chernobyl and more recently in Japan can cause damage to both thyroid structure and function. (See thyroid cancer for further information.)

All such exposed children should have regular thyroid function screening as well as ultrasound surveillance. Increasing use of I^{131} ablation as a therapeutic modality for management of Graves' disease in adolescence has led to a need for ongoing surveillance and management of evolving hypothyroidism, with testing every 6–12 weeks until adequate replacement is established.

Thyroidectomy

Partial thyroidectomy for hyperthyroid conditions or adenoma is likely to result in euthyroidism in the short term. However, the natural history of Graves' disease over 15 years may be of gradual evolution to hypothyroidism.

Drugs Causing Hypothyroidism

Amiodarone deserves special mention, as a common treatment for cardiac arrhythmias in infants and children. The molecule is composed of approximately 30% iodine, which causes blockade of uptake into the normal thyroid (unlike adults where it may cause hyperthyroidism). It is both a competitive and non-competitive inhibitor of T_3, binding to the thyroid hormone receptor. Evolution of blockade may take weeks from onset of the drug use, so regular weekly thyroid function tests are required to avoid the possibility of missing profound hypothyroidism. After drug withdrawal it may take weeks to months before the effect of iodine excess has worn off.

- Drugs that impair T_4 absorption are calcium carbonate, ferrous sulphate, cholestyramine and sucralfate.
- Drugs that can accelerate T_4 clearance include rifampicin, carbamazepine and phenytoin.
- Dexamethasone reduces TSH levels during its administration, with a mild rebound effect after drug withdrawal.

Haemangiomas of the Liver

Consumptive hypothyroidism caused by an haemangioma in infants is a rare but well-recognised cause of hypothyroidism which tends to resolve spontaneously as the haemangioma shrinks.

Signs and Symptoms of Acquired Hypothyroidism

Careful evaluation is very important in a child as both symptoms and signs of hypothyroidism are often subtle.

Physical signs and symptoms of acquired hypothyroidism in children and adolescents depend on the severity and the duration of disease. The most common manifestation is slowing of linear growth rate, often observed within a family by other younger children appearing to catch up to the affected child. This is usually accompanied by relative weight gain and the appearance of plumpness. School function is often not impaired and indeed the child may be a 'good' student, labouring slowly and carefully over schoolwork.

The typical features of adult hypothyroidism are far less commonly seen in children but their presence depends on the duration of the complaint and the time to presentation for medical care. Lethargy, excessive sleep, puffiness, dry skin, coarse hair, patchy alopecia and unexplained anaemia may all be presenting features. Typical hypothyroid facies occurs occasionally with severe hypothyroidism. Slowing of mentation and impaired school performance are usually transient and reversible on treatment in acquired hypothyroidism of childhood. Menorrhagia in the older girl with hypothyroidism is a common complaint.

Examination of a child with presumed hypothyroidism can be very helpful. The presence of goitre is common with autoimmune thyroiditis and the thyroid should be carefully palpated. In particular, slow relaxation phase of deep tendon reflexes is easily detected. A careful search should be made for the appearance of pseudohypertrophy of calf muscles in severe hypothyroidism. Muscle weakness is common and the muscle pseudohypertrophy is referred to as Kocher-Debre-Semelaigne syndrome.

Rarely, sexual precocity can occur with premature thelarche, galactorrhoea, menstruation and ovarian cysts in girls and macroorchidism in boys. This occurs due to high levels of TSH being perceived as FSH in the hypothalamus.

Pituitary enlargement secondary to hyperplasia of thyrotrophs, due to persistent increased TSH secretion, may be mistaken for a tumour or adenoma. This pituitary enlargement resolves with adequate thyroxine replacement.

Diagnostic Approach

A clinical suspicion based on a thorough history and examination should prompt investigations.

Investigations that will provide useful evidence of aetiology of hypothyroidism are included but may not be available. Treatment without a definitive causative diagnosis may be needed.

Biochemical Confirmation of Hypothyroidism

Hypothyroidism can be biochemically confirmed by elevated TSH and a low fT_4. The severity of hypothyroidism is usually judged on the basis of the level of T_4 and the degree of delay in skeletal maturation.

An elevated TSH with normal fT_4 suggests subclinical hypothyroidism and requires close follow-up clinically and also by repeat biochemical assays of TSH and fT_4 every 2–4 weeks till a definite diagnosis can be reached. Persistently elevated TSH with subclinical hypothyroidism also requires consideration for treatment with thyroxine. Care should be taken to use age-appropriate values while interpreting the biochemical results.

Skeletal age estimation should be performed to assess the duration and severity of hypothyroidism. The growth chart gives valuable information on the extent of involvement and age of onset.

Aetiological Diagnosis of Acquired Hypothyroidism

In acquired hypothyroidism, ultrasound examination of the thyroid will elucidate the echogenicity and vascularity of the thyroid gland and the presence of cystic lesions and help in arriving at the diagnosis. In autoimmune thyroiditis, US demonstrates a heterogeneous pattern of echoes and an enlarged gland.

A thyroid nuclear scan will be helpful to detect CH missed on screening or a late-onset congenital hypothyroidism, usually in the setting of an ectopic thyroid or dyshormonogenesis.

In older children and adolescents serum antithyroid antibodies should be measured where possible. Antithyroid peroxidase and antithyroglobulin antibodies are positive in Hashimoto's thyroiditis in high titre. Low level thyroglobulin antibodies are not informative. They simply confirm some form of inflammatory attack on the gland.

Chronic autoimmune thyroiditis is common with type 1 diabetes and some chromosomal anomalies, especially Turner syndrome. Autoimmune thyroid disease can also occur with polyglandular autoimmune disorder but is not the usual presenting manifestation of these disorders.

Rationale for Management

Replacement with LT_4 to the physiological range is the primary aim of therapy, to obviate symptoms and to return normal linear growth, physical and intellectual functions. The dosing has to be individualised, based on clinical and biochemical monitoring. LT_4 should be replaced in doses sufficient to normalise TSH and correct fT_4 to the upper half of the normal range.

Moderate to Severe Hypothyroidism

Replacement with L-thyroxine should be commenced as early as possible. The dose of LT_4 varies from 80 to 100 μg/m^2/day. Periodic re-evaluation clinically and biochemically is necessary to optimise outcome of replacement therapy. In the growing child this is usually performed every 4–6 months.

Subclinical Hypothyroidism

In children with mild elevation of TSH (5–10 uU/mL) and who are clinically euthyroid (subclinical hypothyroidism) the decision to treat has been controversial. These children can be followed up every 3–6 months. Persistent elevation of TSH may warrant treatment with thyroxine for 12–24 months, with reassessment after withdrawal of treatment for 6–8 weeks.

Hypothyroidism may revert to euthyroidism in some cases of autoimmune thyroid disease or other forms of subacute thyroiditis. However, long-term progression to permanent hypothyroidism may also occur, mandating regular follow-up.

Goitre usually resolves or reduces in size with LT_4 replacement therapy.

Fine-needle aspiration of a nodule to rule out malignancy should be performed on prominent nodules that persist even after replacement with LT$_4$, especially in patients with lymphocytic thyroiditis. This test is only useful if performed in a setting where competent and experienced histologic examination of the specimen can be undertaken. Spurious results are frequent when this rule is not heeded.

Long-term Outcome

Planning for transition to an adult clinic is necessary for all permanent CH and acquired hypothyroidism.

HYPERTHYROIDISM

Background

Hyperthyroidism results from excessive levels of free circulating thyroid hormones and is characterised by accelerated metabolism and undesirable effects.

Hyperthyroidism is uncommon in childhood. Graves' disease accounts for the majority of cases.[17,18]

Pathophysiology

Mechanisms that can Produce Hyperthyroidism

Hyper-function of thyroid follicular cells can occur via a number of different mechanisms:

STIMULATION OF TSH RECEPTORS BY TSH OR TSH RECEPTOR ANTIBODIES (TRAB)

Graves' disease is characterised by antibodies directed against the TSH receptor (TRAb). TRAb produces the toxic goitre of Graves' disease. It is detected in more than 90% of patients. These stimulating antibodies act similarly to pituitary TSH, thereby stimulating thyroid growth and function. The most likely explanation for the various manifestations of Graves' disease is via cross-reactivity of the circulating antibodies

with thyroidal antigens like TSH-R and the orbital and extra-orbital antigens.[19]

INCREASED TSH PRODUCTION FROM A PITUITARY ADENOMA OR PITUITARY RESISTANCE TO THYROID HORMONES

These can result in hyperthyroidism. This is rare.

ABNORMALLY HIGH LEVELS OF HCG

As with germ cell tumours, these can stimulate the TSH receptors and lead to hyperthyroidism.

THYROID FOLLICULAR CELL DESTRUCTION AND RELEASE OF PREFORMED T$_4$ AND T$_3$

Thyroid follicular cell destruction can follow any inflammatory process of the thyroid and may be of infective or autoimmune cause. There is a release of T$_4$ and T$_3$ secondary to destruction of thyroid cells. The hyperthyroidism tends to be transient and mild and usually lasts for a few weeks or months. It occurs in the context of the following conditions:

- **Sub-acute thyroiditis** is relatively rare in children. It is a self-limited inflammation of the thyroid gland usually associated with a viral illness.
- **Hashimoto's disease.** The thyrotoxicosis results from release of thyroid hormones with extensive autoimmune destruction of thyroid follicular cells. This is also known as Hashitoxicosis and occurs early in the course of chronic lymphocytic thyroiditis. High levels of thyroid peroxisomal (TPO) antibodies are usually seen, although they can be found in other causes of thyrotoxicosis. Thyroglobulin antibodies are frequently positive and represent breakdown of thyroid tissue with release of thyroid hormones.

AUTONOMOUS HYPER-FUNCTION OF FOLLICULAR CELLS

This is rare in childhood and may be due to a toxic adenoma, familial non-autoimmune hyperthyroidism (FNH), McCune–Albright syndrome or a very rarely a hyperfunctioning thyroid cancer.

A gain of function mutation of the TSH receptor is a rare condition which results in constitutive activation of TSH signalling. This causes increased follicular cell growth and functioning. The disease is transmitted as an autosomal dominant trait and therefore, unlike Graves' disease, both males and females are equally affected.

INGESTION OR ADMINISTRATION OF THYROID HORMONES OR IODIDE

This can result in excessive amounts of circulating free hormones and can cause hyperthyroidism. The ingestion can be acute or chronic and may be accidental or iatrogenic.

Administration of iodides oral or parenteral, especially in iodine-deficient individuals, can also cause hyperthyroidism. This phenomenon is known as the 'Jod-Basedow effect'.

Hyperthyroidism has also been reported in children treated with amiodarone, the iodine-rich anti-arrhythmic agent. However, in infants and young children, hypothyroidism is far more likely with amiodarone use.

CLINICAL SETTING

Hyperthyroidism

Clinical Manifestations of Hyperthyroidism

Hyperthyroidism in childhood is relatively uncommon and often presents for care quite late in its course. The onset of thyrotoxicosis is usually insidious, with behavioural abnormalities, emotional lability and declining school performance dominating the clinical picture in the early stages.

Children rarely complain of the typical symptoms of hyperthyroidism experienced by adults such as anxiety, palpitations, tremulousness and weight loss. More often, a parent first notices

a sudden decrease in weight, which has been mistaken as a growth spurt. On questioning, the family has often noticed that the affected child is warmer than the rest of the family, taking off excess clothing when others are cold and sometimes sleeping with minimal covers. The parent may complain that the child cannot keep still, and that his or her concentration is poor and that listening skills have deteriorated. This is often reiterated by school staff with a concomitant reduction in class marks and performance over preceding months or occasionally even years.

Insomnia and nocturia are common and often seen, together with easy fatigability and lethargy during the day. Marked weight loss with increasing appetite, palpitations, tremors, restlessness and muscle weakness may become manifest, as the disease progresses. Myopathy may vary from a complaint of poor strength to periodic paralysis.

Increased linear growth rate may be noted, often appearing more obvious due to concomitant weight loss. If thyrotoxicosis is present, long-term or undertreated, bone mineral accrual is impaired. Infants and children under the age of 3 years may develop craniosynostosis with persistent very high levels of thyroid hormone of any cause. Cardiomyopathy with mitral regurgitation has been reported in children with thyrotoxicosis.

The symptoms and signs of hyperthyroidism are highly variable and tend to be more severe in Graves' disease. In some children cardiovascular manifestations, like palpitations or exercise intolerance, may be prominent while in others neuropsychiatric manifestations may be more obvious.

The Value of Careful History and Examination

Although Graves' disease is the most common of the hyperthyroid conditions of childhood, a careful history may elicit a suggestion of either Hashimoto's thyroiditis or, very rarely, subacute thyroiditis.

A short history of 3–12 weeks together with mild symptoms is more suggestive of the toxic phase of Hashimoto's thyroiditis.

A history of a severe 'sore throat' or marked lower neck tenderness, in association with toxic symptoms, will usually point to subacute thyroiditis.

Sore, gritty or prominent 'staring' eyes immediately suggest Graves' disease.

- Surprisingly, although diffuse goitre, which may be quite large, is often noted at presentation this is commonly missed by both family and attending practitioners.
- During clinical examination attention to presence of a thyroid bruit indicates high vascularity within the gland, usually associated with Graves' disease.
- A firm, gritty texture to a gland is more suggestive of Hashimoto's thyroiditis, although, in a child a fairly smooth, soft enlargement of the thyroid gland is not atypical of the condition.
- Extreme tenderness throughout the gland suggests thyroiditis.
- A single palpable nodule is usually not associated with hyperthyroidism in children and merits careful attention (see thyroid cancer). A toxic thyroid nodule is very rare in childhood.

Specific Conditions Associated with Thyrotoxicosis

Graves' Disease

Graves' disease is the most common cause of thyrotoxicosis in children and adolescents, although rare in infancy. It can occur in the preschool age group through childhood but the incidence rises sharply in the adolescent age group. Girls are affected six times more often than boys. It is a multisystem autoimmune disease with a genetic and familial predisposition (up to 60%), presenting with goitre, hyperthyroidism, and eye manifestations (infiltrative ophthalmopathy).

How a Family Sees the Problem

The condition has profound effects on a child or adolescent and on their family, which extend beyond the classical symptoms of thyrotoxicosis. As diagnosis of the condition can be delayed for months or sometimes even years after the onset of initial symptoms, behavioural disorder as a result of hyperthyroidism can be a marked feature. This may have been diagnosed as attention deficit disorder, in some cases punished for poor attention, deteriorating school performance and sometimes even for poor sporting performance.

Within the family, progressive weight loss in the presence of a normal or increased appetite may suggest a malignant process, which can cause extreme fears which may be difficult to eradicate, even once the correct diagnosis has been made.

Frequent headaches and irritable red eyes are sometimes considered to be due to a perceived need for spectacles.

Examination

Typical signs of hyperthyroidism are outlined in Table 3.5.

Eye signs are much less common in children with Graves' disease than in adults but include eyelid lag, lid retraction, periorbital oedema, chemosis and extra-ocular muscle dysfunction. Proptosis occurs occasionally but usually settles within the first 12 months after diagnosis and treatment. Surgical intervention for thyroid eye disease is rarely needed in children. The use of wrap-around sun glasses and artificial tears to reduce conjunctival irritation is very helpful.

The thyroid is usually symmetrical enlarged, soft and non-tender. A palpable thrill or audible bruit may be felt or seen, reflecting increased blood flow through the thyroid gland.

Diagnosis is confirmed with elevated free T_4 and free T_3, together with a suppressed TSH and positive thyrotropin receptor antibodies. Thyroid ultrasound or technetium scan reveals

TABLE 3.5   Symptoms and Signs of Hyperthyroidism

SYMPTOMS

- Anxiety, hyperactivity, restlessness, altered mood
- Insomnia
- Heat intolerance, excessive sweating
- Palpitations, dyspnoea
- Increased appetite, weight loss
- Increased frequency of stools
- Weakness/periodic paralysis
- Polyuria
- Oligomenorrhoea or amenorrhea
- Pruritis

SIGNS

- Fine tremor, hyperreflexia
- Sinus tachycardia, supraventricular tachycardia (SVT)
- Moist, warm skin, palmar erythema
- High-output cardiac failure
- Hair loss, onycholysis
- Muscle weakness, wasting, periodic paralysis
- Osteoporosis
- Hypercalcemia
- Chorea

diffuse increased uptake throughout an enlarged gland.

Treatment is required for a minimum of 2 years. Graves' disease in childhood and adolescence has a much lower long-term remission rate than the same condition in adults, with 20–30% long-term remission being reported in most series. For those of Southeast Asian extraction the chance of long-term remission in young people with this condition is closer to 5–10% maximum.

(Details of treatment are outlined below.)

Subacute Thyroiditis (de Quervain's Thyroiditis) and Hashitoxicosis

It is relatively uncommon for a child to present for care with these conditions in the acute phase when thyrotoxic symptoms are present. A parent might notice jitteriness or poor attention span and the child may complain of a sore neck. However, symptoms usually are short lived, then they disappear. In retrospect, if the child subsequently becomes hypothyroid, the parent may remember the sequence of toxic symptoms having occurred weeks or months prior.

Features of hyperthyroidism are usually mild. Fever, local pain and tenderness of the thyroid gland may be noticed in de Quervain's thyroiditis for 4–6 weeks. Radioiodine uptake by the thyroid gland will be low or absent, denoting thyroid damage. Recovery occurs without any residual thyroid dysfunction. Treatment includes anti-inflammatory drugs, and in severe cases corticosteroids.

The thyrotoxic phase of Hashimoto's disease may last a little longer (from 1 to 6 months) but is rarely symptomatic in a child. Most recover and require no treatment but subsequent hypothyroidism can occur, months or even years later.[20]

Toxic Nodule

Hyperfunctioning adenomas are rare in childhood and adolescence. Occasionally, the free T_4 will be normal but T_3 will be elevated (T_3 toxicosis). Careful clinical examination of a thyrotoxic child may include the finding of large café-au-lait marks suggestive of McCune–Albright syndrome. In this rare case, a toxic adenoma or T_3 toxicosis is more likely than Graves' disease. If available, radioactive iodine (RAI) thyroid study demonstrates increased uptake of iodine by the nodule. Surgery is the treatment of choice.

Familial Non-autoimmune Hyperthyroidism (TSH Receptor Mutation)

The age of onset is variable and some affected individuals remain asymptomatic for years before developing goitre or thyrotoxicosis. Occasionally, an infant or young child may exhibit symptoms while the affected parent does not.

In older patients the goitre symmetrically enlarges, may evolve into a multinodular goitre and bruits may be audible over the lobes. Eye signs of thyrotoxicosis like stare, lid lag and wide palpebral fissures may be present, but infiltrative ophthalmopathy as in Graves' disease is not seen.

Though the hyperthyroidism responds to antithyroid drugs, it is difficult to manage and subtotal thyroidectomy or RAI ablation is required for permanent remission.

TSH-producing Adenoma

Hyperthyroidism can occur with increased TSH secretion from a TSH- secreting adenoma (TSHoma) of the pituitary. This is extremely rare as a primary presentation in childhood and adolescence; with few cases reported in this age group. Clinical presentation might include visual symptoms due to optic chiasmal compression.

However, a TSHoma may occur in a child as a consequence of extreme and long-standing *hypo*thyroidism. This lesion resolves with treatment of the thyroid deficiency and needs no specific intervention.[21]

Excess Iodine Intake

This occurs in the context of a goitre resulting from chronic iodine deficiency. When iodine is introduced, particularly in moderate to large amounts, thyrotoxicosis can occur.

Exogenous Thyroxine Intake

Acute or chronic ingestion of excessive quantities of thyroid hormone resulting in thyrotoxicosis is termed thyrotoxicosis factitia. In children this ingestion may be accidental or iatrogenic. It is rare for parents to be able to accurately state the amount of overdose, so a guarded approach needs to be taken for safety.

Onset of symptoms with acute ingestion of T_4 is usually 12–48 hours and may be as late as 7 days. Most cases are mild and require only gastric decontamination and a cathartic. Hospitalisation should be considered, with cardiac monitoring if available.

β-adrenergic blockade will help to alleviate most symptoms. Despite an apparently large reported intake of thyroxine tablets and unmeasurably high levels of T_4, children are frequently remarkably asymptomatic. Care must be taken for observation for at least 7 days, as the half-life of T_4 is 6 days.

Iopanoic acid can be used as an excellent short-term option for immediate relief of clinical symptoms and improving biochemical parameters, its action being via blockade of conversion of T_4 to T_3 and are also potent inhibition of type 1 and 2 deiodinases.[22] In life-threatening situations or thyroid storm due to acute ingestion, exchange transfusion may be helpful.[23]

With chronic ingestion of thyroid hormones, symptoms of hyperthyroidism are similar to those with other pathology, but thyromegaly will be conspicuously absent. The problem is most commonly seen in adolescents or adults attempting to lose weight via excess thyroid hormone intake. It is rare in children. Low or absent serum thyroglobulin level may be helpful in differentiating this disorder from other causes of thyrotoxicosis.

Thyroid Storm

Thyroid storm can occur with any cause of hyperthyroidism but is most reported in patients with Graves' disease. It is rare in children but can be seen in adolescents with poor compliance with antithyroid medication or rarely as a first presentation of long-standing disease.

Precipitating factors include infection, trauma, surgery, withdrawal of antithyroid drugs, radioactive iodine therapy and simultaneous consumption of sympathomimetic agents.

The classical manifestations of thyroid storm are:

- fever, usually over 38°C
- tachycardia, high-output cardiac failure

- neurological features of confusion, seizure or coma
- gastrointestinal dysfunction with vomiting, diarrhoea and jaundice.

Thyrotoxic Periodic Paralysis (TPP)

TPP is a sudden acute onset of reversible weakness or paralysis occurring with thyrotoxicosis. There is a preponderance with Asian race and male gender.

Episodes of TPP can vary from mild weakness to complete paralysis. The weakness usually involves the limbs with the proximal muscles more affected than the distal.

Precipitating factors include strenuous exercise, high carbohydrate intake, infection, trauma and emotional stress. A typical description is of the affected patient developing weakness after eating a rice meal.

Laboratory results demonstrate thyrotoxicosis and hypokalaemia.

The weakness responds to potassium supplementation and antithyroid therapy.

Severe cases may require β-adrenergic blockade and glucocorticoids.

Diagnostic Approach

- Where resources are limited, diagnostic skills become more important, as with every aspect of medicine.
- The taking of an adequate history, which includes duration of symptomatology and specific features such as thyroid pain and tenderness or the presence or absence of thyroid eye disease, along with a complete family history, is likely to give a major clue to the type of thyroid disorder.
- An examination which includes not only the cardinal signs of thyrotoxicosis but which checks the presence of a thyroid bruit, evaluates the texture of the thyroid gland and tenderness if any and pays attention to eye disease, will further hone the clinical diagnosis.

- Where available, a totally suppressed TSH is of more diagnostic value in confirming thyrotoxicosis than the absolute value of thyroid hormone levels.
- Treatment with carbimazole can be commenced, as described, with clinical judgement of resolution of thyrotoxic symptoms and signs. If Graves' disease is considered the appropriate diagnosis then treatment for 2 years will increase the likelihood of a long remission. If available, free T_3 and TSH measured at 4–6 monthly intervals should be sufficient to give a reasonable confirmation of clinical accuracy as to medication dose.

Biochemistry

A simple feedback loop between the hypothalamic pituitary axis and the thyroid ensures that biochemical diagnosis of thyrotoxicosis is simple. Hyperthyroidism is usually suspected on clinical grounds or rarely may be picked up on routine tests.

- The diagnosis of hyperthyroidism is confirmed with elevated levels of T_4 and free T_4 or T_3 with suppressed levels of TSH. Elevated T_3 levels without free T_4 elevation constitutes T_3 toxicosis.
- Elevated levels of serum T_4 with normal free T_4 and TSH is seen with TBG excess or familial dysalbuminaemic hyperthyroxinaemia.
- Patients with isolated pituitary resistance to thyroid hormones present with clinical hyperthyroidism, but the TSH levels are elevated or normal with elevated free T_4. This has to be differentiated from TSH-producing pituitary adenomas.
- A low or undetectable TSH alone is also not absolutely diagnostic of hyperthyroidism, as this can be seen in central hypothyroidism. However, the symptoms are completely different and the two diagnoses are unlikely to be mixed!

Further Tests that May Be of Value

BIOCHEMISTRY

- If free T_4 is unavailable, a total T_4 can be performed but it must be remembered that this is dependent on circulating levels of binding proteins.
- The presence of TRAb establishes the cause as Graves' disease. This test may take weeks to be performed if available at all and is thus unhelpful in establishing a definitive cause prior to commencement of treatment. Clinical history and examination are far more important.
- Thyroid peroxidase and thyroglobulin antibodies are strongly positive in Hashitoxicosis but are usually seen also in Graves' disease. These antibodies are negative when the cause is of excess thyroxine intake.

IMAGING

Imaging may be utilised to look at structure and function of the thyroid.

- Ultrasound will provide evidence of single or multiple nodules, may show generalised increased gland vascularity suggestive of Graves' disease or the toxic phase of Hashimoto's disease or a patchy appearance suggestive of thyroiditis.
- A technetium scan provides further evidence of function. It is of more use in an adult, where a single toxic adenoma or a functioning nodule if multinodular goitre is present. Its major use in a child is to demonstrate the difference between high uptake, as seen in Graves' disease, and zero uptake as seen (rarely) in subacute thyroiditis.

The presence of precocious puberty, café-au-lait pigmentation or polyostotic fibrous dysplasia, suggest autoimmune hyper-functioning of the thyroid with McCune–Albright syndrome.

Management of Thyrotoxicosis

As the vast majority of hyperthyroidism needing treatment during childhood and adolescence is Graves' disease, the following management will refer to Graves' disease only. The reader is referred to recently published management guidelines[24]

Antithyroid drugs are the treatment of first choice, with a duration determined in part by wishes of the patient and family and in part by compliance.

For any child or adolescent with Graves' disease, treatment must be supervised by a parent or carer at all times, particularly when the child is thyrotoxic. Short-term memory and attention span are both significantly impaired in the presence of thyrotoxicosis, severely reducing compliance. By far the most common reason for relapse, enlarging goitre and difficult management is due to treatment omission.

General Advice

In addition to medical management of Graves' disease, the child's school must be informed about the condition and its management. A written statement to the school principal is required, and must include the fact that the child may have sustained months of poor concentration prior to diagnosis. What may have been perceived by school staff as inattention and poor behaviour has probably been related to the underlying condition and will resolve rapidly with treatment. The child may require assistance with extra tuition to catch up on lost schooling.

In addition, all sporting activities should be restricted until euthyroidism is achieved.

Antithyroid Drugs

Antithyroid drugs remain the first-line treatment for children and adolescents with Graves' disease. Available drugs include carbimazole (CMZ), propylthiouracil (PTU) and methimazole (MMI). MMI has 10-fold more potency than PTU and has a longer half-life.

SIDE EFFECTS

Side effects occur with both groups of drugs, but are lesser with MMI. They are unpredictable and can occur after any duration of therapy. They are usually mild and reversible on stopping the drug, but can be life-threatening also. Most serious side effects are hypersensitive and include agranulocytosis, hepatitis, hepatic failure and antineutrophil cytoplasmic antibody (ANCA)-positive vasculitis.

Propylthiouracil has been linked to a large increased risk of hepatic toxicity and occasionally to fulminant hepatic failure. It is therefore contra-indicated as first-line treatment except in two extenuating circumstances:

- Allergy to carbimazole or methimazole.
- Where a pregnancy is desired in the immediate future. Carbimazole has not been shown to be safe in pregnancy and has potential for *teratogenicity*, particularly with cutis aplasia of the scalp but also with other head and neck anomalies. It is therefore contra-indicated for use in pregnancy and propylthiouracil should be substituted in this special case. Although not applicable to the treatment of most adolescents, propylthiouracil has been shown to be safe for breastfeeding mothers, although it is excreted in small quantities in breast milk. Consideration should be given to methimazole or carbimazole for this circumstance in view of recent toxicity data for PTU.

Any patient commencing treatment must be informed of possible side effects and told to attend a medical practitioner should there be any evidence of a rash or of oral thrush and a sore throat. Twenty percent cross reactivity between carbimazole and propylthiouracil exists so that the patient continues to need close monitoring to avoid the possibility of a similar reaction to the second drug.

TREATMENT PROTOCOLS

Recommended starting doses are:

- CMZ: 0.5–1 mg/kg/day in 8-hourly doses
- PTU 5–10 mg/kg/day in 8-hourly doses
- MMI: 0.5–1 mg/kg/day in 12-hourly doses.

Clinical responses to PTU and MMI are seen in 4 to 6 weeks. Until then, the symptoms and signs of hyperthyroidism may be controlled with β-blockers. Propranolol (0.5–2 mg/kg/day in divided doses) is effective for symptom control but should not be used or should be ceased if asthma occurs.

The dose of the antithyroid drug has to be titrated to achieve a euthyroid state. Progressive dose reduction to minimal levels may be easy to achieve. Sometimes, however, even a tiny dose change can cause widely varying hormone control. In this case a 'block and replace' approach can be adopted. This involves giving higher doses of antithyroid drugs and adding levothyroxine to counter the hypothyroidism that develops with the higher doses of ATD. The 'block and replace' approach results in potentially more side effects from the antithyroid drugs, due to the higher amount of drug dosing required.

There is always a time lag between commencing treatment and achieving a euthyroid state because the biosynthetic block is not complete and stores of preformed hormone must be discharged. A patient with a small thyroid gland is likely to respond more quickly than one with a large goitre. TSH levels may remain suppressed for several months despite clinical euthyroidism and are therefore not the only guide to treatment initially.

It is usual to treat a thyrotoxic child for around 2 years before attempting to discontinue medication. Treatment for any less time is almost certain to result in rapid relapse. Remission rate for children with Graves' disease is far lower than that for adults, between 10 and 30% and even lower chance of remission in those of Chinese or Vietnamese origin. Relapse usually occurs within 3 to 6 months of discontinuation of therapy and therapy can be resumed after a relapse. The chance of a second remission is reduced. Male gender, age over 13 at diagnosis, a small goitre and mild disease are all associated with a higher chance of remission.

Decision making about when to undertake a trial off treatment is very important for an adolescent in the later years of school. An overactive thyroid has a major effect on concentration skills and attention. It may be more sensible to continue treatment until the end of schooling, to reduce relapse risk at an important time.

Radioiodine Therapy

Radioiodine is an effective and relatively safe therapy for Graves' disease in children and adolescents when adequate medical therapy with antithyroid drugs have failed to achieve remission, when serious side effects precludes further use of antithyroid drugs or when the patient wants definitive treatment. Radioiodine is trapped in the thyroid cells which are ultimately destroyed by internal radiation.

The aim of treatment should be to ablate the gland with later addition of long-term thyroxine replacement.

This has been shown to provide the most effective and most stable outcome. Hypothyroidism usually occurs 2 to 3 months after the treatment. If hyperthyroidism persists, a second or third dose of radioiodine may be required, but should not be considered for a minimum of 6 months after a first dose, to allow time for effect to occur.

Dosing with I^{131} requires minute attention to detail, with antithyroid drug withdrawal for 4 days before and after the dose and with a negative pregnancy test checked 24 hours prior to dose in all girls after menarche. Details of a treatment schedule are beyond the scope of this article. This type of treatment should be undertaken with specialist care. School exclusion is necessary for 12 days after a dose of I^{131}, as a public health and safety measure.

Aggravation of thyroid eye disease has been linked in the past to radioactive iodine administration. More recently this has been challenged. A short course of corticosteroid as prednisolone with rapid tapering from 50 mg/day over 3–4 weeks may be advised if there is any sign of aggravation of eye symptoms after a dose of I^{131}.

Surgery

Surgery is no longer commonly used for definitive management of Graves' disease. Occasionally, an adolescent who has been non-compliant with antithyroid drugs over many months will develop a very large goitre which does not shrink even when euthyroid status is achieved. Surgery is the only option available for these patients.

Rarely, a family will want a definitive procedure, to resolve the need for taking medication for years.

Surgery may be offered if radioiodine is refused. Any potential surgical candidate must be aware of possible risks for postoperative hypoparathyroidism, permanent or transient, and vocal cord paralysis.

Near-total thyroidectomy is now advocated to avoid recurrence of hyperthyroidism and should only be performed by an experienced team. Surgery is performed after a euthyroid state is achieved with antithyroid drugs. Lugol's iodine is sometimes added to the treatment 2 weeks prior to surgery to reduce gland vascularity.

Toxic Nodular Thyroid Disease

See section on nodular thyroid disease below.

Neonatal Hyperthyroidism

Transient neonatal hyperthyroidism may occur in a baby born to a mother with Graves' disease, due to transplacental transfer of TRAb to the fetus, with activation of TSH receptors and increased thyroid hormone secretion in the fetus. It is quite rare, occurring only in around 3% of infants whose mothers are or have been thyrotoxic.[25]

Thyrotoxicosis can continue until maternal antibodies disappear from the bloodstream, around 6—12 weeks postpartum.

Women at risk are not limited to those with active disease, but also those in remission following antithyroid drugs, surgery or radioactive iodine in the past.

Clinical Presentation

The clinical presentation depends on the net effect between the stimulatory action of the TRAb and the inhibitory action of the TSH receptor-blocking antibodies and whether or not the mother has been using antithyroid drugs during the last trimester of pregnancy. In this case symptoms may not be present until a few days of birth, as the effect of the transplacentally transferred antithyroid drugs disappear from the newborn.

Clinical manifestations vary in severity and course. It is relatively easy to diagnose if considered a risk and where the attending paediatrician is aware of the maternal state.

However, a past history of Graves' disease in the mother may have been omitted in the taking of a neonatal history or a thyrotoxic mother may not have had regular antenatal care and may herself be extremely unwell. This is very important to consider, in assessing the capacity of the mother to care for her infant.

For the mother, immediate care of her toxic state must be sought from an adult physician, so that she is in a fit condition to feed and care for her infant.

For the infant who is jittery and unwell, sepsis or some form of cardiovascular problem is often considered, long before thyrotoxicosis is recognised as the cause for the clinical state of the infant.

Prematurity, IUGR, fetal tachycardia and goitre are common in these babies. These infants appear restless, hyperactive with an anxious and alert look. Increased appetite,

poor weight gain, fever, diaphoresis, diarrhoea and erythema also occur in some infants. Tachypnoea, tachycardia, cardiac failure and hypertension are other common findings. Other findings may include hepatomegaly, splenomegaly, jaundice, thrombocytopenia, microcephaly secondary to craniosynostosis and advanced bone maturation.

Diagnostic Approach

Fetal tachycardia and goitre on fetal ultrasound may alert the paediatrician to the possibility of this problem before birth. All neonates clinically suspected to have hyperthyroidism should have plasma levels of free T_4, T_3 and TSH estimated to confirm the hyperthyroid state, where at all possible.

Awareness of normal thyroid hormone levels in a neonate is necessary. This can be complicated in a preterm infant, where T_3 levels should be low and T_4 levels vary widely depending on the gestational age and health of the infant. In this case extreme suppression of TSH is the most reliable indicator of neonatal thyrotoxicosis, because a preterm infant's TSH should be well above 3—4 mu/L in the first few days of life.

For the term infant, neonatal ranges for T_4 and T_3 are considerably higher than those for an older infant. A free T_4 of 30 pmol/L is quite normal for a neonate.

Rationale for Treatment

- Prompt and adequate treatment of neonatal hyperthyroidism is essential for a good outcome. Propylthiouracil should be administered at a dose of 5—10 mg/kg/day in three divided doses. PTU has a mild advantage over methimazole or carbimazole in that it also blocks the conversion of T_4 to T_3 but given recent toxicity concerns its use has become restricted.
- Lugol's iodine 1—3 drops per day may be added in severe cases to block thyroid hormone secretion.

- Propranolol, treatment of heart failure and additional supportive measures with adequate calories and fluid should be instituted whenever required.
- Antithyroid drug doses should be titrated to achieve a euthyroid state or if necessary a 'block and replace' approach must be adopted.

Treatment may only be required for 2–4 weeks but can go on as long as 3 months, until maternal antibody levels disappear.

Breast feeding is encouraged, even if the mother is taking antithyroid medications. These are excreted in breast milk at a low level and do not interfere with infant thyroid status.

Long-term Outcome of Neonatal Hyperthyroidism

Untreated or inadequately treated neonatal hyperthyroidism results in developmental delay, craniosynostosis and microcephaly. Early recognition and prompt treatment confers a good prognosis with normal neurodevelopmental outcome.

PERMANENT NEONATAL HYPERTHYROIDISM

Persistent neonatal hyperthyroidism occurs with constitutive activation of TSH signalling either due to dominantly inherited mutations in TSH receptors or mutations in GNAS (McCune–Albright syndrome). These are extremely rare conditions. They should be suspected in the absence of maternal antibodies. Therapy consists of long-term antithyroid drugs as tolerated or total thyroidectomy or iodine ablation as definitive treatment.

PRETERM HYPERTHYROIDISM

Prenatal thyrotoxicosis occurring in the third trimester of pregnancy is extremely rare. If diagnosed, this may be on the basis of persistent fetal tachycardia or poor growth in the third trimester even though the mother may be biochemically euthyroid. The treatment should be undertaken in a specialised unit. Maternal propylthiouracil may be considered even in an euthyroid mother, to reduce toxicity in the fetus.

THYROID NODULES

Thyroid nodules in childhood are uncommon. When present they are usually solitary. Up to 30% of such lesions in children and adolescents are malignant, a far higher percentage than in adults. Definitive diagnosis therefore must be undertaken. (See below for thyroid cancer management.)

Pathology

A nodule may be solid or cystic, single or part of a multinodular goitre.

A single nodule may be a cyst, adenoma or carcinoma. Rarely, a parathyroid adenoma might be palpable in the neck and mistaken for a thyroid mass. Lymphadenopathy is unlikely to be mistaken for a thyroid lesion. However, careful examination for associated lymphadenopathy must be sought when a thyroid nodule is found, in case of metastatic spread of malignancy.

Multinodular goitre occurs commonly in the presence of chronic iodine deficiency or with dyshormonogenesis.

Thyroid lymphoma is rare but occurs in Hashimoto's thyroiditis.

History

It is uncommon to see a functioning thyroid adenoma with thyrotoxicosis in this age group. Presentation is usually made because a painless lump is noticed in the neck.

Family History

- History of familial goitre should be sought and parental necks should be observed. Knowledge of local areas of iodine deficiency is helpful and the family should be questioned as to use of iodised salt.

- Endocrine neoplasia – MEN 2A, succinate dehydrogenase (SDH) mutation, familial medullary or papillary cancer.
- Past radiation exposure during pregnancy, childhood (usually related to cancer treatments) or environmental hazard.
- Duration of presence of a nodule is usually unhelpful as most will present for care as soon as they are noticed. Sudden increase in size may indicate haemorrhage or malignancy.
- Associated hoarseness, pressure symptoms may indicate malignancy.

Examination

This includes evidence of:

- hyperthyroidism or hypothyroidism
- nodule size and consistency of nodule
- tenderness to indicate trauma or haemorrhage
- presence of other nodules
- cervical lymphadenopathy, tracheal shift
- other evidence for a systemic disorder such as MEN 2A with a Marfanoid appearance and ganglioneuromata of lips and eyelids.

Investigations

Thyroid function is likely to be normal.

Ultrasound will differentiate solid from cystic lesions.

Technetium scan can provide evidence of a hot or cold nodule but is of less value than ultrasound, because very few nodules are 'hot' in childhood and thyroid function will define overactivity.

Fine needle aspirate (FNA) is only helpful with an experienced pathologist for histology. In particular, a follicular lesion cannot be defined as benign or malignant based on FNA histology. The definition is based solely on capsule invasion which can only be established on excision histology.

Treatment

Surgical excision is usual, for diagnosis, with the exception of a nodule which is 'hot' to scan, with suppression of the remaining thyroid tissue. In this case an ablative dose of radioactive iodine could be considered, as the radionucleotide is taken up solely into the hot area, while the remainder of the gland is usually unaffected. If malignant, follow-up is as described below:

- If benign and solitary, the remaining thyroid tissue should retain normal function.
- If dyshormonogenesis with multinodular goitre is seen, suppressive thyroxine is needed to prevent regrowth of residual tissue.

THYROID CANCER IN CHILDHOOD

Background

With increasing survival after treatment of childhood thyroid cancer, the face of thyroid cancer in childhood has changed.[26] In the past it was a relatively rare condition, to be suspected where a child presented with a single lump or nodule in the area of the thyroid gland or in adjacent cervical lymph nodes. Then, as now, a history of past radiation exposure is important as a potential risk factor for thyroid cancer. Other risks include unusual chromosomal abnormalities such as a BRAF mutation, RET rearrangements (in particular MEN 2A and 2B) and possibly SDHD mutations.[27] Environmental radiation hazard has also increased thyroid cancer risk in communities so exposed.[28]

Many modern childhood cancer regimes involve ionising radiation exposure as whole brain radiation, targeted radiation for brain tumour, spinal radiation, chest or neck radiotherapy, or total body radiation, prior to bone marrow transplant. All these events pose potential threats to the thyroid.[29]

A dose of 2-5 Gy radiation exposure to the thyroid in infancy or childhood increases the risk of thyroid nodularity, at a calculated rate of around 2% per annum nodule formation, with a peak incidence 15–20 years after radiation exposure. After stem cell transplantation, the risk for thyroid malignancy rises rapidly 8–10 years after radiation exposure, with the highest risk for the younger patient, particularly if age at the time of exposure was less than 10 years. It is therefore mandatory in all children and adolescents who have been exposed to ionising radiation of any source that thyroid surveillance be carried out.

In the past, thyroid cancer in both children and adults had a marked female preponderance. With radiation exposure as part of cancer protocols in childhood now being a major risk factor, the preponderance of females is no longer present.

In children, up to 30% of excised solitary nodules are malignant. Overall, thyroid cancer accounts for around 1.5% of total childhood cancers and 3.5% total childhood solid malignancies with an increasing prevalence and a prolonged duration of risk, in excess of 40 years.

In general, thyroid cancer, particularly in the first decade, is thought to be more aggressive than that seen in adults, with a high risk for disease progression and recurrence.[30] Local invasion and the presence of cervical lymphadenopathy are both frequent with distant metastases reported between 8 and 30%.[31] Despite these features, mortality is less than that in adults with 98–99% total survival over 25 years reported.[32]

Pathology

Solitary thyroid nodules are uncommon in children and adolescents and may have either increased or decreased uptake of radionucleotide when scanned. A nodule cold to scanning material is non-functional. If it is also solid to ultrasound examination, it has an increased risk for malignancy in comparison with a hot nodule, where thyrotoxicosis is the rule. It is, however, rare but possible to have a functioning (hot) thyroid cancer.

History

A careful history should be sought for a source of past ionising radiation exposure. This includes maternal exposure to irradiation in the latter part of pregnancy, perhaps related to scanning procedures which might be inadvertently administered for suspected pulmonary embolus. Extremely early and brief maternal radiation exposure in the first 2–6 weeks of a pregnancy is less likely to cause harm, as the thyroid has not yet formed. However, due to possible retention of ionising material in maternal tissues, surveillance for the exposed infant must be performed for several years.

Examination

Detection of a thyroid nodule less than 1 cm in size is unlikely clinically. With increasing reports of invasive papillary thyroid cancer after radiation exposure during cancer treatment in childhood, even in nodules as small as 5 mm diameter, ultrasound is now recommended, with repeated evaluation every 2 years.

Diagnosis

Diagnosis of likely thyroid cancer can be made prior to surgical excision in children as well as in adolescents and adults. If a technetium scan and ultrasound reveal a solid nodule then fine needle aspiration can be undertaken. A child or young adolescent will usually require some sedation for such a procedure to be performed successfully. FNA should be performed by a skilled radiologist with ultrasonographic identification of the lesion. Most importantly, the aspirate must be examined by a pathologist skilled in reporting of fine needle aspirates.

Even in the best hands there is a 1/10 chance of missing a malignancy on FNA.

The majority of thyroid cancer seen in children is papillary. In the unusual circumstance that follicular carcinoma is considered, it is important to remember that fine needle aspirate cannot differentiate benign from malignant follicular disease and removal of the thyroid nodule surgically is required to make that distinction. The difference between benign and malignant follicular thyroid disease hinges on vascular invasion and capsule invasion.

Management

Protocols for childhood thyroid cancer are less clearly defined than those for adults.

With an isolated single nodule and no history of radiation exposure, as a low-risk category, lobectomy with removal of the thyroid followed by use of suppressive thyroxine may be sufficient, aiming to keep TSH below 0.4 mIU/L.

Most affected children are in a high-risk category due to known radiation exposure. Primary treatment involves total thyroidectomy with central lymph node clearance followed by an ablative dose of I^{131} and then suppressive thyroxine long term.

Post-surgical hypocalcaemia, if present, usually resolves over days or weeks and rarely requires long-term management with calcium and calcitriol.

Management of thyroid cancer should be undertaken in a specialist facility. The following gives a brief overview of management only. For details of general adult management of thyroid cancer the reader is referred to recent publications.[33] Details of paediatric management for this previously rare disorder generally follow these guidelines. However, despite a relatively good prognosis and more frequent and severe early metastatic presentations in youngsters than adults, the duration and extent of follow-up for children is less well defined.

I^{131} administration for thyroid remnant ablation and for any possible metastatic disease requires complex protocols. If a diagnostic scan reveals more than 3–5% residual uptake in the neck, completion thyroidectomy must be performed prior to radio iodine administration, to avoid radiation burns to adjacent structures.

Distant metastases are detected by iodine scans but local neck disease is not, due to the small size of lymph nodes and thus minimal ability to take up scanning material. Therefore in order to detect cervical lymph nodes affected by metastatic disease, it is necessary to concomitantly undertake a neck ultrasound. The metastatic neck node has a clearly abnormal and identifiable pattern of vasculature.

Following remnant ablation, thyroxine is reinstituted at a dose to suppress TSH.

Follow-up involves 6-monthly neck ultrasound, stimulated thyroglobulin levels (by thyroxine withdrawal or rTSH if available) as a marker of residual or new abnormal thyroid tissue and annual iodine scan, for at least 10 years. For a more extensive review the reader is referred to new reviews.

References

1. Hunter I, Greene SA, MacDonald TM, Morris AD. Prevalence and aetiology of hypothyroidism in the young. *Arch Dis Child* 2000;**83**:207–10.
2. Huang SA, Tu HM, Harney JW, et al. Severe hypothyroidism caused by type 3 iodothyronine deiodinase in infantile haemangiomas. *N Engl J Med* 2000;**343**: 185–9.
3. Rose SR, Foley T, Brown RS, et al. Update on newborn screening and therapy for congenital hypothyroidism. *Pediatr* 2006;**117**:2290–303.
4. Golbahar J, Al- Khayat H, Hassan B, et al. Neonatal screening for congenital hypothyroidism: a retrospective hospital based study from Bahrain. *J Paediatr Endocrinol Metab* 2010;**23**:39–44.
5. LaFranchi SH. Newborn screening strategies for congenital hypothyroidism: an update. *J Inherit Metab Dis* 2010;**33**(Suppl. 2):S225–33.
6. Van Vliet G, Grosse SD. The continuing health burden of congenital hypothyroidism in the era of neonatal screening. *J Clin Endocrinol Metab* 2011;**96**:1671–3.

7. Devos H, Rodd C, Gagne N, et al. A search for the possible molecular mechanisms of thyroid dysgenesis: sex ratios and associated malformations. *J Clin Endocrinol Metab* 1999;**84**:2502–6.

8. Grasberger H, Retetoff S. Genetic causes of congenital hypothyroidism due to dyshormonogenesis. *Curr Opin Pediatr* 2011;**23**. http://dx.doi.org/10.1016/10.1.1097MOP.0b013e32834726a4.

9. Van Vliet G, Larroque B, Bubuteishvili L, et al. Sex-specific impact of congenital hypothyroidism due to thyroid dysgenesis on skeletal maturation in term newborns. *J Clin Endocrinol Metab* 2003;**88**:2009–13.

10. Castanet M, Polak M, Bonaiti-Pellie C, et al. Nineteen years of national screening for congenital hypothyroidism: familial cases of thyroid dysgenesis suggest the involvement of genetic factors. *J Clin Endocrinol Metab* 2001;**86**:2009–14.

11. Olivieri A, Stazi MA, Mastroiacovo P, et al. A population based study on the frequency of additional congenital malformations in infants with congenital hypothyroidism: data from the Italian registry for congenital hypothyroidism. *J Clin Endocrinol Metab* 2002;**87**:557–62.

12. Brown RS, Bellisario RL, Botero D, et al. Incidence of transient congenital hypothyroidism due to maternal thyrotropin receptor-blocking antibodies in over one million babies. *J Clin Endocrinol Metab* 1996;**81**:1147–51.

13. LaFranchi SH, Austin J. How should we be treating children with congenital hypothyroidism? *J Paediatr Endocrinol Metab* 2007;**20**:559–78.

14. Bongers-Schokking JJ, De Muink Keiser-Schrama SM. Influence of timing and dose of thyroid hormone replacement on mental, psychomotor and behavioural development in children with congenital hypothyroidism. *J Pediatr* 2005;**147**:768–74.

15. Rallison ML, Dobyns BM, Meikle AW, et al. Natural history of thyroid abnormalities: prevalence, incidence and regression of thyroid diseases in adolescents and young adults. *Am J Med* 1991;**91**:363–70.

16. Roberts CG, Ladenson PW. *Hypothyroidism. Lancet* 2004;**363**:793–803.

17. Weetman AP. Graves disease. *N Engl J Med* 2000;**343**: 1236–48.

18. Cooper DS. *Hyperthyroidism. Lancet* 2003;**362**:459–68.

19. Duprez L, Parma J, Van Sande J, et al. Pathology of the TSH receptor. *J Pediatr Endocrinol Metab* 1999; **12**(Suppl. 1):295–302.

20. Nabhan ZM, Kreher NC, Eugster EA. Hashitoxicosis in children: clinical features and natural history. *J Pediatr* 2005;**143**:533.

21. Shomali ME, Katznelson L. Medical therapy for gonadotroph and thyrotroph tumors. *Endocrinol Metab Clin North Am* 1999;**28**:223.

22. Braga M, Cooper DS. Oral cholecystographic agents and the thyroid. *J Clin Endocrinol Metab* 2001;**86**:1853.

23. Lehrner LM, Weir MR. Acute ingestion of thyroid hormones. *Pediatr* 1984;**73**:313.

24. Bahn Chair RS, Burch HB, Cooper DS, et al. Hyperthyroidism and other causes of thyrotoxicosis: management guidelines of the American thyroid association and American association of clinical endocrinologists. *Thyroid* 2011;**21**:593–646.

25. Skuza KA, Sills IN, Stene M, et al. Prediction of neonatal hyperthyroidism in infants born to mothers with Graves disease. *J Pediatr* 1996;**128**:264–8.

26. Hameed R, Zacharin M. Changing face of paediatric and adolescent thyroid cancer. *J Paediatr Child Health* 2005;**41**:572–4.

27. Nikiforova MN, Nikiforov YE. Molecular genetics of thyroid cancer: implications for diagnosis, treatment and prognosis. *Expert Rev Mol Diagn* 2008;**8**:83–95.

28. Cardis E, Krewski D, Boniol M, et al. Estimates of the cancer burden in Europe from radioactive fallout from the Chernobyl accident. *Int J Cancer* 2006;**119**: 1224–35.

29. Sigurdson AJ, Ronckers CM, Mertens AC, et al. Primary thyroid cancer after a first tumour in childhood (the Childhood Cancer Survivor Study): a nested case-control study. *Lancet* 2005;**365**:2012–23.

30. Rachmiel M, Charron M, Gupta A, et al. Evidence-based review of treatment and follow up of pediatric patients with differentiated thyroid carcinoma. *J Pediatr Endocrinol Metab* 2006;**19**:1377–93.

31. Lazar L, Lebenthal Y, Steinmetz A, et al. Differentiated thyroid carcinoma in pediatric patients: Comparison of presentation and course between pre-pubertal children and adolescents. *J Pediatr* 2009;**154**:708–14.

32. Shapiro NL, Bhattacharyya N. Population-based outcomes for pediatric thyroid carcinoma. *Laryngoscope* 2005;**115**:337–40.

33. Cooper DS, Doherty GM, Haugen BR, et al. Revised American Thyroid Association management guidelines for patients with thyroid nodules and differentiated thyroid cancer. *Thyroid* 2009;**19**:1167–214.

4

Adrenal Disorders

Martin Ritzén, Margaret Zacharin

O U T L I N E

The discussion on adrenal disorders below is meant for a clinical setting where resources for expensive laboratory or imaging studies are limited. The reader is referred to standard textbooks when it comes to very rare conditions that require extensive and expensive tests. Also, detailed descriptions of methods used in clinical investigations of endocrine disorders can be found in such textbooks, and will not be described below. Instead, emphasis will be

Practical Pediatric Endocrinology in a Limited Resource Setting
http://dx.doi.org/10.1016/B978-0-12-407822-2.00004-9

put on the possibilities of arriving at a diagnosis that is close enough to allow suggestions on rational treatment by means of thorough history taking, physical examination and limited laboratory analyses.

In countries where access to medical care is difficult, related in part to educational, financial and travel restrictions, disorders of adrenal function pose special problems that are less commonly encountered in Western medical practice. These issues may relate to problems of late diagnosis of inherited disorders of adrenal gland function, consequent family and social distress, isolation and possible societal exclusion. Major problems also arise due to limited or intermittent access to medications that are essential for life and maintenance of health.

A detailed analysis of the social and family issues consequent upon and related to a diagnosis of a disorder of sexual development (DSD), of all causes and including those due to heritable disorders of adrenal enzyme biosynthesis, is beyond the scope of this chapter.

(See Chapter 5 on Disorders of Sexual Development for further information.)

It is, however, important to take into account that when these issues occur, adequate and ongoing management planning for a causative medical condition may be infinitely compounded by social and emotional complexities arising from late diagnosis and suboptimal circumstances for management.

This chapter will confine discussion to practical aspects of medical diagnosis and management strategies.

BACKGROUND: PATHOPHYSIOLOGIC CONSIDERATIONS

The human adrenal produces two major classes of hormones: steroid hormones from the adrenal cortex and catecholamines (primarily epinephrine = adrenaline) from the adrenal medulla. Although the cortex and the medulla develop from different embryological tissues, the adrenal medulla is dependent on the neighbouring secretion of glucocorticoids, both for its development and its function. The following physiologic events are of importance in understanding abnormalities of adrenal structure and function.

Foetal Development of Adrenal Hormones

The first steroidogenic adrenal cells appear close to but distinct from the genital ridge at around 6 weeks gestation, at the time of sex determination and the development of labioscrotal fusion. Abnormalities in adrenal enzyme function with resultant excess androgen production thus affect genital development at this critical stage. Cortisol production by the foetal adrenals shows marked variations throughout gestation. It is high during the latter part of the first trimester, then decreases markedly, only to increase again at the end of the third trimester. The start of cortisol production, as shown by the emergence of expression of the necessary enzymes involved in steroid synthesis, coincides with adrenocorticotrophic (ACTH) appearance in the foetal pituitary at week seven. Transfer of maternal cortisol to the foetus is probably of minor importance, since it is inactivated by placental 11β-hydroxysteroid dehydrogenase type 2 (11βHSD2). Rapid changes in requirement for adrenal steroids occur at birth with the involution of the foetal adrenal cortex, mandating an intact adrenal cortex and medulla for adequate function, although mineralocorticoid requirements are slower to rise.

Hypothalamic-Pituitary-Adrenal Axis Development

Hypothalamic regulation of ACTH secretion occurs via corticotrophin-releasing hormone

(CRH) and arginine vasopressin (AVP). Regulation of fluid balance in disorders of impaired adrenal mineralocorticoid secretion occurs via stimulation of AVP. This in turn stimulates ACTH production.

Cortisol Regulation

- Cortisol production has a diurnal variation, under the influence of ACTH and CRH, established after the first few months of life. This is relevant when assessing *cortisol production*, for conditions of either high or low levels.
- Importantly, cortisol is metabolised in the liver by P450 enzymes. Anti-tuberculosis drug treatment involves liver enzyme induction with increased *cortisol metabolic rate* and can precipitate adrenal crisis. (See below.)
- Conversely, in conditions of *cortisol excess*, as a catabolic agent it has adverse effects on linear growth, bone metabolism and osteoblast function, and vitamin D metabolism; it also suppresses immune function.

Mineralocorticoid Regulation

Aldosterone action occurs via the mineralocorticoid receptor, *to regulate sodium excretion and fluid balance*. 11β hydroxysteroid dehydrogenase type 2 (11βHSD2) inactivates cortisol to cortisone, maintaining selectivity of the receptor. Deficiency of this enzyme results in low renin hypertension because of elevated intrarenal cortisol that binds to the mineralocorticoid receptor.

Aldosterone regulation occurs via the renin angiotensin system, with excess resulting in hypertension and hypokalaemic alkalosis and deficiency in salt loss with polyuria, dehydration, hyponatremia, hyperkalaemia and metabolic acidosis.

Pathways for Adrenal Steroid Production: Normal and Abnormal

The adrenal cortex produces three different classes of steroid hormones: glucocorticoids, mineralocorticoids and androgens (Figure 4.1). Thus, the various disorders will have symptoms that depend on whether there is a deficiency or excess of one or several of these hormones.

Both the normal steroid synthesis in the adrenal cortex, and the enzymes involved, are depicted in Figure 4.1A.

Cholesterol is transferred into the mitochondria of steroidogenic cells via the StAR (steroid acute regulatory protein) with subsequent conversion to steroid hormones via activity of a series of P450 enzymes. The changes that are found in the most common form of CAH, 21-hydroxylase deficiency (21-OHD), are highlighted (Figure 4.1B).

In the absence of the 21-hydroxylase activity of P450c21, three pathways lead to androgens. First, the pathway from cholesterol to DHEA remains intact. Although much DHEA is inactivated to DHEA-sulfate, the increased production of DHEA will lead to some DHEA being converted to testosterone and dihydrotestosterone (DHT). Second, although minimal amounts of 17-OHP are converted to androstenedione in the normal adrenal, the huge amounts of 17-OHP produced in CAH permit some 17-OHP to be converted to androstenedione and then to testosterone. Third, the proposed backdoor pathway depends on the 5α and 3α reduction of 17-OHP to 17OH-allopregnanolone. This steroid is readily converted to androstanediol, which can then be oxidised to DHT by the reversible 3α-HSD enzyme. Although first discovered in marsupials, mass spectrometric examinations of human urinary steroid metabolites indicate this pathway may also occur in the human adrenal.[1]

After the involution of the foetal adrenal cortex during infancy, endogenous production rates for adrenal steroids are constant at

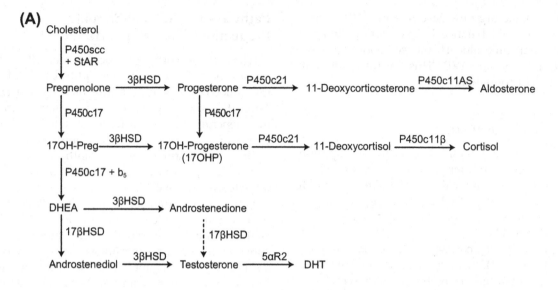

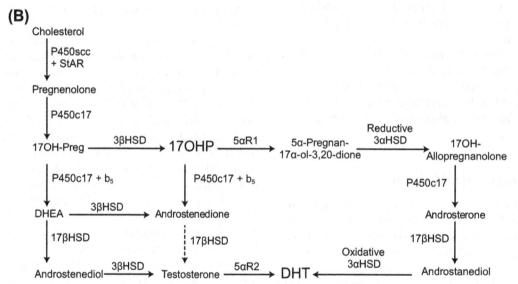

FIGURE 4.1   Foetal steroidogenesis: (A) normal foetal adrenal steroidogenesis; (B) most common enzymatic defects of adrenal steroidogenesis.

Note: **(A)** Because the foetal adrenal has low levels of 3β-HSD, most steroidogenesis is directed towards DHEA (and thence to DHEA-sulphate), but small amounts of steroid enter the pathways towards aldosterone and cortisol. The adrenal 21-hydroxylase, P450c21, is essential in both these pathways. The adrenal can make small amounts of testosterone via 17β-HSD. **(B)** Where an inborn error of glucocorticoid synthesis is present (e.g. congenital adrenal hyperplasia [CAH]), the adrenal medulla is morphologically abnormal and cannot produce adrenaline in normal amounts. Adrenaline deficiency is of minor clinical importance, but might increase the risk of hypoglycaemia, especially if cortisol and growth hormone deficiency are also present as occurs with hypopituitarism. *Reprinted with permission from Congenital adrenal hyperplasia due to steroid 21-hydroxylase deficiency: an Endocrine Society clinical practice guideline. JCEM 2010 Sep;95(9):4133-60. Copyright 2010, The Endocrine Society.*

approximate levels for cortisol of 6–9 mg/m^2/day, DHEAS 4–6 mg/m^2/day and aldosterone 0.1 mg/m^2/day. Knowledge of this production rate assists in understanding treatment requirements in various disorders.

CLINICAL SETTING

Since each hormone produces characteristic clinical effects, a carefully performed medical history taking and physical examination will in most cases lead to the most probable diagnosis – even if hormone assays are not available.

When hormone confirmation of clinical suspicion is not possible in the medical situation, it is worth considering trying to organise a reliable link with facilities elsewhere that are able to provide definitive confirmation of a diagnosis. This may sometimes save months or years of concern and confusion for families and practitioners alike. For example, dried filter paper blood or urine samples can be used for diagnosis of several forms of adrenal hyperplasia (see below).

Conditions with Glucocorticoid Deficiency

Glucocorticoid deficiency is the result of an impaired function of one or several links of the hypothalamic-pituitary-adrenal (HPA) axis. Conventionally, diseases of the adrenal cortex itself are called primary, those of the hypothalamus or pituitary secondary adrenal insufficiency.

Primary Adrenal Insufficiency

Primary adrenal insufficiency is due to an absent or impaired function of the adrenal cortex itself. Acquired primary adrenal insufficiency is rare, but may be caused by an autoimmune process, infection (e.g. tuberculosis) or, rarely, bleeding within the adrenals. More common causes of impaired function are inborn enzymatic defects that prevent or decrease synthesis of some or all of the adrenocortical hormones. If cortisol deficiency is marked, the elevated ACTH levels will cause adrenal hyperplasia (congenital adrenal hyperplasia, CAH). In addition to subnormal levels of the end products cortisol, aldosterone and/or testosterone, a deficiency in a specific enzyme will lead to accumulation of precursor steroids which in its turn can give rise to characteristic symptoms (see further below).

Secondary Adrenal Insufficiency

Secondary adrenal insufficiency (ACTH deficiency) is most often part of a multiple pituitary hormone deficiency that can be congenital ('idiopathic') or due to an acquired condition such as a pituitary or hypothalamic tumour, hydrocephalus, or (rarely) caused by autoimmune hypophysitis. An abnormal ACTH receptor, as in the rare familial isolated glucocorticoid deficiency, will mimic isolated ACTH deficiency, except that the excess ACTH production will cause hyper-pigmentation.

PRINCIPLES AND PROBLEMS OF TREATMENT PROVISION

Availability of corticosteroids for replacement treatment varies widely in different countries. This chapter provides information for use of standard replacement medications with hydrocortisone or prednisolone. Due to the dangerous consequences of medication omission in conditions of adrenal insufficiency, every effort to provide a constant supply of drugs for treatment of these conditions should be made in each country. This is usually most effective if addressed through government policy changes.

Attempts by families to conserve medication, for reasons of cost or availability, by inappropriate dose reduction or infrequent dosing can have catastrophic effects on general health and growth, together with unwanted virilisation in the case of congenital adrenal hyperplasia. Parental understanding of the nature of the disorders and need for constant treatment often requires patient and repeated information and reinforcement, to prevent serious illness and risk of death for an affected individual.

For disorders associated with androgen excess, this type of intermittent or repeated medication omission will lead to virilisation, with further confusion, possible social exclusion and a consequent high risk of depression and possible suicide.

In some parts of the world, until recently there have been no boys detected as being born with severe salt-losing adrenal disorders and few girls, due to multiple early deaths either in the home environment or even in local or village hospitals where access to diagnosis is limited. This situation is changing, with better information and easier access to testing but diagnosis and management of these conditions is still a major challenge for medical and para-medical staff and for families.

Provision of widely disseminated, clear and comprehensive information to families, local medical facilities and educational establish-ments, regarding the need for constant careful, treatment, with institution of emergency action plans during times of ill-health, will remain an essential component of care, to reduce the burden of these disorders in communities around the world.

CONGENITAL ADRENAL HYPERPLASIA

Inheritance

CAH is caused by a variety of enzyme defi-ciencies in the adrenal cortex. The various enzymes are indicated in Figure 4.1 — each one of them will result in clinical signs and symptoms that depend on whether the enzyme deficiency results in abnormally low or high production of glucocorticoids, mineralocorti-coids or androgens.

It is estimated that about 95% of all CAH is caused by 21-hydroxylase deficiency (21-OHD). The incidence is quite similar around the world, 1/10,000–1/15,000. The incidence of 11β-hydroxylase deficiency (11β-OHD) varies among ethnic groups, reaching 2–15% of the overall CAH incidence. In places where consan-guinity is common, incidence of rarer forms of CAH increases.

The 'classical' 21-OHD patient is character-ised by subnormal cortisol and, if the enzyme deficiency is severe, low aldosterone produc-tion, while accumulation of cortisol precursors cause elevated androgen levels (androstene-dione, testosterone and dihydrotestosterone). Conventionally, the classical form is subdivided into 'salt losing' and 'simple virilising' forms. However, there is no sharp demarcation line between the two; a patient with a simple virilis-ing form may show salt loss during severe illness. 'Non-classical' CAH patients maintain enough glucocorticoid and mineralocorticoid production to escape diagnosis at birth, but the moderately elevated androgen production will eventually cause symptoms of hyperandrogen-ism later in life.

CAH is inherited as an autosomal recessive trait. Thus, parents are generally asymptomatic carriers of the mutated genes, but siblings should be examined for signs and symptoms of CAH. Generally, a good genotype/phenotype correlation is found in 21-OHD. However, if the two alleles carry different mutations, one causing mild and one causing severe enzyme deficiency, the best functioning allele will deter-mine the phenotype. Therefore, it is not unusual that a parent who carries one mild and one severe allele gives birth to a child with a severe form, because the other parent is a non-symptomatic carrier of one allele with a severe mutation.

A comprehensive guideline to the diagnosis and management of 21-OHD has recently been published by the Endocrine Society.[1] The reader should consult that publication for detailed information of management in a setting where up-to-date laboratory and imaging facilities are available. In the following, some practical information will be given on how diagnosis and management can be achieved even without sophisticated laboratories.

DIAGNOSTIC APPROACH TO THE NEWBORN WITH SUSPECTED 21-HYDROXYLASE DEFICIENCY (21-OHD)

Clinical Presentation

The clinical presentation at birth depends on the sex of the child; a girl with a severe ('classic') form of 21-OHD is born with variably virilised genitalia. The virilisation may be so severe that the child is thought to be a boy.

The finding of genital ambiguity at birth is a medical and social emergency. Parents are shocked, distressed and confused and are often subjected to poor and ill-informed comments as to the supposed sex of the child. Competent assessment by a well-informed clinician, with accurate and clear communication to the family, will help allay anxiety and reduce stress. Serious long-term adverse consequences can occur if these needs are not attended.

Symptoms in the form of salt loss, dehydration, vomiting and failure to thrive do not appear until 5–15 days of life, when the child has already been discharged from the maternity ward. Therefore, in most Western countries, newborn screening for elevated levels of 17-hydroxyprogesterone (17-OHP) on the second or third days of life is used to detect CAH before serious salt loss has appeared.

This test is not available in many countries. Furthermore, in some countries the majority of births occur at home. For those who attend a hospital, discharge home frequently occurs within 24 hours of birth. Ability to trace a patient may be limited and loss to follow-up is likely.

Family History

Typically, parents are healthy carriers of mutated CYP21A genes; the carrier incidence of 21-OHD is about 1/50. Consanguinity may or may not be noted. When a diagnosis of CAH is made, growth and pubertal development of all siblings, male and female, should be investigated. Many boys with severe salt-losing CAH die undetected, by the end of the second or third week of life. A family history of early neonatal deaths should immediately alert the paediatrician to the possibility of a salt-losing condition.

Physical Examination

A girl with classical forms of 21-OHD will be more or less virilised; findings of clitoral enlargement, displacement of the vaginal opening towards or into the urethra, posterior fusion of labiae, scrotalisation of the skin of the labia majora and variable pigmentation of this area are common, with the key finding of absence of gonads in the scrotal folds or labia.

A boy with CAH has apparently normal male genitalia at birth, although an astute observer may detect a relatively large phallus and, in a pale-skinned infant, the appearance of abnormally dark scrotal pigmentation. This is much less easy to detect in populations with darker natural skin tones.

Careful palpation to confirm or exclude palpable testes is very important in the newborn with ambiguous genitalia. Identification of one or both testes strongly suggests that it is an XY child rather than a virilised girl with CAH. However, CAH due to 21 hydroxylase deficiency is the most common cause of ambiguous genitalia.

Presence of a uterus may be confirmed by very careful rectal examination for the presence of a cervix, but only with a small finger used for examination.

After the first few days of life, both boys and girls with salt-wasting forms will gradually develop dehydration, failure to thrive, hypotension, vomiting and eventually death, if not diagnosed and treated.

Important Differential Diagnoses in the Neonatal Period

- CAH in a 46,XX girl should always be ruled out in the case of a 'boy' born with non-palpable testes.
- Causes of ambiguous genitalia other than CAH should be considered. The key dividing finding on physical examination is the finding of palpable testes. Their presence excludes all forms of disorders of sex development (DSDs) with virilisation of 46,XX individuals.
- Any newborn boy who maintains good urine production in spite of dehydration and salt loss should alert the doctor to the possibility of CAH. Since girls with classic CAH will be virilised, they are less likely to be missed at birth.
- Salt loss and dehydration with maintained urine production may be caused by low urinary tract obstruction, irrespective of adrenal function. Therefore, in boys with normal genitalia, this condition might be mistaken for CAH.

11-HYDROXYLASE DEFICIENCY (11β-OHD)

A deficiency in the 11β-hydroxylase enzyme (P450c11β, see Figure 4.1) will also cause cortisol deficiency. However, deoxycorticosterone, a precursor of aldosterone, will accumulate.

Since this steroid has mineralocorticoid activity the child will not show salt loss and dehydration after early infancy, as occurs in 21-OHD. However, a newborn with 11β-OHD deficiency does not usually exhibit hypertension and indeed may lose salt in the first months of life and thus be clinically indistinguishable from a child with 21-OHD deficiency.

Sodium concentrations in blood and blood pressure will be normal or elevated, with hypokalaemic alkalosis. Since glucocorticoid production is impaired, the low cortisol levels will raise ACTH secretion and cause overproduction of androgens that will virilise the female foetus or, in cases of partial 11β-OHD, cause signs of androgen overproduction in childhood or later.

Other rare forms of CAH may be considered where consanguinity is common.

3β-DEHYDROGENASE DEFICIENCY

3β-dehydrogenase deficiency demonstrates DHEAS accumulation prior to the enzyme deficiency (see Figure 4.1). It is rare, with inconsistent salt loss, and presents as an undervirilised male with perineo-scrotal hypospadias and/or cryptoorchidism or as a slightly virilised female, due to excess DHEAS. If severe, it presents in the neonatal period. In a partial form it can present as hyperandrogenism in an adolescent girl.

17α-HYDROXYLASE DEFICIENCY

17α-hydroxylase deficiency occurs with a block in production of glucocorticoid and androgen, resulting in an undervirilised male with female genital appearance in both sexes. Mineralocorticoid excess, via DOC accumulation, results in hypertension and hypokalaemia. Presentation is often in later childhood or adolescence, with genital ambiguity and hypertension.

LABORATORY INVESTIGATIONS OF CAH IN THE NEONATAL PERIOD

With Minimal Laboratory and Imaging Resources

- Serum sodium, potassium for salt loss.
- Urea, creatinine to exclude renal disorders.
- Ultrasound for presence of uterus and gonads, either as ovaries or for possible inguinal gonads where partial testicular descent is considered. Experience of pelvic ultrasound examination of infants is important. If the radiologist is unfamiliar with neonatal examination it is likely that both uterus and gonads will be missed.
- Genitogram can be helpful for delineation of internal structures but is often poorly performed and is of no value if radiologic expertise is unavailable.
- Buccal smear may be done for early confirmation of likely female infant, if karyotype is unavailable, with the finding of Barr bodies (X chromatin). This test is easy to perform, with results available within 24 hours. However, it is unreliable in the neonatal period, and needs an experienced examiner even later in life. False negative results are notorious even in qualified labs.

With Optimal Laboratory and Imaging Resources

- 17-hydroxyprogesterone (17-OHP): This test may be diagnostic, if performed on day two of life or later. However, many infants are discharged from hospital after 12–24 hours, making a very early test less valuable and harder to interpret even if it is performed. Presence of maternal 17-OHP may interfere with reliability of the test within the first 24–48 hours after birth. Some screening laboratories accept to analyse 17-OHP from dried blood on filter paper. This is an inexpensive assay that can also be used for follow-up visits.
- If salt loss: As above, aldosterone, renin, androstenedione, testosterone, DHT, DHEAS can be considered. However, these hormone values are difficult to interpret in the neonatal period.
- A urinary steroid profile can be performed on fresh urine or on a lab grade filter paper sample, air dried and sent to a specialised laboratory, and can provide invaluable early, accurate diagnosis of 21 and 11 hydroxylase deficiencies. Isolated assay of pregnanetriol is also diagnostic, except for the first month of life. Establishment of links with available laboratories for diagnosis of rare disorders is essential in countries where resource availability is constrained.
- Karyotype.
- Ultrasound and genitogram. In preparation for future surgery, cystoscopy to define location of the vaginal opening into the urethra.
- Mutation analysis is optional. It is generally not needed for diagnosis but it is of value for genetic counselling.

DIAGNOSTIC APPROACH TO 'SIMPLE VIRILISING' FORMS OF CAH LATER IN CHILDHOOD

Clinical Presentation

Patients with impaired but not abolished 21-hydroxylase activity may escape salt loss during basal conditions, but may develop hyponatraemia during periods of physical stress, such as severe infections or at a time of sustaining injury. While girls with classic forms of 21-OHD or 11β-OHD will most often be diagnosed during the neonatal period because of virilisation, some may present for the first time later in childhood because of early pubarche, tall stature and increased linear growth rate.

Boys may escape diagnosis until they show very marked symptoms such as increased growth rate, premature pubarche, acne, oily skin and increased penile size at any age after 1–2 years, or, in case of 11β-OHD, increased blood pressure.

Family History

A family history of other affected children or early and possibly recurrent neonatal death does not exclude this diagnosis, as a more severe allele may have caused a prior salt-wasting neonatal disorder in the same family.

Relevant Previous Medical History

Documentation of growth rate should be sought. If previous measurements are not available, comparisons with sibling growth rate or that of age-matched peers may be informative.

- The tempo of development of pubarche or other signs of 'skin puberty' (all the signs of androgen effects on skin, like axillary hair, apocrine sweat odour, oily skin and/or acne) is important, in CAH. These signs typically progress slowly.
- Does the child become sicker than peers during long-standing high fever? Has he or she sustained surgery and general anaesthesia well?
- In suspicion of 11β-OHD: has he or she ever been found to be hypertensive?

Physical Examination

At the first examination, as well as at all subsequent visits, height and weight must be recorded, using a growth chart, to provide accurate information as to growth velocity. Blood pressure, pigmentation and all signs of androgen action (skin puberty, muscle and penile development, voice level) should be documented.

Other causes of androgen excess should be kept in mind during follow-up. Adrenal tumours can sometimes be found through careful palpation of the abdomen. Where accurate diagnosis is not available and differential diagnosis includes possible adrenal tumour, at follow-up visits during treatment, distribution of body fat should also be noted: looking for possible clues to corticosteroid excess as an alternative diagnosis (Cushingoid body habitus as compared to 'simple' obesity?).

Investigations at First and Subsequent Visits

With Minimal Laboratory and Imaging Resources

- At first visit, for diagnosis: serum sodium and potassium. Both may be normal in both 21-OHD and 11β-OHD, but sometimes sodium is elevated in 11β-OHD.
- Bone age.
- Abdominal ultrasound to exclude adrenal tumour.
- For monitoring treatment: At each 3–6-monthly follow-up visits: height, weight and other physical signs must be recorded, aiming for slowing of growth rate.

With Optimal Laboratory and Imaging Resources

At first visit, for diagnosis:

- As above, plus serum 17-OHP.
- 11-deoxycortisol may be performed but availability is likely to be extremely limited.
- If baseline 17-OHP is only slightly elevated, a short ACTH stimulation test with measurements of 17-OHP and cortisol is needed for diagnosis of 21-OHD. A stimulated level of more than 30 nmol/L suggests 21-OHD. Note: Some immunoassays for 11-deoxycortisol cross-react with 17-OHP.
- DHEAS: very high DHEAS suggests adrenal tumour, most often carcinoma.

- Further adrenal imaging (ultrasound, MRI or CT scan) to rule out adrenal carcinoma.

Follow-up visits for management after diagnosis of CAH should occur every 6 months or more frequently, depending on findings at the preceding visit and possible changes in medication. While investigations may be of value to optimise management, cost and availability may preclude their use.

The most important feature of good control in CAH is linear growth rate, followed by examination findings of lack of further virilisation (and normal BP for 11 hydroxylase deficiency). Added confidence as to effectiveness of treatment can be gained by bone age review, where bone age advance should be consistent with chronologic age or have slowed significantly if late institution of effective treatment has occurred.

If methods for assay of 17-OHP in blood filter paper spots (as used in many neonatal screening programmes) or in saliva are available, repeated sampling during one day every 3—6 months gives valuable information about the diurnal rhythm during treatment.

DIAGNOSTIC APPROACH TO NON-CLASSICAL CAH IN CHILDHOOD

Patients carrying 'mild' mutations in both CYP21A alleles (or one mild and one severe mutation) will most often show symptoms of hyperandrogenism later in childhood or in adulthood. Thus, non-classical CAH should be suspected in children with increased growth rate and/or signs of androgen excess: premature pubic hair, acne, oily facial skin.

Family History

A positive family history may or may not be noted, as described above for classical CAH. Mild, non-classical forms of 21-OHD are very common in some populations; it is estimated to have a prevalence of 1/130 in Mediterranean countries, while it is much less common in Northern Europe. If similar symptoms are found among siblings, CAH rather than adrenal carcinoma is a much more likely possibility.

Physical Examination and Differential Diagnosis

Not all children presenting for the first time with premature pubarche have 21-OHD.

Girls with apparently non-classical CAH are born without virilisation, but precocious pubarche may appear later during childhood. In both sexes, the spectrum of symptoms varies from non-symptomatic to early onset pubic and/or axillary hair, acne, oily skin, accompanied by growth acceleration.

Presence of hypertension (in addition to the above signs of androgen excess) suggests partial 11-hydroxylase deficiency even if the child has not previously presented for care.

Partial labial fusion with clitoromegaly suggests the possibility of an undervirilised male. With the added presence of hypertension, 17α-hydroxylase deficiency should be considered.

Importantly, in girls under the age of 8 years, the presence of pubic hair together with breast enlargement is not a sign of CAH but rather of central precocious puberty.

Similarly, a boy with pubic hair and testicular growth greater than 4 mL volume under the age of 9 years will have central precocious puberty rather than an adrenal cause for his androgenic signs.

Rapid progression of signs of androgen excess indicates adrenal carcinoma.

Laboratory Investigations

With minimal laboratory and imaging resources biochemical measurements may not be required. X-ray for bone age provides a measure of the accumulated exposure to androgens; abdominal and pelvic ultrasound excludes tumour.

With Optimal Laboratory and Imaging Resources

- 17-OHP for possible 21-OHD, 11-deoxycortisol (11β-OHD).
- DHEAS (adrenal carcinoma).
- Testosterone, androstenedione.
- Short ACTH stimulation test, with cortisol, 17-OHP, and 11-deoxycortisol at 0, 60 minutes. If 17-OHP is less than 30 nmol/L 1 hour after ACTH injection, 21-OHD is unlikely.
- Bone age.
- CT scan or MRI of adrenals to search for possible adrenal tumour if the diagnosis remains uncertain after blood tests and pelvic ultrasound.
- Mutation analysis is informative but not standard of care.

Other differential diagnosis in non-classical CAH

Adrenal Carcinoma

See the section on excess adrenal steroid production. Adrenal carcinoma is rare, but early intervention is life saving!

Idiopathic Premature Pubarche

Slow and minimal progression of signs of androgen excess in a child 5–10 years old may be familial. In such a case growth rate is not increased and 17-OHP and 11-deoxycortisol are normal. If DHEAS levels are found to be normal or only slightly elevated, adrenal carcinoma is unlikely.

Early Onset Polycystic Ovarian Syndrome

With a worldwide increase in excess weight gain and early onset obesity, the presence of PCOS and metabolic syndrome is being diagnosed with increasing frequency in childhood and very early adolescence, often with premenarchal acne and hirsutism as the first complaint. Unlike CAH, however, there is no abnormal growth acceleration beyond that seen in the relatively rapid growth of an overweight child. The conditions may thus be difficult to differentiate clinically. Presence of signs of hyperinsulinism with acanthosis nigricans may be of assistance.

MANAGEMENT OF A CHILD WITH CLASSICAL 21-OHD

The goals of glucocorticoid treatment are multiple. The first and most important goal is for effective communication to the parents of an affected child of the need for constant medication with appropriate increases at times of acute deterioration in health. Then, the aims of treatment should be as follows:

- to substitute the deficient cortisol secretion without causing signs or symptoms of over or undertreatment
- to suppress the production of excess adrenal androgens and their precursors
- to provide adequate available treatment for emergency needs during episodes of acute intercurrent illness.

The first two goals are not always easy to reach with current regimens. Although the normal daily secretion rate of cortisol is believed to be 6–9 mg/m^2 body surface area, giving this daily dose of hydrocortisone in 3–4 divided doses is often insufficient for suppression of ACTH secretion and excess adrenal androgen production. Therefore, hydrocortisone doses in the range 11–15 mg/m^2 or more are often needed to avoid hyperandrogenism. Long-acting glucocorticoids like prednisolone (given twice daily) or dexamethasone (once daily) can be used, but they often lead to over treatment, manifested in the long run by suppressed growth and excess weight gain.

If hormone assays are not available to study a child with signs of androgen excess but blood pressure and sodium blood levels are normal, it is not possible to distinguish between 21-OHD and 11β-OHD. However, since both are treated with hydrocortisone, this difficulty is not important for management, except that fludrocortisone or extra salt should not be added until low sodium levels have been documented.

It is important to point out to parents that if the child has some remaining adrenal function at diagnosis (in moderately severe or mild forms), treatment will suppress this spare function. Thus, if treatment is interrupted, the child will be at greater risk for adrenal crises during prolonged stress than he or she was before treatment started!

Emergency Management Plan for All Adrenal Insufficiency of Any Cause

In disorders like 21-OHD, where both glucocorticoid and mineralocorticoid are deficient, the acute treatment of adrenal crisis should aim at simultaneous correction of both. Since hydrocortisone at high doses has potent mineralocorticoid effects, it is generally enough to give intravenous salt as normal saline and IV or IM hydrocortisone alone during the first day. Fludrocortisone is added when the patient can take oral medication. Even patients with non-salt-losing forms of 21-OHD may become salt losers during stress, since the increased level of 17-OHP acts as a competitive inhibitor to aldosterone at the mineralocorticoid receptor level.

Such a plan will prevent most deaths from acute adrenal insufficiency.

To be successful it requires an emergency plan comprising the following, tailored to each individual depending on age:

- availability of parenteral hydrocortisone for administration at home or in a local medical facility; this includes provision of drug, syringes and needles for safe administration
- written and verbal communication of reasons for use and means of delivery
- adequate instructions to parents and carers about method of delivery of preparation to enable confident delivery in an emergency.

Monitoring Glucocorticoid Treatment in CAH Without Hormone Measurements

The dosing of hydrocortisone must be adjusted for an individual patient, in order to avoid over- or undertreatment. Even if hormone measurements are not available, important information can be obtained from careful history taking and physical examination.

The long-term success of glucocorticoid treatment of CAH can be read in the growth chart. Normal growth rate for age is a sign of adequate treatment, while over or undertreatment result in subnormal or increased growth rate, respectively.

Careful physical examination at each visit is important: Elevated androgens result in oily facial skin; a shining nose in a CAH child who should not have reached puberty suggests ongoing undertreatment! Comedomes and acne take longer to develop but are definite signs of elevated androgens. Development of pubic or axillary hair takes months. Bone age acceleration generally goes in parallel with increased growth rate, with a lag time of several months.

The distribution of hydrocortisone over the day is important. Normally, cortisol levels are high in the early morning, then decrease, to reach a nadir at midnight. The administration of hydrocortisone should try to mimic the natural rhythm. A common schedule is to give 50% of the daily dose as early in the morning as possible, 25% at midday and 25% in the late afternoon/evening. It may be preferable to give the second dose immediately after school, to avoid need for medication at school. Some teenagers are very drowsy in the morning;

administering the morning dose at 5 am may help. Late afternoon fatigue suggests that the midday dose is too low.

The first sign of overtreatment with glucocorticoids is a rounded face, with subsequent slowing of growth rate. This is evident before generalised obesity develops. Photos at regular intervals help in detecting these early Cushingoid features.

Careful measurements and plotting height and weight into a growth chart is mandatory to detect evolution of these features.

Laboratory Monitoring of Glucocorticoid Treatment Where Available

In a well child electrolyte measurements are not of value and will be normal.

Morning 17-OHP (in 21-OHD) or 11-deoxycortisol (11β-OHD) gives a spot measurement of the adequacy of glucocorticoid substitution at the time of sampling; in 21-OHD, 17-OHP values above 30 nmol/L should raise suspicions of undertreatment, less than 5 nmol/L the opposite. However, repeated measurements over the day are needed to determine if the divided doses of hydrocortisone are optimally distributed. Note that the levels of 17-OHP are sensitive to stress; if the blood sampling is done from a screaming child, 17-OHP will go up!

Androstenedione and testosterone measurements give direct indications of the androgen levels that should be suppressed. However, elevated testosterone levels are also manifested by clinical signs like oily skin, blackheads and acne, and, in the long run, increased growth rate. Measurement does not add much guidance to management.

Monitoring of Mineralocorticoid Treatment in 21-OHD

For two reasons, addition of 50–200 μg of fludrocortisone (Florinef®) to the treatment with hydrocortisone is recommended for all patients with classical forms of 21-OHD, even if sodium

and potassium levels were normal at diagnosis (so-called simple virilising form). The dose of hydrocortisone can be kept lower with co-administration of fludrocortisone. Even patients with the simple virilising form of 21-OHD may show salt loss during extreme stress.

Long-standing overtreatment with fludrocortisone may induce hypertension; therefore blood pressure monitoring is obligatory. Undertreatment is suspected if salt craving or salt loss during stress is noted.

During the first 3–12 months of life, patients with salt-losing forms of 21-OHD benefit from addition of 1–2 g/day of salt, in addition to fludrocortisone. The salt can be dissolved in multiple portions of breast milk over the day; too concentrated solutions may cause nausea and vomiting. Maturation of the renin angiotensin system is very variable. Careful monitoring of blood pressure is required at 6-weekly intervals, to detect sudden onset of hypertension that indicates the need for reduction in or cessation of salt supplements.

- Electrolyte levels are normal in treated 21-OHD patients and need not to be checked at each visit.
- Renin in serum (or renin activity) is the best laboratory means to monitor mineralocorticoid treatment; if renin is unmeasurable, the dose should be reduced. Levels at or slightly above the upper normal level are acceptable; higher levels should lead to an increased dose.

ACQUIRED DISORDERS OF THE ADRENAL CORTEX

Primary Adrenal Insufficiency (Addison's Disease)

Diagnostic Approach

On a worldwide basis, tuberculosis followed by HIV are the commonest cause of primary adrenal insufficiency. This condition must always be considered in the context of ill health related to these underlying disorders.

Fulminant infection, most often due to meningococcaemia, can present with bilateral adrenal haemorrhage accompanied by severe shock, at any age (Waterhouse—Friderichsen syndrome).

In boys, X-linked adrenoleukodystrophy (ALD) should be considered, especially if the patient shows signs of mental or neurological problems. Evidence for this condition should be sought diligently in a family history, where progressive neuropathy in an affected male may be the only clue. Onset of symptoms may be either neurologic or adrenal and years may separate the two events. Progress to severe deterioration is very likely where neurologic signs are present at less than 8 years, with a better outlook if diagnosis is made at an older age.

Sometimes the development of Addison's disease is preceded by another autoimmune disease such as diabetes mellitus type I, gluten intolerance or hypothyroidism. A history of alopecia, candidosis and/or hypocalcaemia (seizures? cramps?) suggests that the adrenal insufficiency is part of polyendocrine syndrome type 1.

Clinical Presentation

Symptoms and signs of adrenal insufficiency disease appear gradually. It is not uncommon to trace symptoms such as fatigue and salt craving for months or years before diagnosis. A history of increased pigmentation over the past year is frequently noted. As there is a slow, progressive decline of health with this disorder, these symptoms are frequently ignored and presentation for medical attention is more often an emergency, near mortal event, with acute deterioration and collapse due to salt-losing adrenal crisis.

Family History

This may be significant in the occurrence of autoimmune diseases or tuberculosis.

Consanguinity between healthy parents and/or finding of siblings with a similar condition suggests a disorder with recessive inheritance, or, if only males are affected, X-linked recessive adrenoleukodystrophy. Adrenal insufficiency can present at any age in this condition, but is common at some time in childhood. The brain manifestations vary in time of occurrence. If presentation is at age less than 8 years, progress is very likely. The chance of brain deterioration decreases with time, so that a child who remains well to 10—12 years of age is more likely to develop adrenomyelopathy. Girls who are carriers do not develop adrenal insufficiency but can have adrenomyelopathy.

Pertinent Past History

Symptoms can be expected from a combined deficiency in glucocorticoids and mineralocorticoids. Typically, a child or adolescent presents to the emergency room with a history of gradual loss of weight, salt craving and poor appetite for months, followed by dehydration, nausea, vomiting and fever over the past few days. Parents might have noticed increased sun-tan the past year, in spite of being indoors more than the siblings.

A history of exposure to tuberculosis (TB) or HIV must be sought. If TB is present and anti-tubercular treatment to be commenced, adrenal insufficiency should be first excluded. Induction of P450 liver enzymes by rifampicin increases rate of cortisol metabolism and can precipitate an adrenal crisis where adrenal insufficiency has not been suspected.

If the child is male, ALD should be considered. As reduced mentation or confusion is often seen as part of a slow deterioration of health with adrenal insufficiency, these symptoms do not necessarily suggest ALD, although it should be considered in a male.

Acute presentation for the first time in a previously healthy child should raise immediate concerns for endotoxic shock with overwhelming bacterial infection accompanied by adrenal haemorrhage.

Concomitant presence of hypocalcaemia, hypogonadism, diabetes mellitus type 1, pernicious anaemia, candidosis or alopecia suggests that the adrenal insufficiency is due to autoimmune polyendocrinopathy.

Physical Signs

In the acute situation, it is common to find dehydration, hypotension, tachycardia and often fever.

- Weight is reduced more than height. Increased pigmentation is noted at scars, palms, gums, knuckles, elbows and knees.
- Genitalia should be normal for age and sex.
- A lumbar mass may be detectable in a thin child, indicating adrenal haemorrhage.

Specific attention should be given to height plotted on a growth chart, in relation to midparental expectation. Linear growth in height is usually normal with Addison's disease.

Investigations

With acute ill health accompanied by signs of adrenal insufficiency as above, blood electrolytes will demonstrate hyponatraemia and hyperkalaemia.

WITH MINIMAL LABORATORY AND IMAGING RESOURCES

- Serum sodium, potassium, calcium and phosphorus.
- Plasma cortisol. If less than 5μg/dL (less than 20 nmol/L) this is confirmatory for adrenal insufficiency.
- Tuberculin test (Mantoux) or QuantiFERON®-TB gold, if not vaccinated against tuberculosis.
- Consideration for HIV ag/ab status.
- X-ray abdomen for adrenal calcification typical of TB or more rarely as evidence of past adrenal haemorrhage.

WITH OPTIMAL LABORATORY AND IMAGING RESOURCES

As above, plus the following.

- ACTH. Note: ACTH should be collected in a plastic syringe as it is destroyed by contact with glass. It is temperature sensitive and needs transport on ice.
- Very long chain fatty acids (only in boys, to rule out adrenoleukodystrophy).
- 17-OHP if CAH is considered on clinical grounds.
- MRI of brain to search for leukodystrophy (males only).

Additional investigations confirmatory for cause may be sent to a specialist laboratory.

- Antibodies against p450c21 (21-hydroxylase), as found in autoimmune Addison's disease).
- Antibodies against p450scc (side-chain cleavage enzyme, found in polyendocrine syndrome type 1).
- Molecular genetics in search for mutations of the genes, for the above-mentioned enzymes or for AIRE gene for APCED.

If a diagnosis of adrenal insufficiency is considered but unclear, a short synacthen test may be performed, using 0.25 μg synthetic ACTH IV with measurement of plasma cortisol at 0, 30, 60 minutes after administration. A rise of cortisol to at least 500 nmol/L (greater than 18 μg/dL) is a normal response.

Management of Adrenal Insufficiency

ACUTE MANAGEMENT

(Common to all conditions with acute adrenal insufficiency and salt loss.)

- Correct dehydration and salt loss, using intravenous normal saline.
- Give stress doses of hydrocortisone IV or IM.

See **Emergency Management plan for adrenal insufficiency of any cause (Box 4.1).**

BOX 4.1
EMERGENCY PLAN

Extra glucocorticoids should be given under the following circumstances:

- In case of acute ill health such as influenza or any infection with high fever, gastroenteritis or any other medical illness.
- For any surgery requiring general anaesthetic.
- For any significant long bone fracture.
- If the condition is mild to moderate, usual dose of glucocorticoids should be tripled for 3 days then doubled for a further 2 days.
- For more severe conditions, either intramuscular or intravenous injection of hydrocortisone should be administered immediately, to be repeated 6-hourly until recovery is assured, after which oral glucocorticoid dose should be tripled for 3 days then doubled for 2 days.
- The initial parenteral stress dose of hydrocortisone for an infant is of the order of 20–25 mg in the first 2 years, 50 mg from 2–8 years then 100 mg. The following daily dose should be 3–4 times the maintenance dose, divided in 3–4 doses per day.

- After the first day of rehydration, add fludrocortisone orally (Florinef®, 0.05–0.2 mg).

LONG-TERM MANAGEMENT

GLUCOCORTICOID Approximate dose equivalence is given below but steroid effect differs clinically, due to the longer duration of action of prednisolone and dexamethasone. As a general guide, hydrocortisone lasts roughly 8–12 hours, prednisolone 12–18 hours and dexamethasone 24–36 hours.

(7.5 mg prednisolone = 30 mg hydrocortisone = 37.5 mg cortisone acetate = 0.25–0.5 mg dexamethasone)

(1 mg prednisolone = approx 4.5 mg hydrocortisone = approx 5 mg cortisone acetate)

- Continue with hydrocortisone, 8–15 mg/m^2 per day, divided in three daily doses (morning, afternoon after school and bedtime is preferable, to avoid the need for medication within school hours), or an equivalent dose of prednisolone in two daily doses, if hydrocortisone is not available. Dexamethasone may be used if it is the only available corticosteroid but use is limited by difficulty of dosage adjustment and usually results in severe weight gain and growth failure.

MINERALOCORTICOID

- Fludrocortisone, 0.05–0.15 mg/day is given to all patients with primary adrenal insufficiency.

Monitoring of glucocorticoid substitution: dosing can be determined by clinical signs: Afternoon fatigue, early morning hypoglycaemia and continued or increasing hyper-pigmentation suggest undertreatment; Cushingoid features and decreased growth rate indicate overtreatment.

Blood pressure should be normal for age; overtreatment can induce hypertension. Serum sodium and potassium should remain normal. Measurement is not required.

Occasional ACTH and renin measurement can confirm treatment doses but is not mandatory.

EMERGENCY MANAGEMENT PLAN

As for CAH, see Box 4.1.

Secondary Adrenal Insufficiency

Causes

ACTH insufficiency occurs as a result of hypothalamic pituitary disorders and is most commonly due to exogenous administration of moderate to high-dose corticosteroids causing suppression of the HPA axis.

This can occur in the context of:

- a child who sustains acute illness or injury while taking corticosteroids, where the adrenal cannot respond to the increased demands of stress
- after cessation of previously long-term corticosteroid use, where dose tapering has been excessively rapid.

ACTH deficiency is rarely isolated and usually occurs in the context of other congenital or acquired hypothalamic pituitary disorders. These include

Congenital panhypopituitarism:

- on a genetic basis
- in the presence of midline disorders such as septo-optic dysplasia or holoprosencephaly.

Acquired lesions with lesions involving midline structures:

- tumours, cysts: craniopharyngioma, glioma
- infections : TB, histoplasmosis
- autoimmune hypophysitis
- after radiation for intracranial tumours.

Clinical Findings

Lethargy, chronic tiredness, pallor, anorexia and mild weight loss are common features of gradual onset ACTH insufficiency. Excess pigmentation is absent. Signs of concurrent hypothyroidism, diabetes insipidus or hypogonadism (in adolescence) support suspicions of pituitary dysfunction.

A diligent search for clinical signs of underlying causes such as midline tumour must be sought.

Acute presentation with collapse and hypotension is uncommon due to preservation of mineralocorticoid function. An exception may exist in the obvious case of a child who has a history of withdrawal from or long-term intake of corticosteroid. In this case, consideration must be given to other causes for acute collapse, including fulminant infection in an immuno-suppressed state.

Assessment

This can be extremely difficult, particularly as the signs of primary adrenal insufficiency, including electrolyte imbalance and pigmentation, are absent. Sometimes, in the acute setting, the only way to confirm a suspected diagnosis may be to administer a stress dose of parenteral hydrocortisone and await response within 10–20 minutes.

- Electrolytes are usually unhelpful as they are probably normal, unless ADH deficiency is part of the picture.
- Blood should be drawn for plasma cortisol and other pituitary hormones including prolactin, prior to treatment, even if storage and later testing only is available. If possible, thyroid function, with free thyroxine and TSH level, should be checked prior to institution of replacement.
- Consideration for precipitating causes should include possible investigation for infection.
- Imaging may include CT, skull X-ray for abnormality of the pituitary fossa, MRI if available.

Management

If in the setting of suspected or confirmed other pituitary hormone deficits, care must be taken with the order of administering replacement treatment.

Hydrocortisone should always be given before thyroxine is instituted, preferably

24 hours prior. If this is not attended, further decompensation of the hypothalamic pituitary axis with acute collapse and shock may occur.

For more chronic and subtle manifestations a high index of suspicion is required and a trial of oral steroid replacement over 2—4 weeks might be considered, to assess response, particularly in a situation such as after cranial radiation, with evolving hypothalamic pituitary dysfunction.

Long-term management and steroid requirement during situations of stress are similar to primary adrenal insufficiency. Mineralocorticoid is not required.

DISORDERS OF MINERALOCORTICOID FUNCTION

Defects in aldosterone production are rare. As they are often confused with complete adrenal insufficiency making a diagnosis of isolated aldosterone deficiency or resistance is very important. A detailed discussion is found in *Chapter 8, Disturbances of Sodium and Water*.

HYPERFUNCTION OF THE ADRENAL/DISORDERS OF THE ADRENAL CORTEX/EXCESSIVE ADRENAL STEROID PRODUCTION

Clinical Presentation

The presentation of a child with excess glucocorticoids is often different from the typical features seen in an adult with that condition. During prepubertal years, a simultaneous increase in rate of weight gain accompanied by a reduction in height velocity is alarming! However, in the growing child the typical facial features of corticosteroid excess may not be readily apparent and striae are often absent due to better elasticity of a child's skin. Use of family photographs, if available, can help identify subtle changes. Hypertension is not a common feature of childhood corticosteroid excess. Bone pain, muscle weakness, hirsutism, and tiredness are common associated complaints, often accompanied by signs of androgen excess (early 'skin puberty', like pubarche, axillary hair, apocrine sweat odour, acne and oily facial skin) in the absence of testicular or breast growth. Osteopaenia with vertebral fractures is common, when a lesion has been long standing, presenting as back pain.

The most common cause of glucocorticoid excess is iatrogenic. Many children with severe juvenile rheumatoid arthritis, malignancies, nephrotic syndrome, inflammatory bowel disease or severe asthma are treated with large doses of glucocorticoids.

Endogenous over-production of cortisol may be due to either a pituitary adenoma with ACTH production (Cushing's disease), or due to a problem of regulation of cortisol production by the adrenal itself (Cushing syndrome).

The latter is more common in children and includes:

- adrenal adenoma
- adrenal carcinoma
- pigmented nodular hyperplasia in association with Carney complex (a form of multiple endocrine neoplasia)
- McCune—Albright syndrome where macronodular hyperplasia occurs.

Less commonly, pituitary ACTH excess causes a secondary form of Cushing's disease in childhood, usually due to a small 2—3 mm micro-adenoma in the pituitary.

Ectopic ACTH production is rare in childhood but can occur in association with gastrinoma, phaeochromocytoma, carcinoid or islet cell tumours of the pancreas.

Assessment

Diagnosis of glucocorticoid over-secretion can be challenging. Care should be given to looking for an associated lesion that may give a clue to diagnosis.

- Iatrogenic causes of Cushingoid features should be the first to be ruled out. These include excessive use of inhaled fluorinated steroids for asthma and excessive use of topical fluorinated steroids for severe eczema.
- A short duration of symptoms and presence of androgen excess should raise suspicion for adrenal carcinoma.
- Presence of frequent fractures and/or bony deformity may indicate fibrous dysplasia with McCune–Albright syndrome.
- Unusual skin lentigines and blue naevi, atrial myxoma and Leydig cell tumours are all associated with Carney complex.

Investigations

Diagnostic investigations should utilise screening tests for corticosteroid excess prior to radiologic imaging, to avoid pitfalls of finding an incidental pituitary or adrenal lesion and assuming it to be causative for clinical symptoms.

With Minimal Access to Laboratory and Imaging Facilities

To confirm excess cortisol secretion:

- Comparison of morning and midnight cortisol levels in blood should be the next step. Loss of diurnal variation in cortisol is the first sign of cortisol excess, due to disruption of the normal circadian rhythm. A clear diurnal rhythm with low midnight cortisol speaks against both Cushing's disease and Cushing syndrome.
- Measurement of free cortisol in a 24-hour urine collection is the most valuable screening procedure, where available, limited only by difficulty of undertaking timed urine collection in a young child. It is a good screening test but should not be used alone owing to 5–10% false negative rate.

To define causes of cortisol excess:

- As a screening procedure, a short dexamethasone test can be applied; 1 mg of dexamethasone given at 11 pm should suppress cortisol the following morning to very low levels, less than 5 μg/L (less than 30 nmol/L)
- Measuring ACTH in serum is an essential step in differentiating ACTH dependent from peripheral causes of adrenocortical over-secretion. Suppressed ACTH in the face of elevated cortisol points to the adrenal cortex as the primary cause; adrenal carcinoma or adenoma being the next to be ruled out. Note that instructions for sampling in a cold plastic syringe, storage and transportation of the serum on ice to the laboratory should be strictly followed! ACTH is a notoriously sensitive peptide. Before the advent of reliable ACTH assays, suppression with low and high doses of dexamethasone for several days was the method of choice to distinguish between normal variants, pituitary adenomas and adrenal tumours. As accurate ACTH assay may not always be available, these tests are described below (Table 4.1).

With Optimal Access to Laboratory and Imaging Facilities

- As above, with addition of the following.

If midnight cortisol and ACTH are high:

- MRI imaging to look for pituitary adenoma
- If no adenoma is seen, inferior bilateral petrosal sinus blood sampling with determination of ACTH in order to localise a micro-adenoma, prior to surgery. Central to

TABLE 4.1 Low-Dose and High-Dose Dexamethasone Suppression Tests

Test	Low dose	High dose
Dose of dexamethasone	Days 2 and 3 give 0.5 mg orally 6-hourly (20 µg/kg/dose 6-hourly in younger children)	Days 2 and 3 give 2 mg orally 6-hourly (80 µg/kg/dose 6-hourly in younger children)
Blood samples	Plasma cortisol and ACTH on: Day 1 at 9 am and midnight Day 4 at 9 am	Plasma cortisol, ACTH/ACTH precursors on Day 1 at 9 am and midnight Plasma cortisol on Day 4 at 9 am
Interpretation	In normal subjects, cortisol level will be suppressed to less than 50 nmol/L. Patients with Cushing's syndrome lose the normal negative feedback control and thus exhibit detectable plasma ACTH and cortisol after dexamethasone administration. Failure to suppress ACTH level less than 5 ng/L is highly suggestive of an adrenal cause of Cushing's syndrome.	Pituitary-dependent hypercortisolism (Cushing's disease): plasma cortisol usually suppresses to at least 50% of basal values. Approximately 10% of patients with Cushing's disease fail to suppress and approximately 10% of those with ectopic ACTH secretion will suppress cortisol levels.

peripheral gradient of greater than 4:1 indicates pituitary origin.

If midnight cortisol is high and ACTH is low: See section on adrenal tumours below.

ADRENAL TUMOURS/ADRENAL CARCINOMA

In children, most adrenal tumours are malignant and produce both glucocorticoids and androgens. In addition some oestrogen secretion may occur. Clinical signs of hyperandrogenism may dominate, rather than those of hypercortisolism, but there are large variations in presentation. Some tumours are large enough to be found by abdominal palpation. Tumour size is correlated to malignancy and prognosis. Surgery is the only therapeutic option; chemotherapy is generally ineffective in stopping growth of metastases, but block of steroid production and administration of anti-androgens can be of palliative value.

Diagnosis with Minimal Laboratory and Imaging Facilities

- Ultrasonography of adrenals can diagnose an adrenal tumour but is unlikely to adequately identify either macro or micronodular hyperplasia. Bilateral adrenal enlargement speaks for a systemic disease rather than carcinoma.
- Cortisol, testosterone and DHEAS in morning and midnight serum samples.

Diagnosis with Optimal Laboratory and Imaging Facilities

- Addition of MRI of adrenals.
- Addition of gas chromatography/mass spectrometry of urinary steroids. In adrenal carcinomas, a multitude of immature steroids is typically found.

- If results of MRI are not conclusive, catheterisation of both adrenal veins with steroid hormone determination is often helpful to localise the tumour in preparation for surgery.
- PET scan with radiolabelled cholesterol may help identify sites of increased steroidogenesis.

Other Adrenocortical Lesions of Childhood

Single, non-secretory incidentalomas are common in adults but less seen in children.

The most common cause of multiple benign adrenal adenomas is that found in adolescent and adult patients with CAH. The occurrence of these adenomas is linked to long-standing high ACTH stimulation due to insufficient suppression by glucocorticoids and can be compared to 'adrenal rest tumours' that are often found in the testes of CAH patients.

Micronodular pigmented adrenal tumours may be typically suspected where cortisol excess is cyclical. However, cyclical steroid production may also occur with other types of cortisol excess in childhood. These lesions are associated with Carney complex. Diagnosis may be confirmed with a paradoxical rise in cortisol after dexamethasone suppression.

Macronodular adrenal lesions of McCune–Albright syndrome are the results of a genetic defect in the intracellular transduction of the ACTH signal. Diagnosis is more likely where the underlying condition is recognised in association with corticosteroid excess.

DISORDERS OF THE ADRENAL MEDULLA

Phaeochromocytoma

Phaeochromocytoma management requires specialist input and should not be attempted in a limited-resource area. Referral to a major centre should be made.

However, as many of these lesions are familial in origin, a brief description is included here.

Phaeochromocytoma occurs rarely in childhood. A majority of childhood cases have a genetic association and are diagnosed after a proband has been identified in an older family member. Phaeochromocytoma can be missed in childhood because measuring blood pressure in children is not emphasised in paediatric teaching and is very frequently omitted in a clinical examination.

Clinical Features

Typical features of episodic headache, palpitations, sweating, anxiety attacks with a feeling of impending doom are rarely noted by children. Occasionally, a child will have a history of panic attacks, for which psychological help has been sought in the past. Presentation may thus be late, with visual abnormality due to papilloedema with Grade 4 hypertensive changes seen in the fundi.

Family History

A family history of health problems suggesting phaeochromocytoma, hyperparathyroidism or thyroid malignancy should particularly be sought, with the underlying diagnoses of Von Hippel–Lindau syndrome, multiple endocrine neoplasia (MEN) 2A or B or succinate dehydrogenase (SDH) mutations being considered as potentially causative.

If a family history of any of these disorders is already known, genetic screening should be performed early for all possibly affected relatives. All these conditions are inherited in an autosomal dominant manner, most with high penetrance. Genetic screening is justified on the grounds that all of the associated health problems and particularly phaeochromocytoma present in a subtle manner, are dangerous to life and health and have potential for cure, if found at an early stage.

Physical Examination

This is unlikely to reveal hidden major pathology except rarely in the case of a paraganglioma associated with SDH mutation or previously unrecognised NF1.

PARAGANGLIOMATA

Paragangliomata can grow to extremely large size anywhere in the aortic chain before being detected clinically. Careful examination should include surveillance from base of skull to pelvis, due to the extra-adrenal location of the lesions. Those lesions found with Von Hippel—Lindau syndrome or MEN are more commonly contained within the adrenal gland. A phaeochromocytoma associated with neurofibromatosis Type1 is extremely rare in childhood, with a lifetime risk of around 4% for this otherwise common mutation.

VON HIPPEL—LINDAU SYNDROME

This is associated with bilateral adrenal phaeochromocytomata which frequently come to attention in mid childhood, presenting with typical symptoms of headache and paroxysmal anxiety, related to hypertension. Other associations of haemangioblastomas of brain, cerebellum and spinal cord, carcinoma of the kidney, pancreatic and epididymal cysts are more commonly seen in adults. Regular surveillance for these associations is usually not performed in children.

MEN 2A

MEN 2A is associated with hyperparathyroidism, medullary carcinoma of thyroid and phaeochromocytoma and is caused by germline mutations of the RET proto-oncogene. Medullary thyroid cancer in association with MEN 2A is universal and can present under the age of 12 months. It is therefore mandatory that all family members potentially affected by this autosomal dominantly transmitted gene be screened and that prophylactic thyroidectomy is undertaken if gene positivity is found. Some genotypes are associated with a more aggressive pattern of early thyroid cancer.

(See Chapter 3, Thyroid Disorders.)

Phaeochromocytoma in association with MEN 2A is more commonly found in adolescence or adulthood. However, regular annual screening with plasma and urinary catecholamines and metanephrines should be undertaken in children.

MEN 2B

MEN 2B is associated with typical features of a Marfanoid appearance together with ganglioneuromas of the lips, tongue and mucous membranes, particularly seen in the lower eyelids which often have an everted appearance. Very early childhood onset of phaeochromocytoma mandates regular screening from time of clinical or genetic diagnosis along with screening for medullary thyroid cancer. Prophylactic thyroidectomy should be considered in all affected individuals.

SUCCINATE DEHYDROGENASE (SDH) MUTATIONS

SDH mutations, particularly B and D, are now recognised to be causative for 30—40% of all childhood phaeochromocytomata. They are associated with secretory and non-secretory paragangliomata throughout the aortic chain, characterised by a prominent vasculature which can cause major problems with surgical intervention due to the vascular network around the tumour. Early diagnosis is paramount in this condition due to complexity of surgical management where tumours are in advanced state, where possible vascular invasion of and adherence to adjacent structures makes surgery very difficult.

Screening investigations should include urinary and plasma metanephrines as well as catecholamines, as a measure of production rate as well as excretion rate. Imaging should include annual screening every 1–2 years by MRI from base of skull to pelvis. Careful imaging of the carotid area at base of skull is required to detect small lesions.

CARNEY COMPLEX

Carney complex consists of various endocrine manifestations including phaeochromocytoma, schwannoma, atrial myxoma and spotty pigmentation of the skin and the Carney triad of phaeochromocytoma (functioning extra-adrenal paragangliomas and pulmonary chondromas).

A similar surveillance for phaeochromocytoma is undertaken for this condition. With the risk of atrial myxoma even during childhood, it is imperative that echocardiography is undertaken to detect such a lesion early as it can result in a ball valve obstruction if undiagnosed.

Management

Surgery for phaeochromocytoma should only be performed in a specialised unit, with facilities for peri-operative intensive care.

Pre-operative management for all phaeochromocytomas is similar, utilising alpha and beta-blockade. Alpha-blockade with phenoxybenzamine is most commonly used, commencing with 10 mg per day and increasing to a maximum of between 80 and 120 mg/day of phenoxybenzamine, depending on the weight of the child. Once fully alpha-blocked, beta-blockade with propranolol can be commenced together with a high fluid intake, either oral or intravenous, to fill the intravascular pool.

Nitroprusside should be available in case of hypertensive crisis at the time of manipulation of the tumour during surgery. It is usual for the vasculature to be clamped prior to tumour handling to minimise this risk.

Post-operatively, any residual tissue in the tumour bed may potentially release catecholamines/metanephrines in the week following surgery. Some alpha-blockade is therefore usually continued for 5–7 days post-operatively.

If adrenal-sparing surgery has been possible, long-term steroid replacement may not be needed. If bilateral adrenalectomy has been performed, replacement treatment in the peri-operative period should be commenced intra-operatively, using stress doses of between 25 and 100 mg of IV hydrocortisone every 6 hours, depending on the size of the child, with addition of mineralocorticoid replacement post-operatively. Doses can be weaned to maintenance levels within 3 days after surgery.

Metastatic phaeochromocytoma or paraganglioma are particularly associated with SDH mutations. Lesions may be slowly growing but their presence indicates a poor prognosis. Early metastasis under the age of 18 is associated with 70% 5-year mortality. Long-term surveillance is necessary for these lesions, using metanephrine measurement and imaging. Treatment with chemotherapy to date has had relatively little success.

Mineralocorticoid-Secreting Tumours

These are very rare in childhood, contrary to adult presentation.

Reference

1. Speiser PW, Azziz R, Baskin LS, et al. Clinical practice guidelines: congenital adrenal hyperplasia due to steroid 21-hydroxylase deficiency: an Endocrine Society Clinical Practice Guideline. *J Clin Endocrinol Metab* 2010;**95**:4133–60.

Further Reading

Ishimoto H, Jaffe RB: Development and function of the human fetal adrenal cortex: a key component in the feto-placental unit. *Endocr Rev* 2011;**32**:317-55.

Joint ESPE/LWPES working group (Clayton P, Miller WL, Oberfield SE, Ritzén EM, Sippell WG, Speiser PW): Consensus statement on 21-hydroxylase deficiency from the European Society for Paediatric Endocrinology and the Lawson Wilkins Pediatric Endocrine Society. Jointly published in *J Clin Endocr Metab* 2002;**87**:4048–53, published simultaneously in Hormone Res 2002;58: 188–95.

National High Blood Pressure Education Program Working Group on High Blood Pressure Children and Adolescents. The fourth report on the diagnosis, evaluation, and treatment of high blood pressure children and adolescents. *Pediatrics*. 2004;**114**:555–576

Nimkarn S. New MI: steroid 11 beta-hydroxylase deficiency congenital adrenal hyperplasia. *Trends Endocrinol Metab* 2008;**19**:96–99.

Warne GL, Grover S, Zajac JD. Hormonal therapies for individuals with intersex conditions: protocol for use. *Treat Endocrinol* 2005;**4**:19–29.

Disorders of Sexual Development in Resource-Limited Settings

Iroro Yarhere, Syed Faisal Ahmed

INTRODUCTION

The safe delivery of a newborn is usually accompanied by a question about the sex of the child. In some settings in Africa, the mother is made to scream the sex to notify relatives who are outside the delivery room. In most cases, the question is easily answered, but for a few families, it is the beginning of a long and often challenging life. When the external genitalia of a child cannot be assigned as male or female by the immediate carers, the child is often referred to as having ambiguous genitalia. In this situation, sex assignment is often delayed, in case the early assignment is incorrect. However,

concerns about sex development exist in other newborns with atypical genitalia, too. These conditions, including those with an abnormality of chromosomal, gonadal or anatomical sex, are collectively referred to as disorders of sex development (DSD).

Children with complex DSD are difficult to manage even in the most advanced care centres and though management guidelines have been proposed for different diagnoses, an individualistic approach is a most appropriate means of management while referring to the standard guidelines. Genetic studies, surgical expertise and many other specialist management techniques may be difficult to source in

Practical Pediatric Endocrinology in a Limited Resource Setting
http://dx.doi.org/10.1016/B978-0-12-407822-2.00005-0

resource-limited societies, but even the basic understanding of aetiology and pathophysiology of these conditions can prove to be a useful guide for optimal management.

This chapter aims to provide the reader with an update on the field of DSD and places its management from the perspective of a clinician practising in a resource-limited setting. In addition, it includes some issues that are specific to countries in Africa, but many of these may also apply to other regions of the world.

THE IMPORTANCE OF THE LOCAL SETTING

Applying the standards of clinical practice that have been stipulated in publications such as the consensus document in 2006[1] or, more recently, in 2011,[2] may be difficult in resource-limited regions for a number of reasons. Some of these are attributable to generic weaknesses in the healthcare system in such regions and include the low level of education of the general public as well as restricted opportunity for education of the healthcare workers, particularly those who work outside major centres. In combination with poor levels of education, many members of the general public have strong traditional values and beliefs which play a very crucial role in influencing the management of many health conditions, including sexual issues which are taboo subjects in many societies.

Identification of any variation in genital development and the extent of abnormality and its subsequent management depends on the experience, knowledge and attitudes of the immediate carers of the newborn. In most resource-poor settings, the local traditional birth attendants are often the commonest professionals who are present at the birth and subsequent management of infants seems to be very variable. The affected infants may occasionally be referred to specialist care centres but are often immediately stigmatised and treated as unusual. Information about the genital difference is either not given or mythological explanations are proffered. Those children with DSD and apparently normal external genitalia are missed and some die in the early newborn periods without being investigated, and a family may lose children in numbers and the diagnosis will not be made until a specialist makes a key observation. There are many early neonatal deaths in both rural and urban areas in resource-limited countries that may have been due to DSD, but as they are not fully investigated, the question remains unanswered.

There is very little scope in the already restricted health budget to address illnesses other than those which are public health priorities such as infections and malnutrition. The burden of a chronic condition in childhood on long-term health is not deemed of a high enough priority, particularly when the population has a high fertility rate. With the priority set on acute conditions, the healthcare infrastructure is poorly equipped to care for the child and the family who need frequent input in a private setting from an expert. Social mores in some regions such as South Asia and the Middle East are such that there is enormous premium placed on being a man rather than a woman Despite the fact that the man may be infertile he will still be the breadwinner for the extended family, whereas an infertile woman may be viewed as a burden for her family.

SEX DEVELOPMENT

In humans, sex development describes the complex path the fertilised egg takes as it develops through fetal life, infancy, childhood and adolescence into a man or woman. Differences between males and females at these life stages can be manifested through a range of features including chromosomes, genes, gonads, hormones, anatomy and psychosocial behaviours. Sex development can be simplistically divided into two processes, gonadal determination and sex differentiation, and generally speaking factors that influence the first process are transcriptional regulators, whereas factors that are important for the second process are hormones and their receptors. Gonadal determination starts in week 3 of gestation and the testes and ovaries are histologically different by 6–8 weeks. The first sign of sex differentiation of the genitalia is evident by about 7–8 weeks when in the presence of testes that secrete anti-Müllerian hormone (AMH), the paramesonephric ducts (also known as Müllerian ducts) which develop next to the mesonephric ducts (also known as Wolffian ducts) start to regress. The testosterone that is secreted by the Leydig cells of the testes augments the Wolffian ducts which differentiate into the epididymis, vas deferens and prostate and it starts to virilise the external genitalia which become distinctly male by 8–12 weeks. Absence of testes results in a lack of external virilisation, regression of the mesonephric ducts and the differentiation of the paramesonephric ducts into the fallopian tubes, uterus and the upper third of the vagina.

Thus, gonadal determination is often considered the key turning point in the pathway to sex development. Until recently it was generally believed that in the absence of a functioning sex-determining region of the Y chromosome (SRY) gene, an indeterminate gonad would *automatically* develop into an ovary. With increasing knowledge about ovarian development, it is becoming clear that there are crucial genes that may act as ovarian-determining factors which in turn may also exert a restraining effect on testes development.[3]

Epidemiology and Classification

Prevalence of genital anomalies may be as high as 1 in 300 births, but the complex anomalies leading to extensive investigations are estimated at 1 in every 2000–4500 live births. Congenital adrenal hyperplasia due to 21-α hydroxylase enzyme deficiency is the commonest known cause of DSD in girls. In Africa, the prevalence is largely unknown, and this is because there are no collective and comparative data, investigations of deaths/post mortems are rarely conducted, and children with such disorders are kept hidden for fear of stigmatisation and possibly being cast away from society. Some conditions such as 5α reductase deficiency are said to be common in the Dominican Republic, Eastern Highlands of Papua New Guinea, and Southern Lebanon.

The following classification as originally proposed in 2006[1] encompasses all forms of DSD and is aimed at reducing the stigmatisation that was associated with the old nomenclature. While the proposed term DSD is now widely used and accepted, some advocates prefer that the first 'D' stands for 'differences' and some still prefer the phrase 'intersex', thus avoiding the connotation of it being described as a disorder.

The 46,XY DSD are characterised by ambiguous or external genitalia, with or without salt wasting, and are caused by incomplete intrauterine masculinisation, and the presence or absence of Müllerian structures. There are many pathologies in this category and they include the following.

Disorders of Gonadal Development

a. Complete gonadal dysgenesis (Swyer syndrome)
b. Partial gonadal dysgenesis
c. Gonadal regression
d. Ovotesticular DSD.

Disorders of Androgen Synthesis or Action

a. Androgen biosynthesis defect, e.g. StAR mutation, 17-hydroxysteroid dehydrogenase deficiency, 5α reductase deficiency
b. Defect in androgen action, e.g. PAIS, CAIS
c. LH receptor defect

d. Disorders of AMH and AMH receptor (persistent Müllerian duct syndrome).

Others, e.g. severe hypospadias, cloacal exstrophy.

In the classification above, all will present as ambiguous external genitalia, except the CAIS or StAR mutation, which will present as females with no ambiguity. The 46,XY with 21 hydroxylase deficiency will not present with ambiguity but may have precocious puberty in early childhood.

The 46,XX DSD are characterised by ambiguous external genitalia, with or without salt wasting, and are caused by masculinisation or overvirilisation of the XX female. The disorders include the following.

1 Androgen excess:
   a. Fetal, e.g. 21-hydroxylase deficiency, 11-hydroxylase deficiency
   b. Feto-placental, e.g. aromatase deficiency, POR
   c. Maternal, e.g. exogenous androgen exposure, ovarian tumours
2 Disorders of gonadal development:
   a. Ovotesticular DSD
   b. Testicular DSD, e.g. SRY+, dup SOX9
3 Others, e.g. cloacal exstrophy, vaginal atresia.

CLINICAL ASSESSMENT

The history should include details of the pregnancy, in particular the use of any drugs that may cause virilisation of a female fetus and details of any previous neonatal deaths (which might point to an undiagnosed adrenal crisis). As important as drug history is, it may not yield much as many people self-prescribe and take across-the-counter drugs. A history of maternal virilisation may suggest a maternal androgen-secreting tumour or aromatase deficiency. A comprehensive family history should be taken, including whether the parents are consanguineous (which would increase the probability of an autosomal recessive condition) or if there is a history of genital ambiguity in other family members. Some endocrine conditions such as congenital adrenal hyperplasia and 5α reductase deficiency have an autosomal recessive inheritance pattern and their incidence may be particularly high in those societies where consanguinity is prevalent such as South Asia. Detailed guidance on the initial approach to a child with suspected DSD has recently been published.[2]

- The general physical examination should determine the general health of the baby and whether there are any dysmorphic features.
- Affected infants, particularly those who have XY DSD, are more likely to be small for gestational age and may display other developmental anomalies.
- In addition to a systematic examination, the affected infant should be examined for midline defects, which may point towards an abnormality of the hypothalamo-pituitary axis.
- The state of hydration and blood pressure should be assessed as various forms of adrenal steroid biosynthetic defects can be associated with differing degrees of salt loss, varying degrees of masculinisation in girls or under-masculinisation in boys, or hypertension (Figure 5.1). Although the cardiovascular collapse with salt loss and hyperkalaemia in congenital adrenal hyperplasia does not usually occur until the second week of life (with salt loss usually evident from day 4) and so will not be apparent at birth in a well neonate, it should be anticipated in a suspected case and salt and steroid replacement should start before these signs develop.
- Jaundice (both conjugated and unconjugated) may be observed in cases of hypopituitarism or cortisol deficiency.

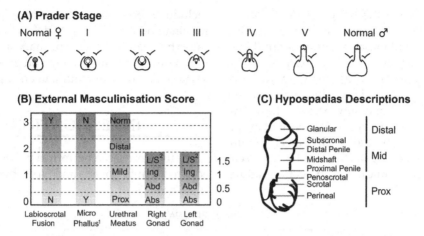

FIGURE 5.1 Scoring external genitalia.
Note: (A) The external genitalia can be objectively scored using the Prader staging system which provides an overall score for the appearance of the external genitalia. (B) Alternatively, each individual feature of the genitalia (phallus size, labioscrotal fusion, site of the gonads and location of urethral meatus) can be individually scored to obtain the External Masculinisation Score (EMS). For the EMS, the site of the urethral meatus is based on C. [1]. Microphallus refers to a phallus below the male reference range; [2]. L/S — labioscrotal. *Adapted with permission from Ahmed SF et al. BJU Int. 2000;85:120—24.*

- The urine should be checked for protein as a screen for any associated renal anomaly (e.g. Denys—Drash/Frasier syndromes).
- A pre-feed blood glucose should be checked for hypoglycaemia (suggestive of hypopituitarism, or occasionally in congenital adrenal hyperplasia (CAH), e.g. 3βHSD deficiency).

Although physical examination is useful, a diagnosis should not be made solely on examination findings. However, the following information is useful in determining what investigations are required, although the possibility of arriving at a diagnosis in all cases of DSD is approximately 40—50% even in the most equipped institutions.

1 Are gonads palpable?
  a. Twenty-five percent of infants with undescended testes and hypospadias have a DSD disorder.
  b. Gonads palpable in the perineum almost always indicate a male karyotype.

2 Is the penile length normal?
  a. Measure stretched length with a spatula from the symphysis pubis to the stretched tip (not foreskin) of the penis.
  b. Normal stretched length is greater than 3 cm at term.
  c. Less than 2.5 cm at term indicates a microphallus.
3 Is there reasonable penile girth on palpation?
4 Is the phallus straight or is there chordee present?
5 How many orifices are present?
6 Is the scrotum hypoplastic?
7 Are there any other physical abnormalities?

The first step of physical examination is the most important in the sequence and guides the steps that follow. The presence of gonads in the labioscrotal folds, the size of the phallus or clitoris, fusion of the labioscrotal folds and the site of the urethral meatus are important details to document when examining a patient with suspected DSD. The absence of a palpable gonad still does not make the baby female as severe testosterone deficiency can cause undescended testes. The external masculinisation score (EMS) is an individualised scoring system which provides an aggregate score for babies and allows the endocrinologist to know which baby should be evaluated further and how extensive the investigation will be. Other important aspects of examinations are state of hydration, the blood pressure and general well-being of the baby. Later presentations in older children and young adults include: precocious puberty in a girl or boy, inguinal hernia in a girl, delayed or arrested puberty in a boy or girl, primary amenorrhoea, breast development in a boy, and gross and occasionally cyclical haematuria in an apparent boy.

INVESTIGATIONS

Many centres can perform a pelvic ultrasound scan to identify gonads and types, but the yield is

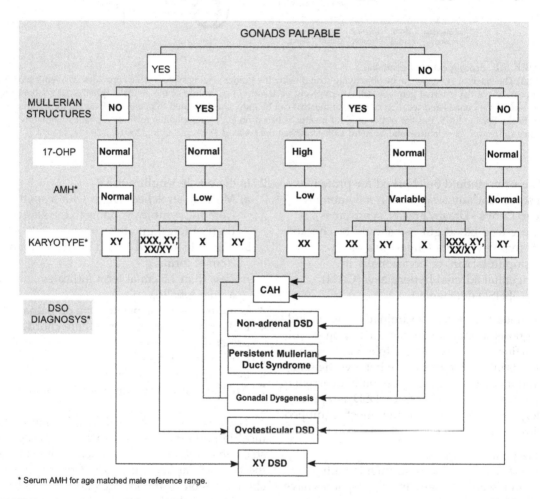

* Serum AMH for age matched male reference range.

FIGURE 5.2 The use of first-line investigations in a newborn suspected of a DSD. *Reprinted with permission from Elsevier from Best practice & research clinical endocrinology and metabolism, 24, Ahmed SF and Rodie M, Investigation and initial management of ambiguous genitalia, 197-218, Copyright 2010.*

very low especially if the radiologist is not specialised in DSD. Recent UK guidance recommends the use of a genitoscopy to visualise the internal organs but a genitogram is still used commonly in many resource-constrained settings. However, genitography also requires proper technique to be able to define the anatomical relationships of the urogenital sinus.[4] A full micturating cystourethrogram should be performed first where possible. All orifices should be imaged — this is usually possible by inserting a small-gauge Foley catheter with a partially inflated balloon to occlude the orifice and then injecting contrast with slight pressure. A correctly performed genitogram should provide information with regards to the size and position of the vagina, the length and morphology of the urethra and the position of the sphincters.

Complete documentation of findings should include as a minimum the size of gonads, type of gonads, length of urogenital sinus, Müllerian structures present and their relationship to the urethra and other structures. In centres where genetic and chromosomal tests are lacking, a tissue biopsy can be done to identify the type of gonad that is present in the pelvis. It should be stressed here that only a piece and not the entire gonad should be biopsied. Finding Barr bodies in a buccal smear means that the baby's karyotype is not a 'normal' male and it is a simple test that gives a result within 24 hours. This test is frequently used in resource-limited settings but its reliability needs further exploration.

Plasma glucose and serum electrolytes, including sodium, potassium, bicarbonate, and chloride, are performed to detect the commonest life-threatening cause of ambiguous genitalia, CAH due to 21-hydroxylase deficiency. Measuring 17-OH progesterone is often the first biochemical step in diagnosing CAH and can be followed by genetic and detailed biochemical tests to confirm the diagnosis. Detailed biochemistry including a urine steroid profile can also help to identify other rarer forms of CAH. Serum AMH and hCG stimulation test are important tests for the identification of functioning testicular tissue.

There are clear limitations in access to diagnostic tests, but some of these issues can be overcome by awareness of the technological advances and the increasing move towards working within clinical and research networks. Samples can be sent either as urine, serum or as blood dried on filter paper to specialist labs. Karyotype that was traditionally performed by cell culture and staining can now be quickly and more cheaply performed by using PCR for X and Y-specific probes. Such technology provides the opportunity to many centres in resource-restricted regions to leap over cumbersome techniques which would be expensive to develop locally.

Availability of drugs is the final obstacle in caring for the child with DSD. Developing countries rely on international advice from organisations such as the World Health Organization in setting priorities for their Essential Medicines List (http://whqlibdoc.who.int/hq/2011/ a95054_eng.pdf), which is a list of medicines that WHO considers should be freely available to populations. Until quite recently oral hydrocortisone and fludrocortisone had not been included on this list. In addition, the cost of a drug may also influence choice, and this needs to be borne in mind when discussing long-term therapy with a family. In the field of rare diseases, there is a need for greater networking and the use of common resources for communication and data collection and sharing. Developments such as the European DSD Register (https://tethys.nesc.gla.ac.uk/) allow clinicians to develop closer links with each other as well as with research groups.

MANAGEMENT

The establishment of a DSD team comprising the geneticist, paediatric surgeon, urologist, psychologist, endocrinologist, neonatologist, and nurse is essential for comprehensive management of the child with DSD. The parents of individual children are included in each team as they cannot be isolated and are pivotal in decision making. It may be difficult to find all of these specialties in a centre, and it has been proposed that they can be located in regional centres and called up when a baby with ambiguous genitalia is born. This will help in developing centres of excellence in various regions in a country and continent. The team is responsible for developing plans for diagnosis, sex assignment and treatment modalities before making recommendations to the parents. This is probably most important in resource-constrained settings so as not to waste the limited funds available to the family. It is unfortunate that many of the families with these conditions are very poor and have almost no access to health insurance to reduce the burden they may face.

Difficult decisions must be made relating to sex of rearing, hormonal therapy and surgery. These decisions are often made over many months, especially in settings where investigations have to be done over time and results may be inconclusive. The delays cause difficulty in making decisions about sex of rearing, and about appropriate hormone therapy or surgical interventions. As discussed by Raza and Warne,[5] there are six principles guiding decision-making in management of babies with DSD.

1 **Minimising** *physical risk* **to child**
   a. Preventing adrenal crises by managing of electrolyte and glucose derangement
   b. Reducing risk of gonadal malignancy
   c. Genitourinary obstruction
2 **Minimising** *psychosocial risk* **to child**
   a. Wrong gender assignment leading to later gender dysphoria
   b. Risk that baby will be unacceptable to parents leading to impaired bonding

   c. Risk of socio/cultural disadvantage to baby
   d. Risk of social isolation, embarrassment
3 **Preserving potential for** *fertility*
   a. Having gonadal structures that are functional
   b. Having viable gametes, or means of shedding these
   c. Being able to carry pregnancy
4 **Preserving or promoting capacity to have satisfying** *sexual relations.*
5 **Leaving** *options open for the future*, **e.g.**
   a. Not removing gonads or phallus except when absolutely necessary
6 **Respecting the** *parents' wishes* **and beliefs.**

In following these principles, many questions are raised and the answers at various stages guide further management approaches. The first step is to know if, in the short term, the baby's life is in danger as occurs in adrenal crises in CAH. Shock and hypoglycaemia can be treated using standard protocols, with immediate commencement of hydrocortisone and fludrocortisone (see Chapter 4, Adrenal Disorders). If there is no danger of adrenal crises, the risk of a urologic complication is assessed and managed. The decision to remove gonads early will depend on the underlying diagnosis and the risk of malignant transformation.[6] Although there is rarely a need for the gonadectomy to be performed in infancy, in many resource-limited settings, the decision to postpone gonadectomy needs to be balanced with the risk of loss to follow-up. This decision should only be undertaken after a careful evaluation of the condition, including the functional potential of the gonads.

- In 46,XY girls with gonadal dysgenesis, the risk of tumour development is more than 30% whereas in girls with confirmed CAIS, the risk is lower than 1%.
- In 46,XY boys with gonadal dysgenesis and gonads in the abdominal or inguinal position, the risk is also high at more than 30%. Boys with a severe degree of undervirilisation (e.g.

born with ambiguous genitalia) probably have a higher risk than boys with only mild undervirilisation at birth. Orchidopexy early in life will probably reduce the risk, especially in those with mild undervirilisation at birth. The risk of tumour development in 46,XY boys with gonadal dysgenesis and gonads in the scrotum at birth is unknown, but probably much lower than those with more proximally sited gonads.

- 45,X/46,XY girls who do not have clitoromegaly have a relatively low risk, estimated at 1–5%, whereas 45,X/46,XY girls who have an enlarged clitoris, and 45,X/46,XY boys with ambiguous genitalia or undescended testes, have a higher than 30% risk.
- In 45,X/46,XY boys with (nearly) normal genitalia at birth, and testes in the scrotum, the risk is unknown, but probably low.

There are numerous personal accounts of gender dysphoria in endocrine practice in the authors' personal experience. A 46,XX DSD baby with CAH who has had multiple clitoroplasty and vaginal reconstruction surgery may be raised as female. Knowing the risk of loss to follow-up, this baby may not receive hormonal replacement and in puberty may develop secondary male sexual characteristics because of adrenal androgens. A 46,XY DSD baby with 5α-reductase deficiency runs the risk of being raised a male, but with inactive testosterone later in life, causing gender dysphoria. Children and families have been ostracised from communities because of DSD, and the risk of suicide and homicide are real. A retrospective review of psychiatric inpatients in a hospital in Saudi Arabia over a 6-year period revealed that among the patients under 18 years old, ambiguous genitalia was one of the common co-morbidities.[7]

Early support for the parents will allow them to examine and understand their early emotional reactions as well as explore present and future worries, adjust to the period of uncertainty during the diagnosis process and facilitate inclusion in informed decision making about themselves or their child. The need for steroid replacement in cases of congenital adrenal hyperplasia and the life-threatening implications of lack of adherence to therapy need to be clearly explained. Discussions with parents need to occur on multiple occasions in a quiet and peaceful setting, with enough time for the family to develop a shared understanding of investigations, results, diagnosis, treatments and the value of ongoing psychological support for both themselves and/or their child. The pace of how information is shared should be set by the family, and issues of confidentiality discussed and respected. Parents' and young people's initial recollections of conversations with professionals may have a long-lasting effect and the use of phrases such as 'differences' or 'variations' in sex development may help to introduce the concept of the range of variation that may occur in sex development. Use of audio-tapes, drawings and written material with details of web sites of support groups are useful aids for families. Parents and young people need to be aware that the management of the condition will require a stepwise approach that first targets short-term goals and then long-term goals that achieve optimal long-term well-being.

It is very likely that families' decisions will be shaped by their own expectations, experiences and their understanding of sex and gender roles within the religious and cultural context of their own social networks. Parents may have a number of concerns which they may have difficulty in voicing. They may be concerned that the child may reject the assigned sex, the child may divulge the disorder to peers, increasing the possibility of stigmatisation, or that the child's future sexual orientation may be different from expected. Generally, people have a very poor understanding of gender development and sexual orientation and a careful discussion, preferably with a health professional with an expertise in this area, will be helpful.[8] These discussions need to occur in a culturally sensitive way. For instance, parents in African society may unknowingly assign gender roles to their children by calling them 'Mummy' for the girl child and 'Daddy' for the boy child. In the Indian subcontinent, parents may equate their child with ambiguous genitalia with a hijra. Although, in popular belief, hijra are people who were born with a DSD and who choose to live apart in separate communities, in reality a large proportion of them do not have any disorder of sex development; often they are homosexual or transsexual individuals who join the group because their lifestyle is otherwise prohibited in the society. Some are boys who have been castrated and others may be simply earning a living as street criminals or drug addicts.

Many families have fertility high up in the scheme of needs and become worried when fertility is questioned. There is always the concern of fertility in conditions of genitourinary origin and parents worry even when the child is an infant. The ability of the surgeons to preserve functions of genitalia is sought for and occasionally requested. The risk of gonads undergoing malignant transformation may be downplayed by the parents and this raises the ethical dilemmas that DSD teams face in decision-making. Parents nonetheless make their decisions based on societal norms and values, and their wishes need to be respected.

Sexual satisfaction is a measure of psychological well-being and may be the basis for future psychosocial and emotional imbalance. While some say they are sexually satisfied, others argue that penile erection and subsequent ejaculation or vaginal stimulation and orgasm do not feature prominently in their measures of sexual satisfaction. Sex is discussed more freely than before in many societies but

still remains a taboo subject in many others. There is, therefore, a need to develop culture-specific innovative methods to deal with issues around sexuality. Sexual satisfaction in females is not necessarily vaginal orgasm but may be all encompassing. The ability of the surgeon to perform vaginoplasty and/or clitoral reduction and still leave these organs sensitive must be discussed prior to surgery. Surgeons in Africa have succeeded in vaginoplasty but are yet to document success of functionality (sexuality and fertility) especially as most patients are lost to follow-up. It is still recommended that these surgeries be performed if the expertise is available and, like the industrialised nations, centres in developing countries should actively work towards developing centres of clinical excellence. The more difficult penile enlargement is most sought after and the functionality of this is rarely achieved.

SPECIAL CONSIDERATIONS IN AFRICA

Many of the problems and current issues described here have application to other countries, in terms of developing strategies to improve health outcomes for DSD.

Newborn Screening

In Western nations where newborn screening is readily available, early detection and diagnosis of children with DSD is made. This allows for prompt and effective management, and prevents complications associated with delays. In all of Africa, and many other resource-constrained countries, newborn screening is unavailable. Screening is done for conditions that are relatively common, and can be treated, even if potentially fatal. Lack of funds, early discharge from hospital following birth, deliveries by traditional birth attendants and, ultimately, lack of government will are reasons these screenings are not done in Africa. Even in areas where the schemes are supposed to have started, logistics prevent proper implementation.

All administrative bottlenecks need to be removed for proper implementation and success of screening procedures. Incorporating screening into the national health insurance scheme in various countries will reduce the cost and increase uptake. With the world shifting focus to non-communicable diseases (NCD) now, Africa and the rest of the developing world cannot be left behind. There are calls for the development of guidelines on management of many NCDs, and these will improve the chances of survival of children. One school of thought has advocated the incorporation of human immunodeficiency virus (HIV) with other screening tests, as this may also increase uptake.

National Health Insurance

This is a scheme that allows all contributors access to proper healthcare. The scheme is still foreign to many and suspicion about the motives behind it prevents individuals from participating. Well-established parastatals and industries have employees that contribute to the health insurance schemes and some communities have also been incorporated by health management organisations (HMO). Such a scheme discriminates against chronic diseases. Affected patients have to pay without government supports, in most countries. Investigations are expensive and often not available, thus prompting referral to other countries, with consequent costs to be borne by families. The drugs and surgical interventions that are needed are expensive. Profit-oriented HMOs are not willing to incorporate them into their schemes. It is therefore left to the medical team to act as advocates and make recommendations on how these items can be incorporated into various schemes.

Support Groups

The risk of stigmatisation prevents formation of support groups, as most of these children are kept hidden away from society. However, support groups can play an important role in providing support for patients and families, improve knowledge of the condition through web sites, and build self-confidence in daily activities. They can help parents better understand the management suggestions of the DSD team, and the short and long-term outcomes of treatments. Another benefit of the support group is that members can meet in places outside the hospital where they do not have to feel like patients, and this can also improve their psychosocial well-being. This has been achieved in the area of HIV/AIDS, where mothers visit each other and encourage themselves, and the method can be adapted into DSD.

Male Gender Preference

In many African societies, male children are preferred to female children. One very common reason for this is the propagation of the 'name'. A man is said to be forgotten if he does not have a male heir. The male marries a woman into the family while the female is married off and deemed to be gone from the family. The male child is the only one entitled to inheritance of his father's properties and if there is no such heir, the father's properties are given to the extended family and not his female child. The legacy of such a man is lost forever. Males are given more opportunities for advancement in their chosen field of work and are allowed to hold esteemed positions in the societies, but the Beijing Declaration (of the Fourth World Conference on Women) and the Millennium Development Goals are allowing for gradual change in this mindset as females are becoming more empowered to improve their well-being and lifestyles.

A woman who is unable to bear a child is less accepted than her male counterpart. She is thought to have brought shame to the family and many have committed suicide for this purpose. It is often the woman who is blamed for the lack of fertility when a couple fail to conceive and prayers are still held for these women while the men are even encouraged to try to conceive with another woman. A man who is sterile is 'forgiven', especially if he has other endearing attributes like wealth.

In some other cultures, though, a woman is entitled to her own wealth and she can inherit from her father and, in the case of divorce, part with her own wealth. The westernisation of many African societies has allowed girls the opportunity to attend schools and become self-sufficient. Indeed many households have women as breadwinners, and it is hoped that, with time, parents whose children need to have sexual reassignment will not be averse to the suggestion of female gender.

References

1. Hughes IA, Houk C, Ahmed SF. Lee PA and the LWPES/ESPE Consensus Group. Consensus statement on management of intersex disorders. *Arch Dis Child* 2006;**91**:554–63.
2. Ahmed SF, Achermann JC, Arlt W, et al. UK guidance on the initial evaluation of an infant or an adolescent with a suspected disorder of sex development. *Clin Endocrinol (Oxf)* 2011 Apr 16. e pub.
3. Schlessinger D, Garcia-Ortiz JE, Forabosco A, et al. Determination and stability of gonadal sex. *J Androl* 2010;**31**:16–25.
4. Chavhan GB, Parra DA, Oudjhane K, et al. Imaging of ambiguous genitalia: classification and diagnostic approach. *Radiographics* 2008;**28**:1891–904.
5. Warne GL, Raza J. Disorders of sex development (DSDs), their presentation and management in different cultures. *Rev Endocr Metab Disord* 2008;**9**:227–36.
6. Pleskacova J, Hersmus R, Oosterhuis JW, et al. Tumor risk in disorders of sex development. *Sex Dev* 2010;**4**:259–69.
7. Al-Haidar FA. Inpatient child and adolescent psychiatric referrals in Saudi Arabia: clinical profiles and treatment. *East Mediterr Health J* 2003;**9**:996–1002.
8. Ahmed SF, Morrison S, Hughes IA. Intersex and gender assignment; the third way? *Arch Dis Child* 2004;**89**:847–50.

6

Obesity in Developing Countries

Orit Pinhas-Hamiel, Matthew Sabin

INTRODUCTION

Overweight and obesity represents a major threat to the future health of the world's children. It is associated with short and long-term health complications including an increased risk of heart disease, type 2 diabetes and cancer (Box 6.1). Although obesity has traditionally been thought of as simply reflecting the affluence of a country, it is in fact a problem which affects youth from both developing and developed countries. This is a significant concern given the fact that in developing countries there is also generally good evidence of co-existent malnutrition and stunted growth.[1]

The story around increasing obesity in developed countries is well known and comprehensive evidence of the problem is now available. Data collected from approximately 1.4 million children aged between 2 and 18 across 23 developed countries have demonstrated linear increases in the prevalence of obesity from 1970 to 2008 in 16 of the countries.[2] Less told, however, is the emerging problem of obesity in developing countries despite several excellent reports on the subject.[1,3] It is concerning that the prevalence of obesity in pre-school children is now similar to the US across most countries in Latin America, the Caribbean, the Middle East and North Africa.[1] Similar trends have also

Practical Pediatric Endocrinology in a Limited Resource Setting
http://dx.doi.org/10.1016/B978-0-12-407822-2.00006-2

BOX 6.1

SHORT AND LONG-TERM COMPLICATIONS OF CHILDHOOD OBESITY

Metabolic

- Endocrine
  - Insulin resistance + diabetes mellitus type 2
  - Pubertal advancement
  - Menstrual abnormalities
  - ↓GH secretion ↑GH clearance
- Cardiovascular
  - Hypertension
  - Dyslipidaemia
  - Metabolic syndrome
- Gastroenterological
  - Non-alcoholic fatty liver disease (NAFLD)

Other

- Pulmonary
  - Asthma
  - Sleep abnormalities
- Orthopaedic
  - Slipped upper femoral epiphysis
- Neurological
  - Idiopathic intracranial hypertension
- Socio-economic
  - Low self-esteem
  - Poor school performance
- Cancer
  - E.g. endometrial, prostate and breast (long term)

---

been observed over the past 20 years in India, Mexico, Nigeria, and Tunisia while Brazil, China and India, as well as other developing countries, have also reported increasing rates of obesity in older children and adolescents.[1]

In 2010, the prevalence of childhood overweight and obesity was estimated at 11.7% in developed countries and 6.1% in developing countries. However, these figures reflect an increase of 65% in developing countries over the last 20 years, compared with an increase of 48% in developed countries[4] and it is predicted that the expected continued rise in childhood obesity will now shorten life expectancy at a greater rate than accidents, homicides and suicides combined.[5]

What are the reasons for this increase in childhood overweight and obesity? Likely they simply reflect a combination of increasing urbanisation, a transition in the quality and quantity of food, and reduced physical activity.[1,6] Their effects on fat accumulation and the development

of associated metabolic conditions in these settings, however, are often more marked[7] — an effect thought to reflect an exaggerated metabolic response to environmental factors on a background of 'thrifty' genes.[8,9,10]

The aim of this chapter is to provide practical guidelines for the paediatrician/physician who examines and treats an obese child within the resource-constrained settings often seen in many developing countries. We will outline the routine work-up needed for evaluating an overweight or obese child/adolescent, and discuss exceptional cases where more complex investigations could be considered.

ANTHROPOMETRIC DATA AND CRITERIA FOR DIAGNOSIS

Body composition dynamically changes with normal childhood growth,[11] and measurement of a child's height and weight forms just one aspect of clinical 'best practice' in paediatrics (Appendixes 1, 2). Many underlying conditions may simply present with faltering weight and/ or height long before the development of quanti-fiable symptomatology, and accurate measure-ments are therefore required. Although it would seem logical that simple visual assess-ment should be enough to recognise those who are either overweight or obese, several studies have shown that in fact parents are not reliable in their perceptions.[12] A child may be brought for an opinion relating to something else, and excess weight for age and sex may be an inci-dental finding. It is therefore important not only to measure children and adolescents but also to address the issue tactfully and carefully where the parents/guardians may not have considered overweight or obesity as a problem. The health consequences of being overweight or obese are as concerning as if a child is under-weight, and it is important that the paediatri-cian/physician consider this in their evaluation. Moreover, and perhaps even more concerning, is the finding that even attending paediatri-cians/physicians often fail to diagnose excess adiposity in their young patients,[13] and this is another reason why any child brought for a medical consultation (even for other reasons) has an accurate determination of their weight and height, with subsequent comparison of the values with normal ranges.

Height and weight measurements are useful on their own, but also serve for calculation of the body mass index (BMI). BMI is an inexpen-sive and easy-to-perform method of screening for the higher and lower weight categories, which may have detrimental health conse-quences. BMI is calculated as weight in kilo-grams divided by height in metres, which is then divided again by height in metres, and is expressed in units of kg/m^2. BMI is a useful surrogate marker of adiposity, but it should be remembered that it does not differentiate between muscle and fat, and it is therefore possible to have a high BMI due to a 'solid',

but not fat, build. BMI dynamically changes throughout childhood and therefore, unlike adults, single figure cut-points for overweight and obesity cannot be used. Instead, a child's BMI needs to be adjusted for age and sex-specific population norms, and while it should be recognised that international cut-points have been generated,[14] country-specific gener-ated data lead to substantial variations in reported prevalence.[15] Where possible, collec-tion of data around the incidence and preva-lence of overweight and obesity should use international and country-specific norms, while the use of country-specific norms are preferable in clinical practice. Many devel-oping countries are beginning to report such country-specific data. BMI charts are shown in Appendixes 3 and 4, while BMI status cate-gories and corresponding percentiles are shown in Table 6.1.

For a child with a BMI above the 95th percentile for his or her age and sex, the degree of obesity can be determined in relation to how 'extreme' the BMI is in relation to the normal variation of BMI seen within the population. In statistics, a z-score (or standard deviation score — SDS) is used to compare means from different normally distributed sets of data. The actual score indicates how many standard deviations the BMI is above or below the mean. The z-score is useful in research in utilis-ing statistical analysis because it enables comparison of observations from different normal distributions. In effect, values from different data sets can be transformed into z-scores and then compared. A number of free software programs for calculating BMI z-scores are available, although these generally are based on normative data generated from the analysis of growth data from US or UK children (http://www.phsim.man.ac.uk/SDS Calculator/). As such, interpretation of the findings may be more difficult and country-specific calculators should be used whenever possible.

TABLE 6.1 BMI Status Categories and Percentiles

Weight status definition	BMI percentile range
Underweight	BMI < 5th percentile
Healthy weight	5th ≥ BMI < 85th percentile
Overweight	85th ≥ BMI < 95th percentile
Obese	BMI ≥ 95th percentile

Waist Circumference

BMI is only one anthropometric measure of overweight or obesity and although it is probably the most widely used, it does have limitations — perhaps mainly in terms of requiring calculation and interpretation, as well as the fact that it does not provide information relating to actual body composition. An alternative measure which has been gathering support is the measurement of waist circumference. This is mainly because it is generally simple to do (requiring only a tape measure) and provides an index of visceral (or truncal) adiposity — a parameter which correlates with risk of metabolic complications. In fact, the United States Heart, Lung and Blood Institute guidelines recommend measuring waist circumference to determine abdominal obesity for assessing the likelihood of developing obesity-related diseases (Appendix 5).

Abdominal obesity, a state of excessive accumulation of both central subcutaneous and visceral fat, has been found to predict metabolic complications such as the metabolic syndrome, type 2 diabetes, and cardiovascular disease in adults, children and adolescents. The metabolic syndrome is a clustering of cardiovascular and diabetes risk factors. Definitions vary in children and adolescents, although the International Diabetes Federation have published a standard definition, the use of which is generally encouraged.[16]

Waist circumference is measured at a level midway between the lowest rib and the iliac crest (Figure 6.1).

An easy 'rule of thumb' is that an individual's waist should be less than half of their height, regardless of age or sex.[17]

Other alternatives include bioimpedance measurement, or imaging of fat-mass with CT or MRI. Obviously, however, these are costly and not widely available and are therefore generally used in research settings in developed countries.

BOX 6.2

CALCULATION OF BMI

Calculating and interpreting BMI using a BMI Percentile Calculator involves the following steps.

1. Obtain accurate height and weight measurements.
2. Calculate BMI according to the following formula: Weight in kg/(height in m^2)
3. Plot the calculated BMI on the graph according to country-specific percentiles for age and sex or, if these are not available, then consider using the Internet for a Child and Teen BMI Calculator, e.g. http://apps.nccd.cdc.gov/dnpabmi/. Be careful, however, in the interpretation of these findings as they will make comparisons with US children and adolescents.

Remember that BMI is a useful surrogate marker of adiposity but that it does not differentiate between muscle and fat.

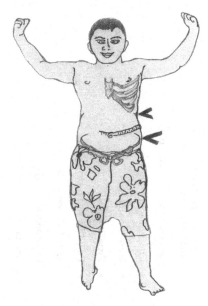

FIGURE 6.1 Measurement of waist circumference. Note: Measure the circumference midway between the top of the hip bone and the bottom of the rib cage at the side of the body. When measuring, the abdomen should be relaxed, the child should be at the end of a gentle exhalation and the tape measure should be held such that a finger of the measurer can be just inserted under the tape measure.

EVALUATION OF POTENTIAL UNDERLYING CAUSES

While the majority of obese children suffer from lifestyle-related obesity, a small proportion will have evidence of an underlying medical, genetic or hormonal cause. A number of endocrine conditions are associated with weight gain, including growth hormone deficiency, panhypopituitarism, hypothyroidism, pseudohypoparathyroidism, Cushing syndrome, polycystic ovary syndrome and hypothalamic obesity. Furthermore, several monogenic obesity syndromes have been identified where obesity is a major feature of the phenotypic appearance, as well as many polygenic conditions where obesity constitutes just one feature of a wider syndrome. The reader is directed to a recent review for a more complete discussion of these conditions,[18] although a summary of these syndromes is provided in Table 6.2.

The measurement of height and weight provides a useful starting point in the evaluation.

The majority of children and adolescents presenting with lifestyle-related obesity tend to be of normal or relative tall stature through childhood, and achieve a final adult height which is within that expected for genetic potential (determined by the mid-parental height). This is, at least in part, likely related to a slightly earlier puberty,[19] but may also be due to the association between obesity and adrenarche which can in some instances advance bone age by a significant degree.[20]

Conversely, children with genetic or hormonal causes of obesity tend to have relatively short stature with a reduced growth velocity for that expected for age and sex. Growth monitoring, with calculation of growth velocity and determination of bone age, can be critically important in this regard in delineating those with an underlying medical cause for their weight gain, compared with those with more simple lifestyle-related obesity. Furthermore, children with genetic causes for their weight gain tend to exhibit a degree of intellectual or developmental delay, and this is therefore an important factor in the assessment of a child with early-onset weight gain.

As with all 'nevers' in medicine, however, there are exceptions to this rule. For example children with an underlying mutation in the MC4R (melanocortin 4 receptor) gene, a genetic condition associated with hyperphagia and weight gain (OMIM #155541), are generally of a bigger build and can exhibit increased linear growth in early childhood (perhaps related to the more severe degree of hyperinsulinaemia seen in these conditions).[21] Likewise, some children with pseudohypoparathyroidism exhibit a degree of increased linear growth in early childhood (although these individuals invariably exhibit short stature in later childhood and

TABLE 6.2 Pleiotropic Obesity Syndromes

Syndrome	Incidence/prevalence	Gene map locus	Characteristic features	Laboratory abnormalities
Prader—Willi (PWS)	1 in 25,000	Deletion or disruption of a genes proximal long arm of the paternal chromosome 15 or maternal uniparental disomy 15 15q12, 15q11-q13	• Severe neonatal hypotonia. Failure to thrive in infancy. • Onset of obesity 6 months to 6 years. Excessive appetite and obsession with eating • Mild to moderate mental retardation • Short stature • Hypogonadotropic hypogonadism • Small penis, scrotal hypoplasia • Hypoplastic labia minora/clitoris	
Laurence—Moon—Biedl	North America and Europe, a prevalence cf 1/140,000 to 1/160,000 newborns. The island of Newfoundland (Canada), 1/17,000 newborns. Bedouin population of Kuwait, 1/13,500 newborns.	A genetically heterogeneous disorder At least 14 different genes involved in the maintenance and function of cilia	• Rod-cone dystrophy, onset 2nd decade • Retinitis pigmentosa, strabismus, cataracts • Left ventricular hypertrophy • Congenital heart defects • Hypogonadism • Renal anomalies • Polydactyly, Brachydactyly • Speech disorder • Developmental delay • Ataxia • Nephrogenic diabetes insipidus	

	Prevalence	Inheritance / Genetics	Clinical features	Laboratory findings
Pseudohypoparathyroidism type Ia (PHP Ia)	In Japan 3.4 cases per 1 million people. No information is available regarding prevalence in other parts of the world.	Autosomal dominant. Inheritance of the mutation on the maternal allele (imprinting). Mutation in the G-protein, alpha-stimulating 1 gene (GNAS1) 20q13.2	• Cognitive deficits • Mental retardation • Hypocalcaemic tetany • Seizures • Basal ganglion calcification • Subcutaneous ossifications • Short stature • Hypogonadism • Hypothyroidism • Blunting of the 4th & 5th knuckles of the hand, most notable when the dorsum of the hand is viewed in flexed position	Hypocalcemia Hyperphosphataemia Elevated PTH Elevated TSH
Alstrom; (ALMS)	Over 450 cases are known worldwide. There are no reliable statistics available.	Autosomal recessive. Mutation in the ALMS1 gene 2p13	• Hearing loss, progressive sensorineural • Cone-rod dystrophy, pigmentary retinopathy • Photophobia & nystagmus (infancy) • Blindness • Subcapsular cataracts • Short stature • Developmental delay • Dilated cardiomyopathy (infancy) • Congestive heart failure • Hypergonadotrophic hypogonadism • Diabetes insipidus • Kidney & pulmonary disease	

(Continued)

TABLE 6.2 Pleiotropic Obesity Syndromes (cont'd)

Syndrome	Incidence/prevalence	Gene map locus	Characteristic features	Laboratory abnormalities
Cohen syndrome AKA hypotonia, obesity and prominent incisors syndrome	Increased frequency in Ashkenazi Jewish population and in Finland. Diagnosed in fewer than 1000 people worldwide. More cases are likely undiagnosed.	Autosomal recessive mutation in the COH1 gene 8q22-q23	• Low birth weight • Short stature • Microcephaly • Chorioretinal dystrophy, myopia, decreased visual acuity, optic atrophy • Mitral valve prolapse • Mental retardation • Hypotonia • Seizures • Delayed motor milestones • Mild lumbar lordosis • Mild thoracic scoliosis • Prominent incisors • Cheerful disposition	

adulthood which is related to the significant advancement of bone age seen in this condition).

A word of caution: the study of human obesity has led to the discovery of novel genes, proteins and molecular pathways relating to energy balance and new 'medical' causes are constantly being described in the literature. In this regard, it is imperative that the assessment of a child with early-onset obesity takes this into account — a child with progressive weight gain despite reported beneficial changes in the child's environment by the parent/guardian may have an, as yet, undiscovered medical cause. It is important, therefore, to consider this when evaluating unusual cases, as well as remembering to keep this on the differential diagnosis list alongside the more thought of situation of social or 'child protection' issues.[22]

SYSTEMIC REVIEW OF MEDICAL HISTORY

Thorough review of organ systems and a complete medical history is required in the evaluation of any overweight/obese child or adolescent. It is important to identify potential medical problems either causing obesity or associated with obesity. Some factors to specifically include in this evaluation are listed below:

- **Perinatal and past medical history:** Was there any evidence of maternal gestational diabetes, and what was the birth weight? There is a 'U' shape curve associating birth weight with risk of later overweight and obesity — big babies tend to be bigger children, as do those who have a low birth weight for gestational age and who 'catch up' in growth during the first few years of life. Was the child breast or bottle-fed? Breast feeding has been associated with lower obesity rates but prolonged breast feeding (particularly combined with early weaning on to solids) can be associated with increased early weight gain.

- **Rate of weight gain:** Increased weight gain in a short time may be secondary to an underlying medical condition, such as Cushing syndrome, or to the use of certain medications, such as antiepileptics or antidepressants. Always think of an underlying medical cause where weight gain has been particularly rapid or extreme.
- **Tiredness, constipation and temperature sensitivity:** These may be secondary to hypothyroidism. Morning tiredness and lethargy may also be secondary to poor quality/quantity sleep, and may indicate obstructive sleep apnoea syndrome. Further questions to probe for this include how propped up the child wants to be to sleep, and whether there is noisy snoring associated with intermittent pauses.
- **Headaches** may be benign in nature but can be secondary to undiagnosed high blood pressure or to idiopathic intracranial hypertension.
- **Shortness of breath:** Reactive airway disease is associated with obesity. In addition, shortness of breath may be secondary to morbid obesity.
- **Enuresis nocturia** may be secondary to obstructive sleep apnoea, or to undiagnosed diabetes mellitus type 2.
- **Irregular menses and hirsutism** may suggest polycystic ovary syndrome (PCOS).
- **Limping, pain in the hips, groin or around the knees** may suggest slipped capital femoral epiphysis (SCFE) or other orthopaedic problems.
- **Snoring may suggest sleeping disturbances:** Obese children tend to suffer from sleep-disordered breathing (SDB), which is characterised by a continuous spectrum from snoring to severe obstructive sleep apnoea syndrome (OSAS).
- **Use of medications:** Glucocorticoids, second-generation antipsychotics such as risperidone, mood stabilisers, tricyclic

antidepressants, anticonvulsants and hormonal contraceptives can all cause increased weight gain.

- **Attention deficit disorder (ADHD) and behavioural problems** are linked to obesity. The causes for this are unclear and may relate to a union of the molecular aetiology of both conditions. Remember, however, that the regular consumption of sugar-containing foods and drinks (and particularly those which also contain artificial colourings, preservatives and/or sweeteners) may potentiate behavioural problems. In these instances, the removal of these types of foods and drinks can often be associated with an improvement in weight status, alongside an improvement or resolution of the behavioural problems.
- **Depression** may be linked to obesity. Obese children are often teased and/or bullied by their peers; this can lead to low self-esteem, poor academic performance and potentially eventual behavioural problems.
- **Family history:** A family history of severe, early-onset obesity may lead to suspicions of an underlying genetic condition. Also, a family history of type 2 diabetes or heart disease confers extra risk to the child/adolescent of developing these conditions in early life.

PHYSICAL EXAMINATION

Blood Pressure

According to the recommendations of the United States Task Force on Blood Pressure Control in Children,[23] blood pressure (BP) should be measured by trained personnel. BP should be measured by auscultation using a mercury sphygmomanometer on the right arm after the patient has been sitting quietly for 5 minutes, with his or her back supported, feet on the floor, right arm supported and cubital fossa at heart level.

It is important that the correct-sized cuff is used — a cuff that is too small for the size of the patient may lead to a spuriously high blood pressure reading. Information on the correct procedures required for the measurement and evaluation of blood pressure in children are regularly published by the American Heart Association.[24] Patients with systolic and/or diastolic blood pressure less than the 90th percentile for age, gender and height are classified as having normal BP (Appendixes 6, 7), while those with systolic and/or diastolic BP greater than the 90th but less than the 95th percentile are classified as having pre-hypertension (Pre-HT). Patients with systolic and/or diastolic BP greater than the 95th percentile are diagnosed as having hypertension (HT).

Buffalo Hump

Buffalo hump, an accumulation of fat on the back of the neck, is associated with the prolonged use of large doses of glucocorticoids or the hypersecretion of cortisol caused by Cushing syndrome.

Moon Face

Moon face, presenting as a rounded red face, is characteristic of Cushing syndrome. Often this sign is absent, however, and only more subtle features of Cushing syndrome may be apparent on careful evaluation.

Acanthosis Nigricans

Acanthosis nigricans is dark, thick, velvety pigmentation of the skin in body folds and creases, most often present in the posterior and lateral folds of the neck, axillae, groin and umbilicus. Acanthosis nigricans in children is associated with insulin-resistance, polycystic ovary syndrome and type 2 diabetes (although in adults but not children is an indication of a concealed underlying malignancy).

Striae

Striae, stretch marks first presenting as pink, thinned skin, enlarge and become reddish purple; finally, mature striae are white, several centimetres long and 1–10 mm wide. They occur in obese children as well as in adolescents undergoing growth spurts, following prolonged use of corticosteroids as well as those with Cushing syndrome.

Abdominal Examination

Abdominal examination may reveal an enlarged liver (with non-alcoholic fatty liver disease (NAFLD)/non-alcoholic steatohepatitis (NASH)), or constipation.

Tanner Stage

Overweight and obese children, as a group, tend to exhibit an earlier puberty than their non-obese peers. Also, body composition and insulin sensitivity dynamically change with the onset and progression of puberty so it is important that pubertal staging is incorporated as part of the routine medical examination. Puberty is associated with significant reductions in insulin sensitivity,[25] leading to decompensation into type 2 diabetes in susceptible obese individuals. It is also worth remembering that some genetic conditions, ranging from common (such as Klinefelter syndrome[26]) to uncommon (e.g. leptin and leptin receptor mutations[21]) are associated with hypogonadism.

Bone Deformity of the Tibia

The overweight child or teenager may compress the bone, causing growth to be affected or even cease one side. The uneven bone changes the natural alignment and can cause curvature or bowing of the tibia, resulting in Blount's disease.

General Signs of Dysmorphism

A number of genetic syndromes, with characteristic dysmorphic features, are associated with obesity.[18] A full review is beyond the scope of this chapter.

Other Features

- **Fingers and toes:** Children with pseudohypoparathyroidism may display short 4th (or 3rd/4th/5th) metacarpals and/or metatarsals, alongside other features such as subcutaneous calcifications. Children with Carpenter syndrome have fused fingers and toes (syndactyly).
- **Eyes:** Eyes are an important part of routine examination — a squint may be associated with difficulties in participating in physical activity sports, visual fields can be abnormal with bitemporal hemianopia present in those with pituitary disease (e.g. craniopharyngioma), and fundoscopy may reveal retinitis pigmentosa in those with conditions such as Bardet–Biedl syndrome. Light sensitivity and blindness due to congenital retinal dystrophy occurs in Alstrom syndrome, as well as childhood obesity.
- **Teeth should be inspected:** Dental caries can be a problem in those where obesity and weight gain is the result of a large consumption of sugar-containing drinks or foods, and the presence of a single central incisor may be indicative of midline problems that can be associated with pituitary abnormalities.
- **Neck:** It is important to examine the neck for the presence of a goitre, as well as looking for acanthosis nigricans.
- **Gynaecomastia:** This is a common finding in peripubescent boys, especially in the setting of obesity. It can be particularly concerning to the individual, limiting opportunities to be involved in team sports etc. In the majority of cases, and particularly with appropriate

weight management, it spontaneously resolves at the end of puberty and further intervention is seldom required. It should be remembered though that gynaecomastia is associated with conditions such as Klinefelter syndrome.

- **Skin:** A careful examination of the skin is required to look for café-au-lait spots or associated changes. Obese children may suffer from intertrigo within their skin folds and may develop secondary infections. As mentioned above, look for striae and acanthosis nigricans.

PRIORITIES FOR LABORATORY FACILITIES

Laboratory work-up is not always required. Where the child is young, there are no concerning features on history or examination, and a lifestyle-related cause is deemed to be most likely then it is reasonable to hold off undertaking any investigations in the initial period, especially when the assessment is being undertaken in settings with limited resources. If attempts to change the family lifestyle do not lead to a stabilisation of weight gain, or if there is the emergence of concerning features during surveillance (e.g. new symptoms or poor longitudinal growth and declining growth velocity) then blood tests can be requested at this stage.

In those who are peripubertal/post-pubertal with significant obesity, a number of investigations are indicated. These are aimed at, first, ruling out an underlying medical cause and/or, second, identifying secondary complications of obesity.

The following are suggestions, although availability of such testing may be limited in resource-constrained settings.

- **Lipid profile:** Mainly elevated triglyceride and low HDL levels are seen in obesity, and reflect an increased risk of future cardiovascular disease — particularly when combined with hypertension.
- **Liver enzymes:** Elevated liver enzyme levels suggest non-alcoholic fatty liver disease.
- **Serum calcium, phosphorus, and parathyroid hormone:** Decreased serum calcium levels in the presence of elevated levels of parathyroid hormone levels can suggest vitamin D deficiency or pseudohypoparathyroidism. Vitamin D levels should be measured, and corrected, before considering a diagnosis of pseudohypoparathyroidism. Furthermore, variations in phenotypic and laboratory features exist within this condition and it is important to understand these when considering this condition a possibility.
- **Fasting glucose level:** Dipsticks for urine testing provide an easy, convenient and relatively cheap measure but may be limited in identifying those with pre-diabetic states such as impaired fasting glucose and impaired glucose tolerance. For identification of the latter, an Oral Glucose Tolerance Test is preferred, although this is often not possible in constrained settings. The author (MS) knows of a number of colleagues, however, who work within limited settings and who use determination of plasma glucose 2 hours after a fast food/high fat meal as an indicator of abnormal post-prandial glucose metabolism.
- **HbA1c:** Determination of HbA1c may be a useful adjunct in the screening for type 2 diabetes.
- **Fasting insulin level** — to determine hyperinsulinaemia. The test is not mandatory for clinical management but, where available, can provide meaningful data on the likelihood to progress to pre-diabetic states or even diabetes type 2. It should be remembered, however, that the test is not widely available in developing countries, that child and adolescent cut-offs are different from those used in adults,[25] and that

controversy still surrounds the issue of whether the determination of fasting insulin is a useful measure.[27]

- **Thyroid function tests**, TSH and fT_4 — where there is clinical suspicion of hypothyroidism.
- **Twenty-four-hour urine collection** to assess cortisol level — this can be a useful measure when there are suspicions of Cushing syndrome. The test is not 100% sensitive or specific, however, and if features persist then repeated determinations may be required. This can also occur in cases where there is cyclical excessive endogenous steroid production such as in primary pigmented nodular adrenal disease (PPNAD) which can occur as part of Carney complex.
- **Iron, ferritin**: Obese children have a tendency towards developing iron deficiency, particularly in settings where nutritional quality is generally compromised such as in developing countries.
- **Vitamin D:** Low vitamin D levels are associated with obesity, and may be related to an increased risk of developing metabolic conditions such as diabetes type 2.

Other laboratory investigations may be required, depending upon the presenting signs and symptoms. At the current time, complex hormonal or genetic testing for rare conditions (such as those looking for mutations in MC4R or determining leptin levels) in severe, early-onset obesity is only available in a few centres across the world. It is expensive, time-consuming and often not appropriate. Only in very unusual cases is it appropriate to approach one of these groups to request genetic testing. Furthermore, genetic testing is unlikely to impact upon management (as conditions like leptin deficiency are extremely rare) and, therefore, within resource-constrained settings, even when an underlying genetic condition is a possibility, often a simple discussion with the parents is all that is warranted.

IMAGING

Bone Age

Advanced skeletal maturation is not an unusual finding in clinically obese children, and a bone age assessment may be helpful in the interpretation of normal versus abnormal growth. Where bone age is advancing rapidly, other conditions (e.g. precocious puberty, congenital adrenal hyperplasia) should be considered.

Ultrasound

For patients with a BMI in the morbidly obese range, an abdominal ultrasound to test for a diffusely echogenic liver can be performed. Often, however, these are difficult studies to undertake due to the patient's body habitus and interpretation of findings can be limited. Ultrasound may also be of some benefit in the diagnosis of PCOS. The distinguishing finding for diagnosing PCOS with ultrasound is the presence of multiple peripheral small cysts in the ovaries (12 peripheral cysts in at least one ovary is sufficient for diagnosis). In addition, there is usually an increase in ovarian volume, and change in ovarian dimensions, with the ovary being more spherical. The diagnosis of PCOS, however, does not rely solely upon the finding of ovarian cysts, and while a review of this condition is beyond the scope of this chapter, the reader is directed to a more comprehensive review of this condition.[28] It should be remembered, however, that severe PCOS-like symptoms and signs (acne, hirsutism, hair growth) may indicate the presence of an androgen-secreting tumour and in these situations hormonal analysis (e.g. DHEAS) and/or adrenal imaging may be required.

DIFFERENTIAL DIAGNOSIS

Most overweight and obese children do not have identifiable disorders other than obesity.

The following conditions should raise suspicions about a possible genetic/organic origin:

- early onset of morbid obesity during infancy
- developmental delay
- new onset excessive weight gain
- decreased growth velocity despite continued weight gain.

TREATING OBESITY

Lifestyle Changes

The basic concept for weight management is simple and logical: the energy balance between intake and expenditure should be negative; in other words, energy intake should be decreased and activity increased. Yet changing habits is a great challenge and often community-based programmes facilitating such changes often fail to show long-term and clinically meaningful changes in weight status. The active participation and support of family members contributes to the success of any intervention, and ideally involvement of the whole family should be encouraged. The aim in young children, and in those where longitudinal growth is still occurring, is to stabilise weight gain such that the weight 'falls back' into normal ranges as the child grows. A stabilisation in weight gain, alongside normal increases in longitudinal growth, will lead to a decline in BMI back to normal over time. In older post-pubertal obese adolescents, a degree of weight loss may be required to achieve a 'normal' weight and BMI.

In essence, goals at reducing dietary intake and increasing physical activity should be individualised and based upon 'common sense' and not extreme recommendations, especially in young children. Here, the key is for the parents to try to change the environment of the child without the child really becoming aware of the parents' actions. Physical activity can be increased by encouragement into fun-based activities, whatever the situation − little

equipment is required for children to become physically active. For example, younger children may only need a football to get more active, while older adolescents who need to train to achieve weight loss will be able to find useful 'equipment' to help them do this in any outdoor environment (e.g. sit-ups, press-ups, chin-ups and the like are all easily attainable in any outdoor parkland environment). Expensive gyms are not required, and even just increasing the amount of walking can often be beneficial in the first instance. Recommendations should be culturally sensitive and appropriate to the local resources.

Dietary Guidelines

The goal is to consume less energy than that required to maintain the current rate of weight gain. For children who are still growing, recommendations should be based on requirements needed for growth and energy expenditure and any attempts at restriction need to ensure that macro- and micro-nutrient intake is not compromised. If possible, it is better for a registered paediatric dietician to be involved in the provision of recommendations, taking into account the child's needs and preferences. However, if a dietician is not available there are several 'commonsense' guidelines which can be provided to parents/guardians. In fact, parent-only treatment may be equally effective as direct consultation with obese children, particularly in young children. The paediatrician/physician can guide in improving parenting skills, such as the following:

- avoid consumption of sugar-sweetened drinks
- establish daily meals and snack time
- never use food as a reward
- decide that the parents will determine what food is offered and when, and the child will decide whether to eat
- offer only healthy options and remove temptations

- eat together as a family whenever possible
- decide that parents will serve as role models
- be consistent
- find ways to praise children's behaviour
- reduce television watching time.

Recommendations need to be culturally sensitive, but can follow general principles around reducing fat and sugar intake.[29,30] The social consumption of energy-dense foods should be limited to special occasions, within the confines of the cultural traditions.

Exercise

Any physical activity is beneficial and should be tailored to the child's preferences and abilities. The essence is to promote activities which are fun-based. Obese children often prefer not to participate in physical activity lessons with 'normal-weight' children as they feel conspicuous and out of place. They may feel uncomfortable with their body size, with sport attire or with their low level of achievement. It is important therefore not to rely on organised sports and to find alternatives which can be encouraged until a time at which the child/adolescent feels more comfortable joining in. Cultural traditions may limit dress code for participation in sports and activities – advice should acknowledge and respect this.

If special programmes for obese children are not accessible, even regular walking for 30 minutes per day, swimming or any ball game can facilitate weight control.

Limit time spent watching television and videos and playing computer games.

Support and Education Programmes

Family-based, lifestyle intervention behavioural and support programmes aimed at changing attitudes and thought processes can be beneficial. However, guiding parents with simple rules can be helpful as well. In the past, community-based approaches have been the mainstay of interventions to address child malnutrition in developing societies. Such community interventions demonstrated effectiveness, feasibility and sustainability. It is thus suggested that community interventions be integrated to reduce obesity, although evidence is still required from these kinds of programmes to support their long-term sustainability.

Oral Drugs

In general, weight loss drugs should not be used in children. Administration of anorectic drugs should be considered only in post-pubertal adolescents who fail to respond to intensive attempts to modify behaviour, diet and family interactions. It is noteworthy that over the last decade three weight-loss drugs, sibutramine, fenfluramine and dexfenfluramine, were withdrawn from the market because of increased risk of morbidity. Currently, the following drugs may be considered in adolescents.

- **Orlistat**, a pancreatic lipase inhibitor that prevents absorption of dietary fat from the gut, is approved for obesity management in adolescents aged 12 or above. It has demonstrated only limited success in maintaining long-term weight loss. Side effects are oily stool (42%), abdominal pain (11%) and faecal incontinence (9%).[31]
- **Metformin** has been proposed as a possible therapy for obese adolescents. Recently, a small but statistically significant decrease in BMI was observed in a long-term controlled study of obese children aged 13 to 18 years treated for 48 weeks with metformin hydrochloride and participating in a lifestyle-intervention programme.[32] In adult studies, however, metformin has been shown to reduce progression to diabetes type 2 in susceptible individuals and it is therefore often used in those with abnormal glucose metabolism or diabetes type 2. The case for using metformin when fasting insulin is raised but glucose

metabolism is normal is not clear at the present time but most would not use it in these circumstances.

Bariatric Surgery for Obese Children

Bariatric surgery is suggested as a possible treatment for adolescents with morbid obesity who have failed all other weight-loss programmes.

Criteria for consideration of bariatric surgery for adolescents include the following:

- BMI greater than 50 kg/m^2
- BMI greater than 40 kg/m^2 with one serious co-morbidity (such as diabetes type 2, obstructive sleep apnoea, severe or complicated hypertension or idiopathic intracranial hypertension)
- attained physiologic maturity
- participation in organised attempts for weight loss for at least 6 months, including nutritional and psychological consulting
- informed consent for surgical treatment

Bariatric surgery is often thought of as a 'last-ditch' attempt but in fact should constitute just one part of a spectrum of management offered to severely obese individuals. Recently published Australian guidelines are available and may act as a guide for those who are considering referral for bariatric surgery in their adolescent patients. Generally, however, resources are limited for these types of operations in developing countries, and it should be emphasised that all such operations should be carried out in centres of expertise who are participating in the long-term collection of longitudinal follow-up data.

SUMMARY

Obesity represents a relatively new, but significant, healthcare problem in developing countries. It is associated with short and long-term detrimental effects on health and practising paediatricians and physicians should be thinking of excess weight issues in their routine clinical practice. Evaluation of an overweight or obese child is a simple and straightforward procedure and can be easily undertaken in resource-constrained settings. Lifestyle-related obesity remains the commonest cause, but evaluation needs to exclude an underlying medical, genetic and/or hormonal cause. Simple recommendations around increasing physical activity and improving the child's diet remain the mainstay of treatment for the majority, and advice and support should be offered within the confines of the cultural traditions and resource limitations.

References

1. Misra A, Khurana L. Obesity and the metabolic syndrome in developing countries. *J Clin Endocrinol Metab* 2008;**93**(11 Suppl. 1):S9–30.
2. Olds T, Maher C. Childhood overweight and obesity in developed countries: global trends and correlates. In: O'Dea K, Eriksen M, editors. *Childhood Obesity Prevention: international research, controversies and interventions.* Oxford: Oxford University Press; 2010. p. 69–83.
3. Prentice AM. The emerging epidemic of obesity in developing countries. *Int J Epidemiol* 2006;**35**:93–9.
4. de Onis M, Blossner M, Borghi E. Global prevalence and trends of overweight and obesity among preschool children. *Am J Clin Nutr* 2010;**92**:1257–64.
5. Olshansky SJ, Passaro DJ, Hershow RC, et al. A potential decline in life expectancy in the United States in the 21st century. *N Engl J Med* 2005;**352**:1138–45.
6. Ramachandran A, Snehalatha C. Rising burden of obesity in Asia. *J Obes* 2010;**2010**. Epub 2010 Aug 30.
7. Misra A, Khurana L. The metabolic syndrome in South Asians: epidemiology, determinants, and prevention. *Metab Syndr Relat Disord* 2009;**7**:497–514.
8. Prentice AM, Hennig BJ, Fulford AJ. Evolutionary origins of the obesity epidemic: natural selection of thrifty genes or genetic drift following predation release? *Int J Obes (Lond)* 2008;**32**:1607–10.
9. Prentice AM, Rayco-Solon P, Moore SE. Insights from the developing world: thrifty genotypes and thrifty phenotypes. *Proc Nutr Soc* 2005;**64**:153–61.
10. Wells JC. Thrift: a guide to thrifty genes, thrifty phenotypes and thrifty norms. *Int J Obes (Lond)* 2009;**33**:1331–8.

11. Veldhuis JD, Roemmich JN, Richmond EJ, et al. Endocrine control of body composition in infancy, childhood, and puberty. *Endocr Rev* 2005;**26**:114—46.

12. Campbell MW, Williams J, Hampton A, Wake M. Maternal concern and perceptions of overweight in Australian preschool-aged children. *Med J Aust* 2006;**184**:274—7.

13. Chaimovitz R, Issenman R, Moffat T, Persad R. Body perception: do parents, their children, and their children's physicians perceive body image differently? *J Pediatr Gastroenterol Nutr* 2008;**47**:76—80.

14. Cole TJ, Bellizzi MC, Flegal KM, Dietz WH. Establishing a standard definition for child overweight and obesity worldwide: international survey. *BMJ* 2000;**320**:1240—3.

15. Reilly JJ. Descriptive epidemiology and health consequences of childhood obesity. *Best Pract Res Clin Endocrinol Metab* 2005;**19**:327—41.

16. Zimmet P, Alberti G, Kaufman F, et al. The metabolic syndrome in children and adolescents. *Lancet* 2007;**369**:2059—61.

17. Garnett SP, Baur LA, Cowell CT. Waist-to-height ratio: a simple option for determining excess central adiposity in young people. *Int J Obes (Lond)* 2008;**32**: 1028—30.

18. Sabin MA, Werther GA, Kiess W. Genetics of obesity and overgrowth syndromes. *Best Pract Res Clin Endocrinol Metab* 2011;**25**:207—20.

19. Wagner IV, Sabin MA, Pfäffle RW, et al. Effects of obesity on human sexual development. *Nature Reviews* 2011.

20. Sopher AB, Jean AM, Zwany SK, et al. Bone age advancement in prepubertal children with obesity and premature adrenarche: possible potentiating factors. *Obesity (Silver Spring)* 2011;**19**:1259—64.

21. Farooqi IS. Monogenic human obesity. *Front Horm Res* 2008;**36**:1—11.

22. Sabin MA, McCallum Z, Gibbons K, et al. When does severe childhood obesity become a child protection issue? Comment. *Med J Aust* 2009;**190**:653—5.

23. The fourth report on the diagnosis, evaluation, and treatment of high blood pressure in children and adolescents. *Pediatrics* 2004;**114**(2 Suppl. 4th Report):555—76.

24. Falkner B, Daniels SR. Summary of the Fourth Report on the Diagnosis, Evaluation, and Treatment of High Blood Pressure in Children and Adolescents. *Hypertension* 2004;**44**:387—8.

25. Goran MI, Gower BA. Longitudinal study on pubertal insulin resistance. *Diabetes* 2001;**50**:2444—50.

26. Bojesen A, Kristensen K, Birkebaek NH, et al. The metabolic syndrome is frequent in Klinefelter's syndrome and is associated with abdominal obesity and hypogonadism. *Diabetes Care* 2006;**29**:1591—8.

27. Levy-Marchal C, Arslanian S, Cutfield W, et al. Insulin resistance in children: consensus, perspective, and future directions. *J Clin Endocrinol Metab* 2010;**95**: 5189—98.

28. Norman RJ, Dewailly D, Legro RS, Hickey TE. Polycystic ovary syndrome. *Lancet* 2007;**370**:685—97.

29. Hu FB. Globalization of diabetes: the role of diet, lifestyle, and genes. *Diabetes Care* 2011;**34**:1249—57.

30. Misra A, Singhal N, Khurana L. Obesity, the metabolic syndrome, and type 2 diabetes in developing countries: role of dietary fats and oils. *J Am Coll Nutr* 2010;**29**(Suppl. 3):S289—301.

31. Chanoine JP, Hampl S, Jensen C, et al. Effect of orlistat on weight and body composition in obese adolescents: a randomized controlled trial. *JAMA* 2005;**293**: 2873—83.

32. Wilson DM, Abrams SH, Aye T, et al. Metformin extended release treatment of adolescent obesity: a 48-week randomized, double-blind, placebo-controlled trial with 48-week follow-up. *Arch Pediatr Adolesc Med* 2010;**164**:116—23.

Further Reading

The Endocrine Society Clinical Guidelines for the Prevention and Treatment of Paediatric Obesity. Available at URL: www.endo-society.org/guidelines/final/upload/FINAL-Standalone-pediatric-obesity-Guideline.pdf

Obesity and the Metabolic Syndrome in Developing Countries: Misra A, Khurana L. Obesity and the metabolic syndrome in developing countries *J Clin Endocrinol Metab* 2008;**93**(11 Suppl. 1):S9—30.

A practical resource for parents of overweight/obese young children (In English): Sabin M. *Is your Child Overweight: what you need to know and what you can do.* Melbourne: Wilkinson Publishing. 2010. ISBN 9781921667510. Available at URL www.wilkinsonpublishing.com.au/index.php?route=product/product&product_id=176.

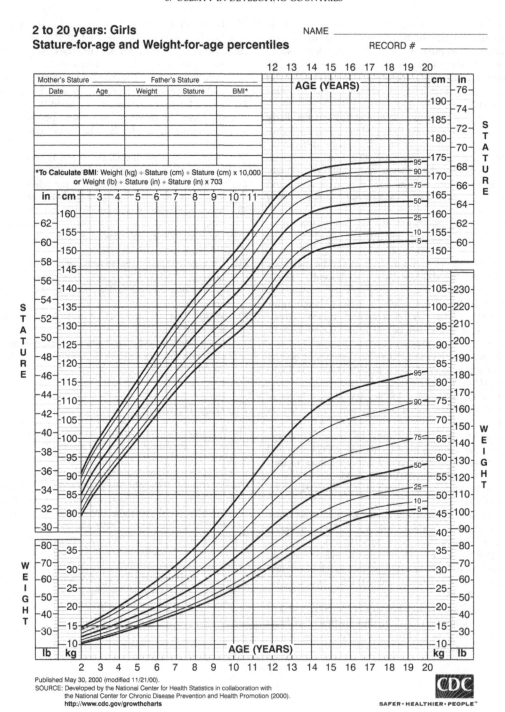

2 to 20 years: Girls
Stature-for-age and Weight-for-age percentiles

NAME _____

RECORD # _____

Published May 30, 2000 (modified 11/21/00).
SOURCE: Developed by the National Center for Health Statistics in collaboration with
the National Center for Chronic Disease Prevention and Health Promotion (2000).
http://www.cdc.gov/growthcharts

APPENDIX 6.1   Girls' weight and height chart.

2 to 20 years: Boys
Stature-for-age and Weight-for-age percentiles

NAME _____

RECORD # _____

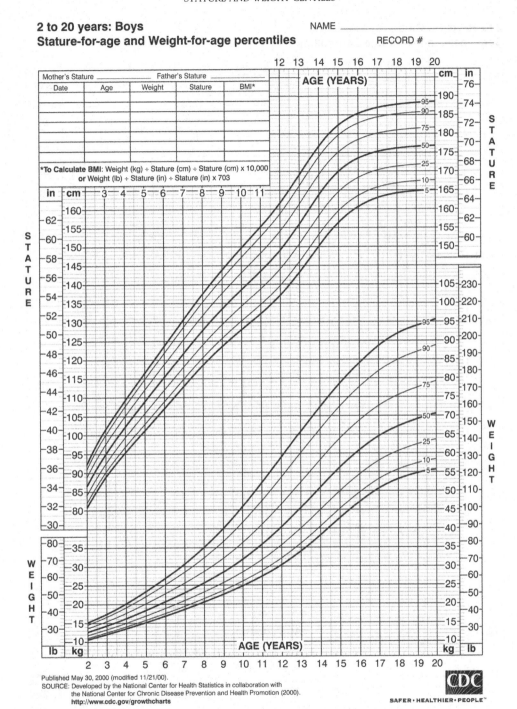

Published May 30, 2000 (modified 11/21/00).

SOURCE: Developed by the National Center for Health Statistics in collaboration with the National Center for Chronic Disease Prevention and Health Promotion (2000).
http://www.cdc.gov/growthcharts

CDC
SAFER • HEALTHIER • PEOPLE™

APPENDIX 6.2   Boys' weight and height chart.

2 to 20 years: Girls
Body mass index-for-age percentiles

NAME _____

RECORD # _____

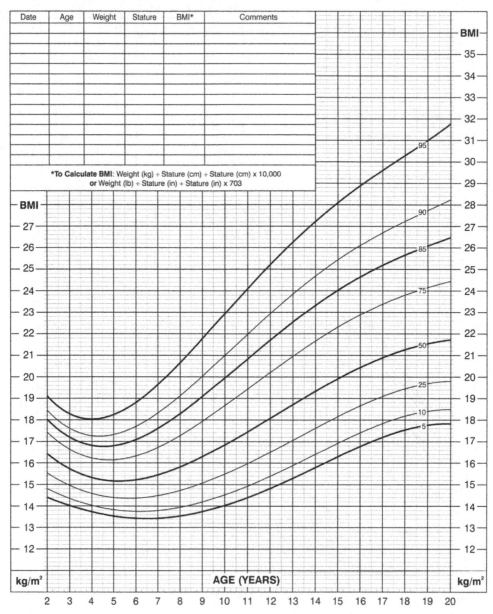

*To Calculate BMI: Weight (kg) ÷ Stature (cm) ÷ Stature (cm) x 10,000
or Weight (lb) ÷ Stature (in) ÷ Stature (in) x 703

Published May 30, 2000 (modified 10/16/00).
SOURCE: Developed by the National Center for Health Statistics in collaboration with
the National Center for Chronic Disease Prevention and Health Promotion (2000).
http://www.cdc.gov/growthcharts

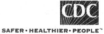

SAFER · HEALTHIER · PEOPLE™

APPENDIX 6.3   Girls' BMI chart.

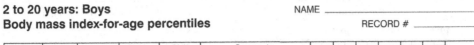

2 to 20 years: Boys
Body mass index-for-age percentiles

NAME _____

RECORD # _____

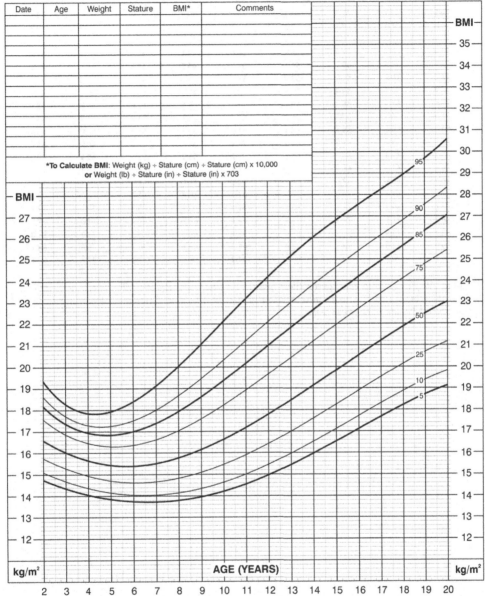

Date	Age	Weight	Stature	BMI*	Comments

*To Calculate BMI: Weight (kg) ÷ Stature (cm) ÷ Stature (cm) x 10,000
or Weight (lb) ÷ Stature (in) ÷ Stature (in) x 703

AGE (YEARS)

Published May 30, 2000 (modified 10/16/00).
SOURCE: Developed by the National Center for Health Statistics in collaboration with
the National Center for Chronic Disease Prevention and Health Promotion (2000).
http://www.cdc.gov/growthcharts

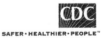

SAFER · HEALTHIER · PEOPLE™

APPENDIX 6.4 Boys' BMI chart.

	Percentile for boys					Percentile for girls				
	10th	25th	50th	75th	90th	10th	25th	50th	75th	90th
Intercept	39.3	43.2	42.9	43.3	43.8	39.9	41.8	43.6	45.0	46.8
Slope	1.8	1.9	2.1	2.6	3.4	1.6	1.7	1.9	2.3	2.9
Age (y)										
2	42.9	46.9	47.1	48.6	50.6	43.1	45.1	47.4	49.6	52.5
3	44.7	48.8	49.2	51.2	54.0	44.7	46.8	49.3	51.9	55.4
4	46.5	50.6	51.3	53.8	57.4	46.3	48.5	51.2	54.2	58.2
5	48.3	52.5	53.3	56.5	60.8	47.9	50.2	53.1	56.5	61.1
6	50.1	54.3	55.4	59.1	64.2	49.5	51.8	55.0	58.8	64.0
7	51.9	56.2	57.5	61.7	67.6	51.1	53.5	56.9	61.1	66.8
8	53.7	58.1	59.6	64.3	71.0	52.7	55.2	58.8	63.4	69.7
9	55.5	59.9	61.7	67.0	74.3	54.3	56.9	60.7	65.7	72.6
10	57.3	61.8	63.7	69.6	77.7	55.9	58.6	62.5	68.0	75.5
11	59.1	63.6	65.8	72.2	81.1	57.5	60.2	64.4	70.3	78.3
12	60.9	65.5	67.9	74.9	84.5	59.1	61.9	66.3	72.6	81.2
13	62.7	67.4	70.0	77.5	87.9	60.7	63.6	68.2	74.9	84.1
14	64.5	69.2	72.1	80.1	91.3	62.3	65.3	70.1	77.2	86.9
15	66.3	71.1	74.1	82.8	94.7	63.9	67.0	72.0	79.5	89.8
16	68.1	72.9	76.2	85.4	98.1	65.5	68.6	73.9	81.8	92.7
17	69.9	74.8	78.3	88.0	101.5	67.1	70.3	75.8	84.1	95.5
18	71.7	76.7	80.4	90.6	104.9	68.7	72.0	77.7	86.4	98.4

APPENDIX 6.5 Waist circumference percentiles. *Source: Fernández JR, Redden DT, Pietrobelli A, Allison DB. Waist circumference percentiles in nationally representative samples of African-American, European-American, and Mexican-American children and adolescents. J Pediatr 2004;145:439—44.*

BP Levels for Girls by Age and Height Percentile

Age, y	BP Percentile	SBP, mm Hg							DBP, mm Hg						
		Percentile of Height							Percentile of Height						
		5th	10th	25th	50th	75th	90th	95th	5th	10th	25th	50th	75th	90th	95th
1	50th	83	84	85	86	88	89	90	38	39	39	40	41	41	42
	90th	97	97	98	100	101	102	103	52	53	53	54	55	55	56
	95th	100	101	102	104	105	106	107	56	57	57	58	59	59	60
	99th	108	108	109	111	112	113	114	64	64	65	65	66	67	67
2	50th	85	85	87	88	89	91	91	43	44	44	45	46	46	47
	90th	98	99	100	101	103	104	105	57	58	58	59	60	61	61
	95th	102	103	104	105	107	108	109	61	62	62	63	64	65	65
	99th	109	110	111	112	114	115	116	69	69	70	70	71	72	72
3	50th	86	87	88	89	91	92	93	47	48	48	49	50	50	51
	90th	100	100	102	103	104	106	106	61	62	62	63	64	64	65
	95th	104	104	105	107	108	109	110	65	66	66	67	68	68	69
	99th	111	111	113	114	115	116	117	73	73	74	74	75	76	76
4	50th	88	88	90	91	92	94	94	50	50	51	52	52	53	54
	90th	101	102	103	104	106	107	108	64	64	65	66	67	67	68
	95th	105	106	107	108	110	111	112	68	68	69	70	71	71	72
	99th	112	113	114	115	117	118	119	76	76	76	77	78	79	79
5	50th	89	90	91	93	94	95	96	52	53	53	54	55	55	56
	90th	103	103	105	106	107	109	109	66	67	67	68	69	69	70
	95th	107	107	108	110	111	112	113	70	71	71	72	73	73	74
	99th	114	114	116	117	118	120	120	78	78	79	79	80	81	81
6	50th	91	92	93	94	96	97	98	54	54	55	56	56	57	58
	90th	104	105	106	108	109	110	111	68	68	69	70	70	71	72
	95th	108	109	110	111	113	114	115	72	72	73	74	74	75	76
	99th	115	116	117	119	120	121	122	80	80	80	81	82	83	83
7	50th	93	93	95	96	97	99	99	55	56	56	57	58	58	59
	90th	106	107	108	109	111	112	113	69	70	70	71	72	72	73
	95th	110	111	112	113	115	116	116	73	74	74	75	76	76	77
	99th	117	118	119	120	122	123	124	81	81	82	82	83	84	84
8	50th	95	95	96	98	99	100	101	57	57	57	58	59	60	60
	90th	108	109	110	111	113	114	114	71	71	71	72	73	74	74
	95th	112	112	114	115	116	118	118	75	75	75	76	77	78	78
	99th	119	120	121	122	123	125	125	82	82	83	83	84	85	86
9	50th	96	97	98	100	101	102	103	58	58	58	59	60	61	61
	90th	110	110	112	113	114	116	116	72	72	72	73	74	75	75
	95th	114	114	115	117	118	119	120	76	76	76	77	78	79	79
	99th	121	121	123	124	125	127	127	83	83	84	84	85	86	87
10	50th	98	99	100	102	103	104	105	59	59	59	60	61	62	62
	90th	112	112	114	115	116	118	118	73	73	73	74	75	76	76
	95th	116	116	117	119	120	121	122	77	77	77	78	79	80	80
	99th	123	123	125	126	127	129	129	84	84	85	86	86	87	88
11	50th	100	101	102	103	105	106	107	60	60	60	61	62	63	63
	90th	114	114	116	117	118	119	120	74	74	74	75	76	77	77
	95th	118	118	119	121	122	123	124	78	78	78	79	80	81	81
	99th	125	125	126	128	129	130	131	85	85	86	87	87	88	89
12	50th	102	103	104	105	107	108	109	61	61	61	62	63	64	64
	90th	116	116	117	119	120	121	122	75	75	75	76	77	78	78
	95th	119	120	121	123	124	125	126	79	79	79	80	81	82	82
	99th	127	127	128	130	131	132	133	86	86	87	88	88	89	90
13	50th	104	105	106	107	109	110	110	62	62	62	63	64	65	65
	90th	117	118	119	121	122	123	124	76	76	76	77	78	79	79
	95th	121	122	123	124	126	127	128	80	80	80	81	82	83	83
	99th	128	129	130	132	133	134	135	87	87	88	89	89	90	91
14	50th	106	106	107	109	110	111	112	63	63	63	64	65	66	66
	90th	119	120	121	122	124	125	125	77	77	77	78	79	80	80
	95th	123	123	125	126	127	129	129	81	81	81	82	83	84	84
	99th	130	131	132	133	135	136	136	88	88	89	90	90	91	92
15	50th	107	108	109	110	111	113	113	64	64	64	65	66	67	67
	90th	120	121	122	123	125	126	127	78	78	78	79	80	81	81
	95th	124	125	126	127	129	130	131	82	82	82	83	84	85	85
	99th	131	132	133	134	136	137	138	89	89	90	91	91	92	93
16	50th	108	108	110	111	112	114	114	64	64	65	66	66	67	68
	90th	121	122	123	124	126	127	128	78	78	79	80	81	81	82
	95th	125	126	127	128	130	131	132	82	82	83	84	85	85	86
	99th	132	133	134	135	137	138	139	90	90	90	91	92	93	93
17	50th	108	109	110	111	113	114	115	64	65	65	66	67	67	68
	90th	122	122	123	125	126	127	128	78	79	79	80	81	81	82
	95th	125	126	127	129	130	131	132	82	83	83	84	85	85	86
	99th	133	133	134	136	137	138	139	90	90	91	91	92	93	93

APPENDIX 6.6 Blood pressure levels for girls. *Source: Reprinted with permission from The fourth report on the diagnosis, evaluation, and treatment of high blood pressure in children and adolescents. Pediatrics 2004;114(2 Suppl. 4th Report):555—76.*

6. OBESITY IN DEVELOPING COUNTRIES

BP Levels for Boys by Age and Height Percentile

Age, y	BP Percentile	SBP, mm Hg							DBP, mm Hg						
		Percentile of Height							Percentile of Height						
		5th	10th	25th	50th	75th	90th	95th	5th	10th	25th	50th	75th	90th	95th
1	50th	80	81	83	85	87	88	89	34	35	36	37	38	39	39
	90th	94	95	97	99	100	102	103	49	50	51	52	53	53	54
	95th	98	99	101	103	104	106	106	54	54	55	56	57	58	58
	99th	105	106	108	110	112	113	114	61	62	63	64	65	66	66
2	50th	84	85	87	88	90	92	92	39	40	41	42	43	44	44
	90th	97	99	100	102	104	105	106	54	55	56	57	58	58	59
	95th	101	102	104	106	108	109	110	59	59	60	61	62	63	63
	99th	109	110	111	113	115	117	117	66	67	68	69	70	71	71
3	50th	86	87	89	91	93	94	95	44	44	45	46	47	48	48
	90th	100	101	103	105	107	108	109	59	59	60	61	62	63	63
	95th	104	105	107	109	110	112	113	63	63	64	65	66	67	67
	99th	111	112	114	116	118	119	120	71	71	72	73	74	75	75
4	50th	88	89	91	93	95	96	97	47	48	49	50	51	51	52
	90th	102	103	105	107	109	110	111	62	63	64	65	66	66	67
	95th	106	107	109	111	112	114	115	66	67	68	69	70	71	71
	99th	113	114	116	118	120	121	122	74	75	76	77	78	78	79
5	50th	90	91	93	95	96	98	98	50	51	52	53	54	55	55
	90th	104	105	106	108	110	111	112	65	66	67	68	69	69	70
	95th	108	109	110	112	114	115	116	69	70	71	72	73	74	74
	99th	115	116	118	120	121	123	123	77	78	79	80	81	81	82
6	50th	91	92	94	96	98	99	100	53	53	54	55	56	57	57
	90th	105	106	108	110	111	113	113	68	68	69	70	71	72	72
	95th	109	110	112	114	115	117	117	72	72	73	74	75	76	76
	99th	116	117	119	121	123	124	125	80	80	81	82	83	84	84
7	50th	92	94	95	97	99	100	101	55	55	56	57	58	59	59
	90th	106	107	109	111	113	114	115	70	70	71	72	73	74	74
	95th	110	111	113	115	117	118	119	74	74	75	76	77	78	78
	99th	117	118	120	122	124	125	126	82	82	83	84	85	86	86
8	50th	94	95	97	99	100	102	102	56	57	58	59	60	60	61
	90th	107	109	110	112	114	115	116	71	72	72	73	74	75	76
	95th	111	112	114	116	118	119	120	75	76	77	78	79	79	80
	99th	119	120	122	123	125	127	127	83	84	85	86	87	87	88
9	50th	95	96	98	100	102	103	104	57	58	59	60	61	61	62
	90th	109	110	112	114	115	117	118	72	73	74	75	76	76	77
	95th	113	114	116	118	119	121	121	76	77	78	79	80	81	81
	99th	120	121	123	125	127	128	129	84	85	86	87	88	88	89
10	50th	97	98	100	102	103	105	106	58	59	60	61	61	62	63
	90th	111	112	114	115	117	119	119	73	73	74	75	76	77	78
	95th	115	116	117	119	121	122	123	77	78	79	80	81	81	82
	99th	122	123	125	127	128	130	130	85	86	86	88	88	89	90
11	50th	99	100	102	104	105	107	107	59	59	60	61	62	63	63
	90th	113	114	115	117	119	120	121	74	74	75	76	77	78	78
	95th	117	118	119	121	123	124	125	78	78	79	80	81	82	82
	99th	124	125	127	129	130	132	132	86	86	87	88	89	90	90
12	50th	101	102	104	106	108	109	110	59	60	61	62	63	63	64
	90th	115	116	118	120	121	123	123	74	75	75	76	77	78	79
	95th	119	120	122	123	125	127	127	78	79	80	81	82	82	83
	99th	126	127	129	131	133	134	135	86	87	88	89	90	90	91
13	50th	104	105	106	108	110	111	112	60	60	61	62	63	64	64
	90th	117	118	120	122	124	125	126	75	75	76	77	78	79	79
	95th	121	122	124	126	128	129	130	79	79	80	81	82	83	83
	99th	128	130	131	133	135	136	137	87	87	88	89	90	91	91
14	50th	106	107	109	111	113	114	115	60	61	62	63	64	65	65
	90th	120	121	123	125	126	128	128	75	76	77	78	79	79	80
	95th	124	125	127	128	130	132	132	80	80	81	82	83	84	84
	99th	131	132	134	136	138	139	140	87	88	89	90	91	92	92
15	50th	109	110	112	113	115	117	117	61	62	63	64	65	66	66
	90th	122	124	125	127	129	130	131	76	77	78	79	80	80	81
	95th	126	127	129	131	133	134	135	81	81	82	83	84	85	85
	99th	134	135	136	138	140	142	142	88	89	90	91	92	93	93
16	50th	111	112	114	116	118	119	120	63	63	64	65	66	67	67
	90th	125	126	128	130	131	133	134	78	78	79	80	81	82	82
	95th	129	130	132	134	135	137	137	82	83	83	84	85	86	87
	99th	136	137	139	141	143	144	145	90	90	91	92	93	94	94
17	50th	114	115	116	118	120	121	122	65	66	66	67	68	69	70
	90th	127	128	130	132	134	135	136	80	80	81	82	83	84	84
	95th	131	132	134	136	138	139	140	84	85	86	87	87	88	89
	99th	139	140	141	143	145	146	147	92	93	93	94	95	96	97

APPENDIX 6.7 Blood pressure levels for boys. *Source: Reprinted with permission from The fourth report on the diagnosis, evaluation, and treatment of high blood pressure in children and adolescents.* Pediatrics 2004;114(2 Suppl. 4th Report):555—76.

Disorders of Mineral and Bone Metabolism

Vijayalakshmi Bhatia, Abhishek Kulkarni, Veena V. Nair

INTRODUCTION

The skeletal system provides the main mechanical support to the body. Structures such as the rib cage, pelvis and skull provide protection to vulnerable internal organs. However, bone is also a metabolically active organ. It is the largest reservoir of two important minerals, calcium and phosphorus, which, along with magnesium, play important roles in intracellular signalling and secretion, neuromuscular excitability and muscular (including myocardial) contractility and function.

Bone is the site of action of hormones such as parathyroid hormone (PTH), PTH-related peptide (PTHrP), calcitriol (1,25-dihydroxycholecalciferol), and calcitonin (although its actions in postnatal physiology are poorly understood), and the site of production of hormones such as fibroblast growth factor 23 (FGF23). These hormones and minerals, coupled with nutrition, exercise, and other hormones such as gonadal steroids and growth hormone, affect bone mass and bone strength of an individual.

Poor bone mass accrued in childhood and adolescence contributes to development of future osteoporosis in the elderly. Several systemic conditions of childhood, such as renal failure, malabsorption, cancer, transplantation and cerebral palsy, to name a few, are associated with significant morbidity in bone health and consequent failure of optimal peak bone mass accrual. The specific genetic aetiologies of several conditions of primary bone fragility and dysplasia have now been discovered, bringing the possibility of new forms of medical therapy.

This chapter deals with mineral metabolism and primary and secondary metabolic bone diseases. Some basic physiology is required in order to understand the nature of these disorders. For a more detailed discussion the reader is referred to standard texts.

NORMAL MINERAL METABOLISM

Calcium Metabolism

Ninety-nine percent of the calcium in our body is present in the skeleton, while the rest is present intracellularly or in plasma. Calcium circulates in plasma either in an ionised form or bound to albumin. The latter is measured as total serum calcium by the chemistry analyser, and its normal value is 8.5–10.2 mg/dL (2.12–2.55 mmol/L) (this range is slightly higher in infancy, and might vary somewhat with the method of estimation).

- Hypoalbuminaemia is associated with lower total serum calcium, which may be corrected by increasing serum calcium by 0.8 mg/dL (0.2 mmol/L) for every 1 mg/dL (0.25 mmol/L) decrease in serum albumin.
- Ionised calcium is about half of total serum calcium, 4.4 to 5.2 mg/dL (1.1 to 1.3 mmol/L).
- Alkalosis decreases ionised calcium by increasing its binding to albumin, and acidosis causes the reverse.

Serum calcium concentration is tightly maintained within a narrow range, with the help of two hormones, PTH and calcitriol. The parathyroid gland cells have a receptor on the cell surface, called the calcium-sensing receptor (CaSR), which senses serum calcium.

Lowering of serum calcium results in PTH secretion by the gland.

PTH restores serum calcium by increasing calcium reabsorption in the kidney, resorption from bone and absorption from the intestine (indirectly by increasing calcitriol production in the kidney).

Activating as well as inactivating mutations of the CaSR are known to cause human disease.[1]

(See also section on hypocalcaemia for more details.)

About 30% of calcium in the gut (dietary or supplements) is absorbed, in the proximal small intestine, both by an active transcellular process and a passive paracellular process. The paracellular absorption through tight junctions is aided by a protein known as a paracellin or claudin. Mutations of this protein result in a syndrome of hypercalciuria, hypomagnesaemia and nephrocalcinosis, as the same protein aids transport across the renal tubule. The transcellular mode of transport is vitamin D dependent and predominates if the calcium intake is below 400 mg/day. When calcium intake is low, there is stimulation of PTH secretion, which results in increased calcitriol synthesis.

Calcitriol, through its receptor, stimulates proteins necessary for transport across the luminal surface (inwardly rectifying calcium channel transient receptor potential, TRPV6); across the cytosol of the intestinal cell (calbindin); and across the basolateral membrane into the blood (via the ATP-dependent calcium-transporting ATPase, PMCA1b).[2]

Factors Affecting Calcium Absorption

- Luminal factors like phosphates, oxalates, phytates and fibre can reduce calcium absorption.
- Human milk, with its higher calcium to phosphorus ratio, provides better bioavailability of calcium than cow's milk.
- Phytates are present in significant amounts in the husk of cereals, and in legumes. Oxalates

are not usually present in diet in significant amounts to reduce calcium absorption.

- The various salts of calcium, like carbonate, lactate, glubionate and citrate, provide the same bioavailability of calcium, except in the rare instance of achlorhydria, where the carbonate salt will not be absorbed if given without meals. The carbonate preparation has the highest proportion of elemental calcium per gram of the salt, and may be the least expensive preparation.

Sources of Calcium

The recommended daily dietary intake of elemental calcium for different age and physiological groups is highlighted in Table 7.1. **The best sources are milk and milk products, many varieties of fish, and to a lesser extent green, leafy vegetables and lentils. Cow's milk (both whole and skimmed) contains approximately 120 mg calcium/100 g.**

Phosphorus Metabolism

Phosphorus, like calcium, resides largely (about 80%) in our skeleton. The remainder is found in visceral organs and muscle. Unlike

TABLE 7.1 Dietary Reference Intake for Calcium Adopted in Different Countries

Age group	UK* (1997)	WHO[†] (2004)	NIH[‡] (2010)
Birth to 1 year	525	300−400	200−260[a]
1−3 years	350	500	700
4−6 years	450	600	1000
7−9 years	500	700	1000
10−18 years	1000 (boys) 800 (girls)	1300	1300
Pregnancy	700	1200	1000
Lactation	1250	1000	1000

Note: [a] = adequate intake.
Sources: * *UK Department of Health 1997;* [†]*World Health Organization 2004;* [‡]*National Institute of Health (Institute of Medicine).*

TABLE 7.2 Serum Phosphorus Levels During Infancy and Childhood

Age	Serum phosphorus (mg/dL)	(mmol/L)
Infant	4.8−7.4	1.55−2.0
Toddler	3.8−6.5	1.23−2.10
Child	3.7−5.6	1.2−1.81
Adolescent	2.9−5.4	0.94−1.74
Adult	2.7−4.7	0.87−1.52

calcium, the phosphorus level in blood is not very tightly regulated. Serum phosphorus is higher in infants and young children as compared to older children and adults (Table 7.2).

Passive absorption via the intercellular route, responsible for half the amount absorbed daily, is dependent on the amount of phosphorus present in the gut. Active absorption is via a vitamin D-dependent sodium-phosphorus co-transport system (Na/Pi co-transporters).

Phosphate as well as calcium deficiency, by stimulating PTH increases 1-hydroxylase activity and calcitriol levels, thus increasing phosphorus absorption. Phosphorus level in blood is mainly regulated by renal phosphorus excretion.

When absorbed phosphorus flux into blood rises, mechanisms which at present are poorly understood activate fibroblast growth factor 23 (FGF23, a hormone derived from osteocytes), which inhibits 1-hydroxylase activity and stimulates excretion of phosphorus (via activation of Na/Pi and other co-transporters and exchangers) in the renal tubule. Conversely, hypophosphataemia inhibits FGF23 secretion and restores serum phosphorus.[3]

Insights into the mechanisms regulating phosphorus metabolism have emerged mainly from the study of metabolic diseases linked with abnormalities of serum phosphorus, such as X-linked hypophosphataemic rickets (XLH).

- Mutations in the FGF23 gene, rendering it resistant to cleavage and degradation, are known in patients with autosomal dominant hypophosphataemic rickets (ADHR).
- Activating mutations of Klotho (a co-factor rendering specificity to the FGF receptor for FGF23) give rise to hypophosphataemic rickets with hyperparathyroidism.
- Mutations in the Na/Pi co-transporter result in hereditary hypophosphataemic rickets with hypercalciuria (HHRH).
- Tumour-induced hypophosphataemic rickets and osteomalacia (TIO) are caused by excessive production of FGF23.
- Conversely, failure of activation of FGF 23 by the protein GALANT3 (due to inactivating mutations in the GALANT3 gene), or of the KLOTHO gene, produce the syndrome of hypophosphataemic familial tumoral calcinosis (HFTC1).

The role of genes such as PHEX (phosphater-egulating gene with homologies to endopepti-dases on the X chromosome), MEPE (matrix extracellular phosphoglycoprotein) and others, are further discussed in the section on hypo-phosphataemic rickets.

Sources of Phosphorus

The daily requirements for phosphorus are similar to those for calcium. Phosphorus is found in most commonly consumed foods, including milk, whole grain cereals and legumes. Thus, its deficiency is not common.

Magnesium

Magnesium is essential for normal secretion and action of PTH, and magnesium deficiency leads to hypocalcaemia. Magnesium in the intestine is absorbed via the help of binding proteins, which are also present in the distal renal tubule, to effect active reabsorption in the kidney. Passive reabsorption in the proximal

tubule and loop of Henle also occur, via the tight junction protein paracellin. Mutations of these and other proteins involved in magnesium transport can cause a variety of hypomagnesae-mia (some with hypocalcaemia and nephrocal-cinosis) and hypermagnesuria syndromes, including Gitelman and Bartter syndromes.[4]

Parathyroid Hormone

Parathyroid hormone (PTH) is an 84 amino acid peptide hormone. It has carboxyl and amino terminal ends. The amino terminal end is biologically active. The intact molecule forms only 5–30% of circulating PTH, the remainder made up by inactive fragments. Assay of intact PTH gives a better estimate of circulating hormone, as in certain conditions such as renal failure, the smaller fragments are found in increased concentrations.

The normal level of PTH is 10 to 55 or 60 pg/mL (1 to 6 pmol/L) in various assays.

PTH is secreted from the parathyroid glands when the calcium-sensing receptor on the parathyroid cells senses low serum calcium.

PTH actions are via a cell surface G protein-linked receptor. Ligand binding to receptor causes dissociation of the $Gs\alpha$ subunit from the trimeric $Gs\alpha\beta\gamma$ complex. The free $Gs\alpha$ stimulates adenyl cyclase, increases intracellular cyclic AMP, and activates various protein kinases.[5]

- Inherited **inactivating** mutations in the PTH receptor cause pseudohypoparathyroidism (PHP). This is an example of imprinting of a gene, wherein the allele inherited from either parent is preferentially expressed in comparison to the allele inherited from the other parent. Thus if the mutated allele is inherited from the mother, PHP1a results, whereas if the mutated allele is inherited from father, pseudo PHP (PPHP) results

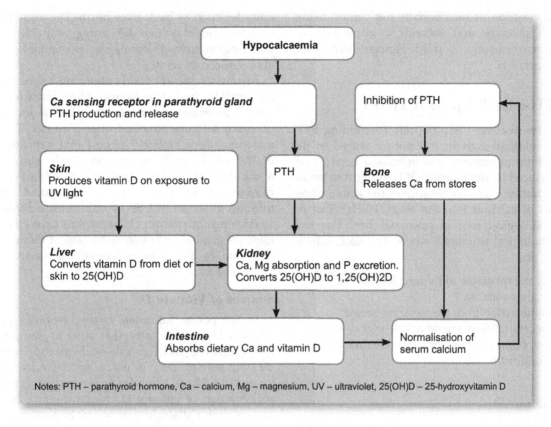

FIGURE 7.1 Overview of calcium homeostasis.

(see section on hypocalcaemia for more details).

- **Activating** mutations of the PTH receptor also causes human disease, in the form of Jansen's metaphyseal dysplasia with hypercalcaemia.

The target organs for PTH action are bone and kidney (Figure 7.1).

In Bone

- During normocalcaemia, PTH acts to bring about bone formation through its receptors on osteoblasts.
- During hypocalcaemia, it brings about resorption, via enhancing osteoclast differentiation.

In Kidney

PTH has three actions:

- In the proximal tubule, it enhances 1-hydroxylase activity and calcitriol production.
- In the distal tubule, it brings about reabsorption of calcium and magnesium, and excretion of phosphorus.

However, if serum calcium is high, the high filtered calcium load at the glomerulus can overwhelm PTH-induced calcium reabsorption at the tubule, resulting in hypercalciuria in absolute terms. Thus hyperparathyroidism paradoxically causes hypercalciuria rather than hypocalciuria. It also decreases reabsorption of bicarbonate and amino acids, both primary and secondary hyperparathyroidism causing a mild Fanconi syndrome (Figure 7.1).

PTH-related Peptide (PTHrP)

The discovery of a peptide resembling PTH in biological activity, but not measured in the PTH immunoassays, was initially in cord blood. Produced by the placenta, it is thought to be the mechanism for maintenance of the active transport of calcium into the fetus. PTHrP has no physiological role in postnatal life. The two pathological situations where its role is important are:

- as the mediator of hypercalcaemia of malignancy, and
- its secretion from the lactating breast, necessitating decrease of calcitriol doses in hypoparathyroid women on treatment, after childbirth.

Vitamin D

Though designated as a vitamin, vitamin D (cholecalciferol, vitamin D$_3$), when metabolised in the body to calcitriol, possesses all the characteristics of a hormone. We obtain our supply of vitamin D mainly from the action of UV energy in sunlight on cholesterol in the dermis, which gets converted to cholecalciferol or vitamin D$_3$. Ergocalciferol or vitamin D$_2$ is the plant source of vitamin D.

Vitamin D Formation

Factors which hinder vitamin D formation in skin include dark pigmentation (darkly pigmented skin requires about five to six times the duration of UV exposure as fair skin to produce the same amount of vitamin D), clothing, sunscreen and older age. The UV energy in sunlight is about four times stronger during summer than in winter, even in low latitudes such as 26 degrees north. The number of hours per day that UV energy capable of inducing vitamin D formation is available is also reduced in winter.

Serum vitamin D levels after sun exposure rise briskly, in a few hours. After consistent daily sun exposure, maximum plateau levels of vitamin D are obtained after 6 weeks. The experiments of Holick[6] suggest that exposure of the whole body to the noon July sun to a minimal erythemal dose of UV (about 20 minutes at 42 degrees north and about 10 minutes in southern USA) would release about 10,000 units of vitamin D. Nature has protective mechanisms against overproduction of vitamin D in skin, by diverting cholecalciferol into inactive isomers.

Sources of Vitamin D

In temperate latitudes, natural sources of vitamin D include fatty fish such as salmon and mackerel, and fish oils such as cod liver oil. Otherwise, food is not a good source of vitamin D. There is evidence for enterohepatic recirculation of vitamin D, due to the fact that patients with disorders of absorption such as cystic fibrosis and chronic pancreatitis are prone to develop vitamin D deficiency.

Vitamin D Metabolism

Vitamin D is hydroxylated to 25-hydroxyvitamin D (25(OH)D) in the liver. Circulating 25(OH)D is the index of sufficiency of vitamin D nutrition. This is further hydroxylated in the kidney, to 1,25-dihydroxyvitamin D (1,25(OH)$_2$D), or calcitriol, which is the potent effector of several calcaemic and non-calcaemic actions of vitamin D. The activity of 1-hydroxylase is enhanced by PTH and also by low concentrations of serum phosphate and calcium. It is inhibited by FGF23.

Actions of Vitamin D

Calcitriol binds to its receptor, which is present in the intestinal mucosa cells (where calcium and phosphate absorption are brought about), in the osteoblast (promotes growth plate mineralisation) and osteoclast precursor, parathyroid glands, and several other organs not related to calcium or bone, for example immune cells as well as skin, breast, colon and prostate. Here it has been demonstrated to have paracrine and autocrine functions, to bring about antimicrobial and anti-cell proliferation functions. Topical vitamin D analogues already have a proven therapeutic role in the treatment of psoriasis. Its role in the pathogenesis of diabetes mellitus type 1 and type 2 and of several cancers is the subject of intense investigation.[7]

Normal Range of Vitamin D

The normal level of vitamin D or 25(OH)D in blood has been the subject of some controversy.[8] Some investigators believe 25(OH)D to be normal at a level below which PTH is stimulated to rise above its normal range. Others believe the level to which calcium absorption in the intestine is enhanceable is the normal cut-off for 25(OH)D. A nomenclature naming less than 20 ng/mL (less than 50 nmol/L) as deficiency and 20 to 30 ng/mL (75 nmol/L) as insufficiency is popular. The upper limit (up till which there is no fear of toxicity) is roughly150 ng/mL.

Paediatricians should bear in mind that many investigators believe that normal levels of vitamin D in children are lower than those in adults (and hence may adopt a cut-off of 20 rather than 30 ng/mL for defining deficiency). Further, toxicity may develop at lower levels than in adults.

Serum vitamin D has been shown to be deficient in all continents and at all latitudes, despite the availability of sunshine, for the reasons described above. Since the implications of vitamin D deficiency are serious, most countries advocate pharmacological prevention of deficiency for people at risk (see also section on rickets).

Calcitonin

Calcitonin is secreted by the C cells of the thyroid gland, in response to hypercalcaemia, and maintains homeostasis by lowering serum calcium. However, its role in calcium metabolism in postnatal life is not remarkable, and its main significance is as a cellular marker of C cells, in the diagnosis and management of medullary thyroid carcinoma. New evidence suggests that neurons in the central nervous system integrate many signals, with the regulation of bone remodelling partly via calcitonin related peptide.

HYPOCALCAEMIA, HYPERCALCAEMIA AND DISORDERS OF THE PARATHYROID GLANDS

Hypocalcaemia

Aetiology

Hypocalcaemia in childhood can be conveniently categorised into neonatal or infantile/childhood hypocalcaemia. The neonatal period has a unique set of factors predisposing the baby to hypocalcaemia. These physiological conditions, when uncompensated, are responsible for 'early' neonatal hypocalcaemia (Table 7.3).

'EARLY' NEONATAL HYPOCALCAEMIA

Abrupt interruption of active transport of calcium across the placenta, coupled with immaturity of the parathyroid glands and delayed initiation of feeding, makes the newborn prone to hypocalcaemia. When the birth is complicated by prematurity, IUGR, asphyxia, sepsis, or if the baby is born to a mother with diabetes, or has received blood transfusions (due to the infused citrate), hypocalcaemia may be precipitated.

TABLE 7.3 Causes of Hypocalcaemia in Infancy and Childhood

NEONATAL HYPOCALCAEMIA

- Early neonatal hypocalcaemia

- Prematurity, intrauterine growth restriction (IUGR)

- Sepsis

- Birth asphyxia

- Infant of diabetic mother

- Blood transfusion

- Late neonatal hypocalcaemia

- Cow's milk feeds

- Maternal hypercalcaemia

- Vitamin D deficiency in mother and infant

INFANT AND CHILDHOOD HYPOCALCAEMIA

Hypoparathyroidism

- Thalassemia, DiGeorge and HDR, Kearns-Sayre, APECED, and Pearson syndromes

- Pseudohypoparathyroidism

- Hypomagnesaemia

- Renal failure

- Vitamin D deficiency

- Familial hypercalciuria hypocalcaemia

- Alkalosis

- Osteopetrosis

'LATE' NEONATAL HYPOCALCAEMIA

The most common cause of 'late' neonatal hypocalcaemia, occurring beyond 4 days of life, is the use of cow's milk, due to its high phosphate load. Maternal hyperparathyroidism, via transplacental transit of calcium but not PTH, results in newborn hypocalcaemia by suppression of fetal parathyroid glands during pregnancy, which then take time to recover postnatally.

Maternal vitamin D deficiency, leading to poor vitamin D stores in the baby, is a common cause of late neonatal or infant hypocalcaemia. This is one situation where vitamin D deficiency may be accompanied by high serum phosphorus rather than the typical finding of hypophosphataemia.[9]

Thus, late or prolonged neonatal hypocalcaemia warrants testing of mother for hypercalcaemia or vitamin D deficiency (see also section on rickets).

INFANT AND CHILDHOOD HYPOCALCAEMIA

The causes of infant and childhood hypocalcaemia overlap.

DiGeorge — velocardiofacial syndrome: parathyroid hormone deficiency may occur due to aplasia of the glands in this condition, associated with microdeletion in the long arm of chromosome 22.

Autoimmune polyendocrinopathy candidiasis ectodermal dystrophy (APECED) syndrome, also known as polyglandular syndrome type 1, can result in autoimmune destruction of the parathyroid glands. This disease is caused by inheritable mutations in the autoimmune regulator (AIRE) gene, and is characterised by the triad of mucocutaneous candidiasis, hypoparathyroidism, and Addison's disease. In addition, the patient may have chronic active hepatitis, gallstones, autoimmune thyroid disease, hypogonadism, malabsorption, obstipation, sicca syndrome, asplenia, and numerous other manifestations.[10]

Pseudohypoparathyroidism (PHP) can cause absent or reduced parathyroid hormone function due to resistance to its action. This condition occurs due to inheritable mutations in the Gsα component of the G protein second messenger gene, downstream of the PTH receptor. It is characterised by the Albright Hereditary Osteodystrophy (AHO) phenotype, consisting of short stature, moon facies, short 4th and 5th metacarpals and metatarsals and mental subnormality. Resistance to thyrotropin-releasing hormone and gonado-tropins may be present, in the patient, or in family members. This gene is characterised by imprinting: the maternally derived allele is expressed in the proximal tubule of the kidney, whereas the paternally derived gene is not. Thus if the maternal allele is mutated, hypocalcaemia results, along with the AHO phenotype (PHP 1a). If the defective allele is inherited from the father, the normal allele from the mother takes care of calcium homeo-stasis, and the only abnormality is AHO phenotype (pseudo PHP or PPHP). PHP 1b is characterised by hypocalcaemia and other hormone resistance, but not the AHO pheno-type. They do not have a mutation in the Gsα gene itself, but perhaps in its regulator. PHP 1c is characterised by hypocalcaemia, other hormone resistance, AHO phenotype, but no mutation in Gsα. There is a variety labelled as PHP II, characterised by hypocal-caemia, hyperphosphataemia, elevated PTH, lacking the AHO phenotype, and showing diminished phosphaturic response to PTH administration, but normal cyclic AMP response. However, since this exact picture is seen in hypovitaminosis D, it remains doubt-ful whether this is a distinct genetic entity or not.

Familial hypercalciuric hypocalcaemia is caused by activating mutations in the calcium-sensing receptor (CaSR) gene, which lower the threshold for PTH release by a hypocalcemic stimulus, i.e. serum calcium has to become very low in order to stimulate PTH secretion. The same mutation in the renal tubule decreases calcium reabsorption. Thus, it is characterised by PTH concentration inappropriately low for the level of hypocalcaemia, hyperphosphatae-mia and hypercalciuria.[11]

Clinical Features and Diagnosis

A careful history and examination, together with basic blood and urine tests, will provide not only evidence for hypocalcaemia but also is likely to reveal a cause, without the need for expensive or complex investigations.

- **Hypocalcaemia in the** neonate presents with nonspecific signs such as jitteriness, lethargy, abdominal distension, poor feeding or apnoea. More serious manifestations include seizure, arrhythmia, laryngospasm and hypotension.
- **The older child** may be able to report circum-oral numbness, tingling of fingers and toes, muscle cramps or carpopedal spasm (adduction of the thumb, flexion at the metacarpophalangeal joints and extension at the interphalangeal joints, also termed tetany).
- **Chronic hypocalcaemia** due to any cause produces dental enamel hypoplasia, subcapsular cataract, basal ganglia calcification, and papilloedema. An ECG will reveal prolongation of corrected QT interval.

Investigations

SAMPLES TO BE TAKEN IMMEDIATELY, BEFORE TREATMENT IS INSTITUTED

- Serum calcium, ionised calcium (iCa)
- Phosphorus, magnesium
- Albumin
- Alkaline phosphatase
- Creatinine.

Care while taking a sample for serum calcium includes always using fresh tubes or vaccutainers (never-washed tubes or vials), and avoiding the use of a tourniquet. If the tour-niquet is essential to finding a vein, it should be released after insertion of the needle, 10 seconds prior to drawing the sample.

FURTHER TESTS THAT ARE OF VALUE AND MAY BE ADDED

- ECG
- Liver function tests
- Venous blood gas picture
- X-ray to look for rickets

- Mother's serum calcium, alkaline phosphatase
- Serum 25(OH)D
- Serum PTH (sample taken during hypocalcaemia, see Box 7.1, page 134, for care while sampling).
- 25(OH)D and 1,25-dihydroxyvitamin D are expensive tests and should be ordered with care
- Urinary calcium: creatinine ratio is useful in the confirmation of familial hypercalciuric hypocalcaemia, with samples from both parents providing valuable information.

NOTE

A secure IV line is mandatory to avoid subcutaneous necrosis from extravasation. Calcium infusions should not be mixed with solutions containing phosphates and bicarbonates, to avoid precipitation.

Treatment

Serum calcium less than 8.0 mg/dL (iCa less than 2.0 mmol/L) in a newborn and less than 8.5 mg/dL in an older child signifies hypocalcaemia.

BOX 7.1

BLOOD SAMPLE FOR PTH

The blood sample for PTH requires special handling, as the molecule is destroyed if kept for long at room temperature. After immediate transportation to the laboratory, the sample should be spun preferably in a refrigerated centrifuge, and stored immediately at $-20°C$ until assay. Assay from a sample already thawed once and refrozen will give erroneous results.

BOX 7.2

CHVOSTEK AND TROUSSEAU SIGNS

Chvostek and Trousseau signs may be elicitable on examination. The former is performed by tapping the face in front of the pinna, below the zygomatic arch, with the patellar hammer. Twitching is observed of the muscles at the angle of the mouth and other facial muscles, due to irritation of the facial nerve. Trousseau sign is elicited by raising the blood pressure 10 mmHg above the systolic pressure, for up to 3 minutes. Production of tetanic spasm of the hand is seen in hypocalcaemia.

- **Immediate treatment of a symptomatic child consists of** IV infusion of 0.2–0.5 mL/kg of 10% Ca gluconate (up to 2 mL/kg in neonates) given over 10–20 minutes while monitoring for cardiac arrhythmias.
- **Maintenance treatment** is by a continuous infusion of 10% calcium gluconate 5 mL (or 50 mg elemental Ca)/kg/day for neonates and 2 mL (or 20 mg elemental Ca)/kg/day for older infants and children.
- **Ongoing treatment:** once hypocalcaemia is controlled, the infusion is tapered and oral calcium supplements (50–75 mg/kg/day of elemental calcium) started. Depending on the aetiology of hypocalcaemia active vitamin D analogues (calcitriol at 15–25 ng/kg/day or alfacalcidol 25–40 ng/kg/day) may be needed pending further investigations.

In case of unresponsive hypocalcaemia, hypomagnesaemia should be suspected. This is treated with $MgSO_4$ (50% solution) in a dose of 0.2 mL/kg intramuscularly, 12-hourly for 24 hours. (For chronic treatment of rachitic states leading to hypocalcaemia, see the section on rickets.)

Monitoring Long-Term Management of Chronic Hypocalcaemia Conditions

- In chronic therapy of conditions such as hypoparathyroidism or PHP, serum calcium is maintained in the low normal range to avoid hypercalcaemia, hypercalciuria, nephrolithiasis and renal failure.
- Oral calcium supplements may be necessary if the child's diet is poor in calcium-rich dairy products.
- **During times of stress** such as fever, patients with chronic hypocalcaemia require higher calcium intake and, sometimes, higher dose of calcitriol. Serum calcium is monitored every 6–8 weeks and urinary calcium every 3 months.
- **Hypercalciuria** can be treated with thiazide diuretics, i.e. hydrochlorothiazide in doses of 0.5–2.0 mg/kg/day if the urinary calcium excretion is greater than 4 mg/kg/day or urinary calcium to creatinine ratio is in the hypercalciuric range for age (greater than 0.2 for older infants and children).

Hypercalcaemia

Hypercalcaemia is less common in the paediatric age group than hypocalcaemia. Presentation is with non-specific symptoms such as constipation, anorexia, vomiting and irritability. Polyuria and polydipsia can result from nephrogenic diabetes insipidus. Chronic hypercalcaemia leading to hypercalciuria will lead to nephrocalcinosis and renal failure.

Aetiology

The causes can be categorised as those caused by increased calcium absorption and those caused by increased resorption from bone or decreased clearance at the kidney (Table 7.4).

INCREASED INTESTINAL CALCIUM ABSORPTION

- **Vitamin D toxicity** due to overdosage results in long-standing hypercalcaemia, as the

TABLE 7.4 Causes of Hypercalcaemia in Childhood

CONDITIONS OF INCREASED CALCIUM ABSORPTION
• Vitamin D toxicity
• Vitamin A toxicity
• William syndrome
• Subcutaneous fat necrosis
• Granulomatous conditions such as sarcoidosis
CONDITIONS OF DECREASED URINARY EXCRETION
• Thiazide diuretic
• Familial hypocalciuric hypercalcaemia
CONDITIONS OF INCREASED RESORPTION FROM BONE
• Hyperparathyroidism
• Familial hypocalciuric hypercalcaemia
• Immobilisation
• PTHrP mediated in malignancy

vitamin gets distributed in the body fat and elimination from the body takes several weeks. This is most commonly found where unregulated and repeated doses of vitamin D are administered by well-meaning parents and/or carers. However, this problem is increasingly seen now that vitamin D deficiency is so widely recognised, where single or multiple medical practitioners may administer repeated stoss (high) doses of vitamin D without checking blood levels.[12]

- **William syndrome** is characterised by hypercalcaemia, elfin facies with a long philtrum, supravalvular aortic stenosis and developmental delay. Hypercalcaemia is due to increased absorption of calcium from the intestine, and is self-limiting after about 3 years of age.
- **Subcutaneous fat necrosis** occurs in newborns who had asphyxia at birth. The

inflamed tissues of fat necrosis probably produce 1,25-dihydroxyvitamin D, causing increased absorption of calcium.

- **Vitamin A toxicity and thiazide diuretic** are two other drugs which can cause hypercalcaemia.

INCREASED BONE REABSORPTION

- **Prolonged immobilisation** causes hypercalcaemia by increasing resorption of mineral from bone. This is commonly seen in association with multiple burns, spinal cord injury or transverse myelitis or Guillain–Barré syndrome, where immobility is acute and very severe.
- **Hyperparathyroidism** presents with hypercalcaemia and pathological fractures due to resorption of bone. In children sporadic parathyroid adenoma is very rare, unlike adults.[13] If hypercalcaemia is found in a child or adolescent together with a raised PTH level, multiple endocrine neoplasia syndromes should be considered. These include MEN 1 syndrome (familial tumours of parathyroid, pituitary and pancreas). Every patient with one of these tumours must be screened for the others, as must their family members. MEN 2A, characterised by phaeochromocytoma and medullary carcinoma of the thyroid, is accompanied by tumours in the parathyroid glands in about a fifth of cases.
- **Jansen's metaphyseal dysplasia** is a rare disorder caused by activating mutations of the PTH receptor. Short stature, features resembling rickets and hypercalcaemia with low PTH characterise this dominantly inherited syndrome.
- **Tertiary hyperparathyroidism** is produced on the background of long-standing secondary hyperparathyroidism, most typically in chronic renal failure and hypophosphataemic rickets. The chronic hyperplasia results in autonomous adenomatous transformation, and hypercalcaemia.

- **Familial hypocalciuric hypercalcaemia** occurs when inactivating mutations of the calcium-sensing receptor are inherited heterozygously. There is an alteration of the set point of PTH secretion, such that a higher serum calcium is required in order for PTH secretion to be blocked. Thus, serum PTH is at high normal or mildly elevated levels, inappropriately high for the high serum calcium. This condition is usually mild and does not require treatment. However, if inheritance is homozygous, it causes severe hypercalcaemia with onset in the neonatal period.

Investigations

Serum calcium, phosphorus, alkaline phosphatase, electrolytes, urinary calcium, plain X-ray hand are the simple investigations needed.

Unless history or examination suggests a clue towards aetiology, PTH will be needed at this stage, to categorise whether it is a PTH-dependent or independent condition.

Depending on whether it is elevated or suppressed, other investigations such as parathyroid scintigraphy and ultrasonography, 25(OH) D and 1,25-dihydroxyvitamin D, PTHrP, among others, will be needed.

Treatment

Besides specific treatment of the underlying cause, the following general principles of management of hypercalcaemia are applicable to many of the conditions.

HYDRATION

Intravenous saline infusion, with increased sodium delivery to the distal tubule, increases calcium excretion. It can be given at greater than maintenance rates, along with a loop (but not thiazide) diuretic (furosemide 1 to 2 mg/kg is suitable).

REDUCTION OF CALCIUM ABSORPTION

In conditions such as vitamin D toxicity and William syndrome, dietary calcium must be reduced to nil (in the former) or about a third of normal (in the latter). Glucocorticoid therapy will decrease intestinal calcium absorption, and also decreases ectopic 1,25-dihydroxyvitamin D production in conditions where this is the mechanism of hypercalcaemia.

DECREASE IN RESORPTION FROM BONE

Bisphosphonates are the most useful category of drugs for this action. Intravenous pamidronate in the dose of 1 mg/kg/day in a 3-hour infusion is given for about 2 to 3 days.

DIALYSIS

Life-threatening hypercalcaemia requires dialysis with a low-calcium dialysate, for immediate treatment.

RICKETS

Rickets is a condition of softening of bones due to inadequate deposition of mineral (a salt of calcium and phosphorus known as calcium hydroxyapatite) in the growth plate cartilage.

Osteomalacia is the term given to softening of bones due to inadequate deposition of mineral in osteoid anywhere in the skeleton, usually after epiphyseal fusion.

The clinical features of rickets are seen in childhood onset of the disease, whereas features of osteomalacia may be seen when the disease is active in adolescence or adulthood. The term osteoporosis is often confused with osteomalacia. The former refers to inadequate amount of tissue laid down in bone, though it is mineralised. The resulting bone is brittle and has a risk of breaking easily, rather than soft, which bends easily as in rickets/osteomalacia (though bone can also break sometimes in rickets/osteomalacia).

Causes of Rickets

Nutritional rickets is caused by deficiency of either mineral component of bone, i.e. calcium or phosphorus, or by deficiency of vitamin D which indirectly leads to deficient mineralisation. Whereas vitamin D and calcium deficiencies are common causes of rickets, phosphorus deficiency is not common except in certain special situations, as it is available in adequate quantities in staple foods like cereal. Deficiency rickets is also seen in malabsorption states such as coeliac disease, regional enteritis or chronic pancreatic disease. There are several errors of metabolism which can give rise to rickets (Table 7.5). They are discussed under the section on metabolic rickets.

Nutritional Rickets

Vitamin D Deficiency

Vitamin D deficiency became rampant in the developed world with the onset of industrialisation, due to inadequate outdoor activity and

TABLE 7.5 Causes of Rickets

Calcipenic rickets	Phosphopenic rickets
Deficiency of calcium and/or vitamin D	Low phosphorus intake
Dietary insufficiency	Prematurity, TPN
Malabsorption — coeliac disease, pancreatic disease	Renal phosphorus wasting
Antiepileptic drug therapy	Hereditary hypophosphataemic rickets
Systemic illness — CRF and liver disease	Fanconi syndrome (proximal RTA)
Distal renal tubular acidosis	Fibrous dysplasia
Vitamin D-resistant rickets type I	Oncogenic hypophosphataemic rickets
Vitamin D-resistant rickets type II	

Notes: RTA — renal tubular acidosis; TPN — total parenteral nutrition.

pollution resulting in poor sun exposure, compounding residence at temperate latitudes where the duration of sunlight is already poor. It thus acquired the name 'the English disease'. Governments of many countries in temperate regions have been fortifying staple food items such as milk or flour with vitamin D. However, due to reports of hypercalcaemia wherein vitamin D toxicity could not be ruled out, some governments have also chosen not to do so. Vitamin D deficiency has made a comeback due to coloured races migrating to temperate lands, less time spent outdoors, obesity (which is associated with lower serum 25(OH)D), inadequate consumption of milk (and therefore of the vitamin D it is fortified with), and the use of sunscreen creams.

In many tropical countries too, vitamin D deficiency is being documented in large segments of the population. The groups at high risk are women (in countries where the modest dress code mandated for women by society precludes adequate exposure of the skin to the sun's rays), and infants and adolescent girls due to the high growth rate and physiological requirements. The baby of a mother who has low vitamin D stores acquires insufficient vitamin D transplacentally as well as in breast milk.

HOW MUCH SUN EXPOSURE IS NEEDED FOR PREVENTION OF VITAMIN D DEFICIENCY?

As discussed above in the section on vitamin D physiology, about 10,000 to 25,000 units of vitamin D are released from whole body exposure of a Caucasian person of light skin colour, to 1 minimal erythemal dose of UV exposure.[14] This would amount to approximately 20 minutes in the peak summer sun at latitude 42 degrees north. A similar minimal erythemal dose for a darkly pigmented person would need approximately 90 to 120 minutes. If the skin is largely covered with clothes, a proportionately smaller amount of vitamin D would be formed.

The cut-off which defines vitamin D deficiency is generally accepted as 20 ng/mL.

However, many investigators believe this may be higher, closer to 30 ng/mL. The toxic level is defined by some authors as 100 ng/mL and others as 150 ng/mL. Data for infants and children is almost non-existent. The Institute of Medicine, National Institute of Heath, USA, recommends 400 units per day of vitamin D to be made available to all individuals from newborn to adulthood, and 800 units per day for those over 50 years.[15] The American Academy of Pediatrics also makes the same recommendation for the paediatric age group.[16]

Calcium Deficiency

In many tropical countries of Africa and Asia, sunshine is available in plenty, but calcium is not (as milk products, the main source of calcium, are prohibitively expensive for poorer people to consume). Serum 25(OH)D has been documented to be around 14 to 16 ng/mL, but calcium intake only 200 mg/day.[17] Rickets in these children is due to calcium deficiency, and healing has been demonstrated with calcium replenishment alone, both radiologically and biochemically, although calcium with vitamin D produced faster healing.[17] For 2010 recommendations on daily reference intake of calcium for various age groups from the National Institutes of Health, USA, the reader is referred to the section on mineral physiology. Milk and milk products, and several fish, are good sources of calcium. During pregnancy and lactation, it may be very difficult to meet these requirements with diet alone, and supplements are generally recommended.

Phosphorus Deficiency

As mentioned already, phosphorus deficiency occurs in certain situations, such as prematurity, malabsorption, and parenteral nutrition (see section on metabolic bone disease of prematurity). In recognition of this, supplements for preterm babies and parenteral nutrition fluids contain the necessary concentration of phosphorus to prevent metabolic bone disease in most but not all infants.

However, in extremely preterm infants, provision of adequate phosphate is near impossible because it requires oral use largely. Especially in those infants who have necrotising enteritis this becomes very difficult. Phosphate deficiency in these infants is common and may last for several weeks. By the time overt metabolic bone disease is clinically apparent in these infants the phosphate deficiency has resolved, and the diagnosis may be obscured by apparently normal biochemistry.

Clinical Features of Rickets

Rickets results in painful, soft bones, muscle weakness and, when severe, in hypocalcaemia. The following are signs of rickets:

- An infant with rickets will be irritable due to incessant pain and will cry when lifted. Sweating is a feature.
- Jitteriness or seizures are particularly common in infancy and adolescence. Hypocalcaemia can result in dilated cardiomyopathy.
- Muscle weakness manifests in the older infant with delayed motor milestones, waddling gait like that of a duck, poor respiratory excursion and abdominal distension.
- Any cause of prolonged hypocalcaemia can result in delayed dentition and dental enamel hypoplasia.
- The softening of bones manifests in infancy as craniotabes (softening of the outer table of the skull, giving a ping pong ball sensation on being pressed) and widening and delayed closure of the anterior fontanelle. The skull looks bossed, with prominence of frontal and parietal bones.
- Depression of the lower part of the chest wall, at the insertion of the diaphragmatic tendons, is known as Harrison sulcus.

- The metaphyseal ends of bones expand, resulting in prominent costochondral junctions ('rachitic rosary'), widened wrists and 'double malleoli' at the ankle. Softening of bone results in deformities such as genu varum (bow legs, commoner in toddlers), genu valgum (knock knees, more common in adolescents), windswept deformity (genu varum in one leg and valgum in the other) and coxa varum at the hip.
- The older child or adolescent can present with short stature.
- Rickets/osteomalacia during adolescence result in deformed, android-shaped pelvis with Looser zones (see below under radiological features) in the pubic and ischial rami. Curvature of long bones may be seen, especially femur and tibia.
- A not uncommon manifestation is anaemia with erythroblasts and myeloblasts, and hepatosplenomegaly, all of which disappear with vitamin D therapy.
- Vitamin D deficiency and rickets are associated with poor immune function, and increased upper and lower respiratory tract infections.

Radiological Features

The typical plain X-ray picture of rickets is seen at the metaphyseal ends of long bone, and consists of cupping, fraying and widening of the metaphyses, with increased lucent space (comprised of unmineralised cartilage) between the metaphysis and epiphysis (Figure 7.2). When treatment is instituted, healing occurs by onset of mineralisation at the edge of the metaphysis, seen as a dense line of healing, which then progresses proximally. Osteomalacia is characterised by Looser zones, which are seen as radiolucent bands running perpendicular to the long axis of the bone, and correspond to areas of unmineralised osteoid. They are typical in certain locations, such as the medial border of the scapulae, upper end of

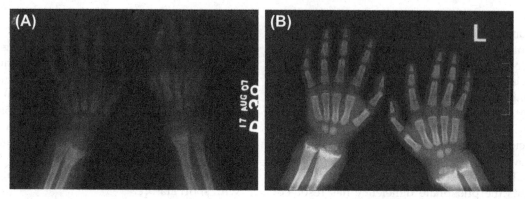

FIGURE 7.2 Rickets. Note: The cupping and fraying at the distal ends of the metaphyses, and widened lucent space between the metaphyses and epiphyses (Figure 7.2A). Figure 7.2B is of a child who received therapy. Healing starts with a zone of calcification close to the epiphysis, and progresses proximally.

humerus, pubic and ischial rami, below the lesser trochanter, and on the upper end of fibula. They normally involve only one cortex, and are not accompanied by callus.

Other features of nutritional rickets/osteomalacia are attributable to the accompanying secondary hyperparathyroidism, and include lytic areas particularly in the metacarpals, pelvis and femur neck. The phalanges show cortical subperiosteal resorption especially on the radial side and intracortical tunnelling.

Biochemical Features

- The earliest stage of rickets is associated with hypocalcaemia. This very quickly is compensated by elevated PTH, in an attempt by the body to bring back normocalcaemia. Thus hypocalcaemia is seen only in severe rickets, when the compensation by PTH proves inadequate.
- Elevated PTH gives rise to phosphaturia, resulting in the hallmark characteristic of hypophosphataemia. However, there are conditions where phosphorus may be high in rickets, including chronic renal failure, and, transiently, during hypocalcaemia associated with vitamin D deficiency.

- Hyperparathyroidism in turn gives rise to generalised proximal tubular reabsorption defects, with bicarbonaturia, metabolic acidosis and aminoaciduria. These revert to normal with normalisation of PTH upon treatment.
- Excessive osteoblastic activity, in an attempt to make more bone, results in elevated alkaline phosphatase.
- Rickets is a disease of growing bone. In the infant or young child whose linear growth is restricted due to chronic disease or malnutrition, the bone changes of florid rickets may be less obvious and alkaline phosphatase may be normal. (Alkaline phosphatase may thus be normal in florid rickets associated with severe malnutrition.)

Serum 25(OH)D would be expected to be low in vitamin D deficiency and normal to borderline in calcium deficiency rickets. Contrary to expectation, $1,25(OH)_2D$ is normal or high, not low. This is due to efficient hydroxylation of any available substrate into the active form, by PTH.

The hallmark of calcium deficiency rickets is low urinary calcium with high $1,25(OH)_2D$.

However, serum 25(OH)D, 1,25(OH)$_2$D and PTH are costly investigations, and are completely unnecessary in the common variety of rickets.

Differential Diagnosis and Approach to a Patient

A suspicion of rickets from clinical features should lead to confirmation of the diagnosis via an X-ray and/or simple biochemistry like serum alkaline phosphatase. Treatment should be instituted and response monitored, as described below.

If clinical features suggest rickets due to the presence of deformity, but alkaline phosphatase is not abnormal and nor is there radiologic evidence of cupping or fraying, differential diagnoses to be considered include:

- Evidence of past rickets which has resolved with time ('burnt-out' rickets) (as deformity takes many years to normalise).
- Blount disease (Figure 7.3), a condition of bowing at the knees due to medial beaking and destruction of the upper tibial metaphyses. It is often seen in male toddlers who are overweight or obese. Most normalise spontaneously, though some with severe disease may need orthopaedic intervention.
- If clinical features are suggestive of deformity, X ray shows abnormal metaphyses, but alkaline phosphatase is normal (without concomitant undernutrition), a skeletal dysplasia involving the metaphyses should be considered.

Treatment

Though vitamin D has been known as the treatment of rickets for more than a century, there is no single uniform dose or regimen used all over the world, to date.

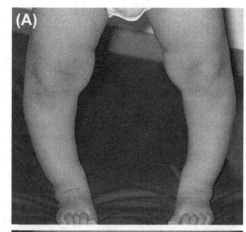

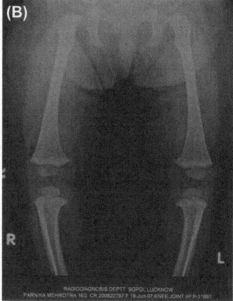

FIGURE 7.3 Blount disease. 7.3A shows bowed legs. 7.3B shows beaking of the medial end of the tibia and absence of the characteristic cupping and fraying seen in rickets.

Some known facts regarding the pharmacokinetics of vitamin D include:

- Vitamin D administered by any route, intramuscular or oral, enters the bloodstream rapidly, and then gets distributed for storage in the adipose tissue, from where it is released gradually, to undergo hydroxylation and become an active hormone. Thus, overdosage can result in toxicity, manifested as hypercalcaemia, which can be life-threatening or cause renal failure.

- Intramuscular administration of a single large dose results in a slow and long-lasting rise of 25(OH)D, with peak reached at about 3 months and plateau lasting beyond 6 months. This route lends itself to administration under observation at infrequent intervals, where compliance with home-based therapy is questionable and the patient does not have easy access to healthcare. On the other hand it brings on all the problems of needle use and disposal, besides being traumatic to a young child.
- Oral administration of a single large dose results in peak 25(OH)D at 1 week, with a plateau till 3 weeks, levels declining thereafter to return to baseline by 2 to 2.5 months.[18]
- Daily smaller doses of 1000 to 5000 units take 2−3 months to achieve stable levels and plateau.[19]

There is no study in children which has addressed all of the following issues together: finding the minimum dose (to minimise cost and toxicity) which raises serum 25(OH)D by 15 to 20 ng/mL, produces quick resolution of elevated alkaline phosphatase, and does not cause hypercalcaemia or hypercalciuria.

Using oral regimens, in 2003, Cesur et al showed that while a single oral dose of 150,000 U could safely heal rickets in infants, hypercalcaemia was present in infants given larger doses of 300,000 U and 600,000 U.[20] Similarly, Markestad *et al* using 3 doses of 600,000 U, Zeghoud et al using 2 doses of 300,000 and 600,000 U and Gordon et al using 50,000 U/week for 6 weeks, orally as prevention in infants, have shown hypercalcaemia or elevated serum 25(OH)D in some of their subjects.[21,22,23]

Intramuscular (IM) use was documented by Soliman et al who studied single-dose injection of 10,000 U/kg (maximum 150,000 U) cholecalciferol IM in infants and toddlers with rickets.[24] Serum calcium, phosphorus and 25(OH)D concentrations normalised at 1 month after injection and alkaline phosphatase and PTH normalised at 3 months. Complete radiological healing occurred in 95% of the children by 3 months. There was no documented hypercalcaemia in any child. Similar treatment efficacy at 3 months was documented in adolescents with severe vitamin D deficiency with a single dose of 10,000 IU/kg (maximum 600,000 IU) IM cholecalciferol.[25] Urinary calcium excretion, which is an early marker of vitamin D toxicity, was not documented in these studies.

Bearing in mind the available information, compliance issues in developing countries, the prohibitive cost of monitoring serum 25(OH)D before and during therapy, the undesirable implications of needle use, and pending more stringent safety and efficacy studies, in regions where vitamin D deficiency is common, it might be safe to use smaller oral stoss doses for *treatment*, such as 30,000 U (in newborns and younger infants) to 60,000 U (in older infants and toddlers) once a month for 3 months, followed by a preventive regimen. For older children there is better evidence for the use of 100,000 units repeated 3 times over 4−6 months, then annual ongoing doses according to need.

Prevention of Vitamin D Deficiency

For *routine prevention*, 400 U daily for newborns and infants (or 4000 to 6000 U daily to lactating mother to increase her breast milk vitamin D to a comparable level) of oral vitamin D for 6 months have been shown to be safe and effective.[26] Similarly, regimens giving 2000 U/day for 6 weeks in older infants and toddlers[23] and 14,000 U/week orally for 1 year in adolescents[27] have also been shown to be safe and effective.

Overall, there is inadequate evidence to support routine stoss dosing of infants for prevention of D deficiency, and smaller daily doses may be preferred until more data is available. However, assessment of need must be made in individual cases, based on likelihood of severe maternal vitamin D deficiency contributing to a vitamin D-deplete infant and to whether clinical review of the patient will be possible. In addition cost is a potential consideration, as daily oral doses of vitamin D may be more expensive for families than stoss oral doses. The doses would have to be tailored to the type of preparations in the market.

For older children, a dose of 60,000 to 100,000 Units given once in 2 to 3 months should be safe.

Who Should Get Routine Preventive Supplementation?

- In light of increasing evidence of vitamin D deficiency in exclusively breast-fed infants, and the serious implications thereof, it is prudent to provide supplementation throughout infancy. A dose of 400 IU per day has been recommended by the American Academy of Pediatrics.[16]
- Beyond infancy, the vulnerable groups are those who will not have sufficient exposure of their skin, and whose physiology demands greater vitamin D and calcium. This includes preterm babies, adolescent girls, women, especially those pregnant and lactating, and the elderly.
- High-risk groups also include those in whom altered vitamin D and calcium absorption and metabolism occur. This includes all children on *anticonvulsant medication* and those with conditions of malabsorption.

Adequate treatment of rickets, occurring due to either dietary calcium deficiency, or vitamin D deficiency, requires provision of generous doses of calcium, generally 1 g daily, for 6 months, along with ensuring age-appropriate daily calcium intake subsequently. All calcium salts have equal bioavailability that is equivalent to that of milk. Calcium carbonate is the cheapest calcium salt with highest amount of elemental calcium (40%).

Vitamin D Toxicity

Intoxication due to excess vitamin D intake is not a rarity.[28] The lipophilic nature of vitamin D and its long tissue half-life (2 months for cholecalciferol) augments the risk of toxicity. Though serum 25(OH)D greater than 100 ng/mL (250 nmol/L) is traditionally considered as a toxic level, hypercalcaemia ensues when the levels are persistently above 150 ng/mL (374 nmol/L) *as seen in adults*.

Intake of doses up to 10,000 U daily *in adults* has been shown to be safe.

Symptoms of acute vitamin D intoxication include nausea, vomiting, constipation, anorexia, polyuria and polydipsia. Severe cases progress to acute fulminant renal failure and cardiac arrhythmias culminating in death.

Therapeutic options include induced emesis and activated charcoal, in acute oral intoxication, saline diuresis, loop diuretics (furosemide), glucocorticoids, phosphate binders, bisphosphonates and calcitonin.

Surgical/orthopaedic treatment of rachitic deformities, if they come in the way of normal ambulation and play, should be undertaken only after complete biochemical and radiological healing of rickets, which may take 18 to 24 months. Mild to moderate deformity normalises over many years with remodelling. Surgery is usually only necessary if deformities interfere with normal ambulation and play.

Effective utilisation of the freely available natural sunshine can be achieved by encouraging outdoor play and activities, adequate culturally acceptable exposure of skin and discouraging overzealous use of sunscreen or avoidance of sun exposure.

Metabolic Rickets

The suspicion that the child we are dealing with does not have simple nutritional rickets should come up when no sign of healing is visible clinically, biochemically or radiologically, after adequate vitamin D and calcium replenishment.

- Though complete radiological healing of nutritional rickets may take 12 to 24 months, alkaline phosphatase should show a downward trend by 1 month.
- If there is no response in another month, after ensuring compliance, one should commence investigation for a metabolic cause of rickets.
- The finding of a clue to the presence of a metabolic condition, such as alopecia or nephrocalcinosis (Table 7.6), may prompt a search for the aetiology right at the initial visit.

Categorisation into two major types of rickets, calcipenic or calcium-deficiency type,

TABLE 7.6 Clinical Clues to the Aetiology of Rickets

Clinical clue	Possible aetiology
Alopecia	VDDR Type II
Bitot spots, corneal ulcer	Malabsorption
Cataract/corneal opacity/KF ring	Proximal RTA
Deafness	Distal RTA
Posterior urethral valve	Distal RTA
Dental abscess	XLH
Delayed dental eruption	Vitamin D deficiency
Enamel hypoplasia	Vitamin D deficiency
Tetany, stridor, seizure	Calcium/vitamin D deficiency, VDDR I and II
Excessive sweating, raised intracranial tension, café-au-lait spots	Fibrous dysplasia

Notes: RTA — renal tubular acidosis; XLH — X-linked hypophosphataemic rickets.

TABLE 7.7 Differentiation Between Calcipenic and Phosphopenic Rickets

Features	Calcipenic rickets	Phosphopenic rickets
CLINICAL		
Proximal myopathy	Present	Absent
Bone pain	Marked	Minimal
Tetany	Present	Absent
Enamel hypoplasia	Present	Absent
Dental abscess	Absent	Present
Osteopenia	Present	Absent (dense bones)
BIOCHEMICAL		
Serum calcium	Low	Normal
Serum phosphorus	Low	Low
Alkaline phosphatase	Markedly elevated	Elevated
PTH	Elevated	Normal/mildly elevated
Osteitis fibrosa	Present	Absent

and phosphopenic or phosphorus-deficiency type, helps in differential diagnosis. The clinical and biochemical characteristics of the two types are highlighted in Table 7.7.

It must be noted that the finding of low serum phosphorus does not necessarily indicate the diagnosis of phosphopenic rickets. This is because all causes of calcipenic rickets, whether nutritional or metabolic, give rise to secondary hyperparathyroidism, which itself is a cause of Fanconi syndrome, leading to phosphate leak from the proximal renal tubule and thus hypophosphataemia. The most useful differentiating test is serum PTH, which is normal to minimally raised in phosphate deficiency rickets and significantly raised in any type of calcium deficiency rickets (Figure 7.4).

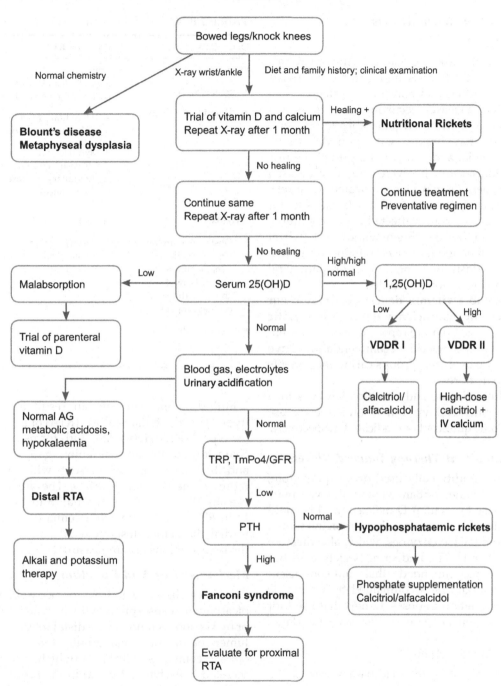

FIGURE 7.4 Approach to resistant rickets.

Calcium Deficiency Rickets

MALABSORPTION

Coeliac disease, regional enteritis or Crohn's disease, cystic fibrosis and chronic giardiasis are some of the conditions in this category.

Coeliac disease, occurring due to gluten intolerance, with raised antibodies to transglutaminase, may present with iron deficiency-type anaemia, abdominal pain, growth failure, short stature, and if severe and unrecognised for long periods may be complicated by rickets. The upper gastrointestinal tract, the site for calcium absorption, is affected in this condition. Once treatment by gluten withdrawal (wheat and all other foods which contain any gluten at all) is instituted, high-dose or parenteral vitamin D is no longer needed.

Fat-soluble vitamin deficiencies may occur in pancreatic insufficiency states such as cystic fibrosis, which require repeated doses of parenteral vitamin D. Specific recommendations have been made by expert groups caring for patients with cystic fibrosis.

Crohn's disease and chronic giardiasis may require parenteral vitamin D until the disease has become quiescent or eradicated, respectively.

Anticonvulsant Therapy Induced Rickets

All the traditionally used drugs, phenytoin, phenobarbitone, carbamazepine and valproate predispose to vitamin D deficiency. This could be attributable to the fact they are activators of cytochrome P450 enzymes, which also metabolise vitamin D. The Endocrine Society USA has recently recommended that anticonvulsant therapy should be accompanied by vitamin D supplementation in doses 3 times that used for other children, i.e. perhaps 1200 units per day.[29]

Renal Tubular Acidosis

Maintenance of the acid-base status of the blood and body is a key function performed by the proximal and distal renal tubules. Any primary or secondary disturbance of these

TABLE 7.8 Causes of Renal Tubular Acidosis

Distal RTA	Proximal RTA
Primary	Primary
• Sporadic	Sporadic (can be isolated or part of Fanconi syndrome)
• Hereditary	• Hereditary (cystinosis, galactosaemia, Lowe
	• syndrome, Wilson disease, tyrosinemia, hereditary fructose intolerance)
Secondary	Secondary
• Obstructive uropathy, vesicoureteric reflux, pyelonephritis, lupus nephritis, medullary sponge kidney, sickle cell nephropathy	• Drugs such as gentamicin, cyclosporine, tacrolimus, heavy metals
• Drugs such as amphotericin B, cisplatin.	

acidification mechanisms can result in distal (type 1) renal tubular acidosis (RTA) or proximal (or type 2) RTA (Table 7.8). Both forms of RTA, characterised by normal anion gap acidosis and hypokalemia, can present with rickets, more so the proximal variety. The anion gap (serum Na + K − Cl) is normal (8 to 12 mEq/L) in RTA due to hyperchloraemia (in contrast to diabetic ketoacidosis or renal failure where the excess anions are unmeasured).

Mechanisms of Acid Excretion

Acid can be excreted from the body either by bicarbonate reabsorption in the proximal tubule or by H+ ion secretion in the distal tubule. In the lumen of the proximal tubule, filtered bicarbonate combines with H+ (which has been secreted in exchange for Na) in the presence of carbonic anhydrase to form carbon dioxide and water. Carbon dioxide diffuses across the luminal membrane, to enter the proximal tubular cell. Here again it combines with water to produce bicarbonate, which then diffuses through the basolateral membrane into the capillary. Thus, there occurs only reabsorption of the filtered bicarbonate in the proximal tubule, no net acid secretion.

Net acid secretion, of about 1 mEq/kg/day, occurs in the distal tubule. H+ ion secretion is brought about by a variety of pumps or exchangers, such as the H+/ATPase pump or the HCO3-/Cl- exchanger. H+ is excreted in urine complexed with bicarbonate, ammonia or titratable acids such as phosphate.

Distal Renal Tubular Acidosis

Inherited genetic defects in these exchangers or their destruction by obstructive uropathy or antibody as in Sjogren syndrome results in diminished or absent function of secretion of H+ ion.

- Kaliuria (leading to hypokalemia) and hypercalciuria are accompanied by polyuria.
- Acidosis results in failure to thrive, resorption of bone and rickets.
- Calciuria, coupled with hypocitraturia, results in nephrocalcinosis and nephrolithiasis, with progressive renal failure if untreated.

Treatment with alkali results in decrease of the polyuria, kaliuria and calciuria, normalisation of acid-base status, regression of failure to thrive and healing of rickets without any high-dose vitamin D therapy.

DIAGNOSIS

The diagnosis is suspected in the setting of rickets not responding to nutritional therapy, or even earlier by the presence of hypokalemia, polyuria and the incidental finding of nephrocalcinosis on ultrasonography. Biochemically, raised alkaline phosphatase and hypokalemia are accompanied by metabolic acidosis with normal anion gap and alkaline urinary pH, and elevated PTH.

If distal RTA is suspected and frank acidosis is not present, it has to be induced by an ammonium chloride loading test.

- Before performing this, absence of urine infection is documented by a simple routine urine microscopy.
- The child is allowed to slowly sip 0.1 g/kg of ammonium chloride, mixed in some juice to make it palatable.
- Induction of acidosis is confirmed by a venous blood gas sample, after 2 hours. Hourly urine pH should be measured for 5 hours after administration of ammonium chloride, using a pH meter, on freshly passed samples.

If all values remain above 5.5, the presence of distal RTA is confirmed.

TREATMENT

Treatment may be given by sodium bicarbonate (0.325 g contains 4 mEq of alkali) (dose of alkali is 1 to 3 mEq/kg/day, to be increased gradually to avoid abdominal distension) or by a solution containing sodium or potassium citrate. These have the benefit of providing citrate, which protects further against nephrocalcinosis, and potassium, which may be needed (1 to 2 mEq/kg/day) to tackle the hypokalaemia. These solutions typically contain 2 mEq/mL each, of alkali and potassium (Table 7.9).

Monitoring is done via serum alkaline phosphatase, potassium, growth and radiological healing. In young children, in addition to deficient H+ ion secretion, some loss of bicarbonate also occurs, necessitating a higher dose of alkali, which diminishes as the child grows older.

Proximal Renal Tubular Acidosis

Proximal RTA may occur due to an isolated defect of bicarbonate reabsorption or may be associated with defective reabsorption of

TABLE 7.9 Composition of Phosphate and Alkali
               Solutions

FOR HYPOPHOSPHATAEMIA:

1. Neutral phosphate tablets in doses of 1 to 4 g/day, in four
   to six divided doses.

2. Joulie's solution: dissolve 136 g dibasic sodium
   phosphate and 58.8 g phosphoric acid in 1 litre of water.
   Concentration of inorganic phosphate is 30.4 μg/mL
   solution. Alternatively, 3.66 g of disodium hydrogen
   phosphate and 1 g sodium dihydrogen phosphate can be
   dissolved in 60 mL of water, to give 1 g elemental
   phosphorus in each 60 mL.

FOR RENAL TUBULAR ACIDOSIS:

1. Sodium bicarbonate tablet: 0.325 g of sodium bicarbonate
   contains 4 mEq of bicarbonate.

2. Potassium citrate solution: generally contain 2 mEq of
   alkali and 2 mEq of K+ per mL solution.

---

potassium, phosphorus, amino acids, uric acid
and glucose (Fanconi syndrome). These could
in turn be due to inherited defects in pumps
and exchangers, or secondary to systemic
diseases (Table 7.4). In contrast to distal RTA,
since H+ ion secretion is normal, urine pH can
become acidic in proximal RTA.

DIAGNOSIS

- Clinical features include failure to thrive,
  hypokalemia, polyuria and rickets. Since
  citrate reabsorption in the proximal tubule
  is affected, urinary citrate concentration is
  high, preventing nephrocalcinosis or
  nephrolithiasis.
- Biochemical features are similar to those of
  distal RTA.
- Confirmation of diagnosis is by
  demonstrating fractional excretion of
  bicarbonate of greater than 15%, by
  measuring simultaneous urine and blood
  bicarbonate during a bicarbonate loading
  test.

If facilities for direct urine bicarbonate estimation are not available, demonstration of

rickets with normal anion gap metabolic
acidosis, hypokalemia, glycosuria, phosphaturia (see below in hypophosphataemic rickets),
in the absence of elevated PTH (which itself
causes Fanconi syndrome) will aid in confirming the diagnosis.

TREATMENT

Treatment is by alkali supplementation, in
doses larger than those used for distal RTA
(5 to 15 mEq/kg/day of alkali). Potassium
supplementation may also be required. If phosphaturia is present, rickets will not heal without
phosphate supplementation (see below for
hypophosphataemic rickets).

Monitoring is by growth rate, cessation of
polyuria, healing of rickets, normalisation of
serum alkaline phosphatase and potassium.

Both proximal and distal RTA are serious
diseases, which can lead to severe morbidity
and even mortality. During stress, there may
be a transient need for higher doses of alkali or
potassium.

Family screening after a proband is diagnosed may help save a life.

Vitamin D Resistance

In many countries, availability of vitamin D
assays is limited and these tests are not
commonly performed at time of presentation
of a child who has rickets. When all the clinical features of rickets are present but the
child fails to respond to standard treatment
regimes, vitamin D resistance should be
considered. A careful family history should
be sought for evidence of a heritable type of
rickets.

Vitamin D Resistant Rickets Type 1
(1 α Hydroxylase Defect)

Mutations of the gene encoding the 1
α hydroxylase enzyme cause rickets which presents in the latter half of infancy, with all the
features of nutritional rickets.

DIAGNOSIS

Serum 25(OH)D is normal, and 1,25(OH)$_2$D is low or inappropriately normal (with normal amount of substrate 25(OH)D and highly elevated PTH, 1,25(OH)$_2$D would be expected to be high, and thus a normal value is actually to be interpreted as 'low').

TREATMENT

The rickets responds to calcitriol (30 to 70 ng/kg/day) or 1α-hydroxyvitamin D (which has to undergo 25 hydroxylation in the liver) in slightly higher than replacement doses initially and later physiological replacement doses. The latter formulation has a longer half-life than calcitriol and can be given once a day. It is also available in tablet form, aiding dosages for newborns and young infants, unlike calcitriol which is available only in soft capsule form. Though it appears less costly than calcitriol, it is also less potent and may need to be given in double the dose.

Vitamin D-Resistant Rickets Type 2 (Calcitriol Receptor Defect)

Mutations in the vitamin D receptor lead to a rare variety of severe rickets presenting during infancy, with hypocalcaemia, seizures and alopecia.

CLINICAL FEATURES

The clinical features show a spectrum, with some patients having milder disease or no alopecia.

TREATMENT

Severely affected patients require continuous IV calcium infusions through a central line, for control of seizures and healing. Once healing is complete, it may be possible in some patients to manage them on high doses of calcitriol and oral calcium.

Phosphorus Deficiency Type of Rickets

Hypophosphataemic rickets typically presents towards the end of infancy, when the child starts to stand erect. Bossing and genu varum (bow legs) are prominent, with very little by way of rachitic signs on the chest or upper extremities. Muscle tone is usually normal, and bone pain is not prominent. The prototype is X-linked hypophosphataemic rickets.

X-Linked Hypophosphataemic Rickets (XLH)

XLH may be sporadic or inherited by X-linked dominant inheritance. Thus, all daughters of an affected father will be born affected, and none of the sons. An affected mother has a statistical risk of passing on her disease to half of her daughters and sons. XLH occurs due to mutations in the PHEX (PHosphate-regulating gene with homologies to endopeptidases on the X chromosome) gene, which result in altered FGF23, a phosphaturic substance.

CLINICAL FEATURES

Hypophosphataemia and inadequate production of calcitriol in the kidney, also a feature of this condition, result in rickets. Since there is no hypocalcaemia, seizures, hypotonia and elevated PTH are not features. In addition to the characteristics mentioned above, dental caries may be observed, and dense bones with coarse trabecular pattern, seen on plain radiology.

DIAGNOSIS

The diagnosis is confirmed by documenting lack of renal phosphate reabsorption in the face of hypophosphataemia. Since phosphaturia is the normal mechanism of the body for keeping serum phosphorus in a normal range, tubular reabsorption simultaneous with a serum phosphorus (TmP/GFR) is needed to confirm the diagnosis.

- Fasting serum phosphorus and creatinine are estimated.
- A simultaneous second void urine (passed about 30 minutes after emptying the bladder) is estimated for urine phosphorus and creatinine.

FIGURE 7.5 Nomogram for deriving urinary phosphate reabsorption linked to glomerular filtration rate (TmP/GFR).

Note: Phosphate clearance is calculated by the formula (urine/serum phosphorus) / (urine/serum creatinine), the tests being performed on morning spot urine and simultaneous fasting serum samples. The clearance, or reabsorption (1 − clearance), can be read off from the diagonal. Serum phosphorus and TmP/GFR are expressed in mg/dL as well as in mmol/L. (*Reprinted with permission from Elsevier: The Lancet 1975; 2:309–10.*)

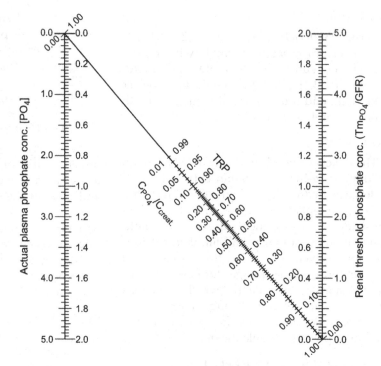

- Phosphate clearance is calculated as [urine/serum P] / [urine/serum creatinine]. The TmP/GFR can be read off on the nomogram given in Figure 7.5. The normal value reflects normal serum P for age, being higher in infants and decreasing in older children. A low value is consistent with the diagnosis of hypophosphataemic rickets.

TREATMENT

- Treatment of rickets is by phosphate supplementation. This is given as a solution of neutral phosphate (Table 7.9), the volume per dose to be very gradually increased over several weeks (to avoid abdominal distension and diarrhoea) to reach a daily dose of 1 g elemental phosphorus.
- Since absorbed phosphorus is not retained for long, doses have to be divided to cover as many waking hours as possible, the first dose

on waking up and the last dose at bedtime. If healing is not achieved radiologically and biochemically (normalisation of alkaline phosphatase) by 1 g phosphate, then doses can be very gradually increased to 2 or 3 g of phosphate.
- Phosphate therapy results in secondary hyperparathyroidism. This is kept in check by calcitriol (20 to 70 ng/kg/day in 2 divided doses).
- Urine calcium: creatinine ratio is kept less than 0.2, to avoid calciuria and nephrocalcinosis.
- Hypercalciuria is treated by thiazide diuretic (hydrochlorothiazide 2 mg/kg/day).

Successful treatment of hypophosphataemic rickets is not easy. Compliance is an issue, due to the distressing abdominal side effects. Even with good compliance and bone healing, short stature remains an unresolved issue in many of these children.

Metabolic Bone Disease of Prematurity

A preterm baby is deprived of the amount of calcium and phosphorus delivered to the fetus transplacentally by active transport during the third trimester. This rich amount of mineral cannot be duplicated in human or other milk. Without it, the baby quickly develops serious bone disease with components of rickets as well as osteoporosis, resulting in serious fractures on normal handling in the neonatal ICU. Serum calcium is usually normal, serum P low and alkaline phosphatase elevated. This condition is well recognised, and prevention is now routine, with human milk fortifiers which can supplement expressed breast milk, and provide about 200 mg/kg/day of elemental calcium and 100 mg/kg/day of elemental phosphorus.

References

1. Brown EM, Macleod RJ. Extracellular calcium sensing and extracellular calcium signaling. *Physiol Rev* 2001;**81**:239–97.
2. Hoenderop JG, Nilius R, Bindels RJ. Calcium absorption across epithelia. *Physiol Rev* 2005;**85**:373–422.
3. Shimada T, Kakitani M, Yamazaki Y, et al. Targeted ablation of FGF23 demonstrates an essential physiological role of FGF23 in phosphate and vitamin D metabolism. *J Clin Invest* 2004;**113**:561–8.
4. Cole DEC, Quamme GA. Inherited disorders of renal magnesium handling. *J Am Soc Nephrol* 2000;**11**:1937–47.
5. Mantovani G, de Sanctis L, Barbieri AM, et al. Pseudohypoparathyroidism and GNAS epigenetic defects: clinical evaluation of Albright hereditary osteodystrophy and molecular analysis in 40 patients. *J Clin Endocrinol Metab* 2010;**95**:651–8.
6. Holick MF. Environmental factors that influence the cutaneous production of vitamin D. *Am J Clin Nutr* 1995;**61**:S638–45.
7. Manson JE, Mayne ST, Clinton SK. Vitamin D and prevention of cancer: ready for prime time? *N Engl J Med* 2011;**364**:1385–7.
8. Rosen CJ. Vitamin D insufficiency. *N Engl J Med* 2011;**364**:248–54.
9. Rao DS, Parfitt AM, Kleerkoper M, et al. Dissociation between the effects of endogenous parathyroid hormone on adenosine 3', 5'-monophosphate generation and phosphate reabsorption in hypocalcemia due to vitamin D depletion: an acquired disorder resembling pseudohypoparathyroidism type II. *J Clin Endocrinol Metab* 1985;**61**:285–90.
10. Perheentupa J. Autoimmune polyendocrinopathy-candidiasis-ectodermal dysplasia. *J Clin Endocrinol Metab* 2006;**91**:2843–50.
11. Lienhardt A, Bai M, Lagarde JP, et al. Activating mutations of the calcium sensing receptor: management of hypocalcemia. *J Clin Endocrinol Metab* 2001;**86**:5313–23.
12. Joshi RR. Hypercalcemia due to hypervitaminosis D: report of seven patients. *J Trop Pediatr* 2009;**55**:396–8.
13. Mallet E. Primary hyperparathyroidism in neonates and childhood: the French experience (1984 to 2004). *Horm Res* 2008;**69**:180–8.
14. Holick MF. Environmental factors that influence the cutaneous production of vitamin D. *Am J Clin Nutr* 1995;**61**:S638–45.
15. Institute of Medicine. *Dietary Reference Intakes for Calcium and Vitamin D.* Washington DC: National Academies Press; 2011.
16. Wagner CL, Greer FR. American Academy of Pediatrics Section on Breast-feeding, American Academy of Pediatrics Committee on Nutrition. Prevention of rickets and vitamin D deficiency in infants, children, and adolescents. *Pediatrics* 2008;**122**:1142–52.
17. Thacher TD, Fischer PR, Pettifor JM, et al. A comparison of calcium, vitamin D, or both for nutritional rickets in Nigerian children. *N Engl J Med* 1999;**341**:563–8.
18. Ilahi M, Armas LAG, Heaney RP. Pharmacokinetics of a single large dose of cholecalciferol. *Am J Clin Nutr* 2008;**87**:688–91.
19. Heaney RP, Davies KM, Chen TC, et al. Human serum 25-hydroxycholecalciferol response to extended oral dosing with cholecalciferol. *Am J Clin Nutr* 2003;**77**:204–10.
20. Cesur Y, Caksen H, Gundem A, et al. Comparison of low and high dose of vitamin D treatment in nutritional vitamin D deficiency rickets. *J Pediatr Endocrinol Metab* 2003;**16**:1105–9.
21. Markestad T, Hesse V, Siebenhuner M, et al. Intermittent high dose vitamin D prophylaxis during infancy: effect on vitamin D metabolites, calcium, and phosphorus. *Am J Clin Nutr* 1987;**46**:652–8.
22. Zeghoud F, Ben-Mekhbi H, Djeghri N, et al. Vitamin D prophylaxis during infancy: comparison of the long-term effects of three intermittent doses (15, 5, or 2.5 mg) on 25 hydroxy vitamin D concentrations. *Am J Clin Nutr* 1994;**60**:393–6.

23. Gordon CM, Williams AL, Feldman HA, et al. Treatment of hypovitaminosis D in infants and toddlers. *J Clin Endocrinol Metab* 2008;**93**:2716—21.

24. Soliman AT, El-Dabbagh M, Adel A, et al. Clinical responses to a mega-dose of vitamin D3 in infants and toddlers with vitamin D deficiency rickets. *J Trop Pediatr* 2010;**56**:19—26.

25. Soliman AT, Adel A, Wagdy M, et al. Manifestations of severe vitamin D deficiency in adolescents: effects of intramuscular injection of a megadose of cholecalciferol. *J Trop Pediatr* 2011;**57**:303—6.

26. Wagner CL, Howard C, Hollis BW, et al. Circulating 25-hydroxyvitamin D levels in fully breastfed infants on oral vitamin D supplementation. *Int J Endocrinol* 2010;**2010**:235035.

27. Maalouf J, Nabulsi M, Vieth R, et al. Short- and long-term safety of weekly high-dose vitamin D3 supplementation in school children. *J Clin Endocrinol Metab* 2008;**93**:2693—701.

28. Joshi R. Hypercalcemia due to hypervitaminosis D: report of seven patients. *J Trop Pediatr* 2009;**55**: 396—8.

29. Holick MF, Binkley NC, Bischoff-Ferrari HA, et al. Evaluation, treatment and prevention of vitamin D deficiency. An endocrine society clinical practice guideline. *J Clin Endocrinol Metab* 2011;**96**:1911—30.

Disturbances of Sodium and Water

Ursula Kuhnle-Kral, Joshua Kausman

INTRODUCTION

Disturbances of sodium and water are among the commonest derangements encountered in hospitalised patients, especially in paediatric patients, due to the prevalence of diseases associated with dehydration. A small proportion of patients will have rarer underlying causes, requiring specialised testing, some of which may be time-consuming or impractical to perform due to lack of local resources. Nonetheless, the initial approach to assessing and safely managing these patients is critical and can be easily performed in most centres.

The purpose of this chapter is to provide an understanding of the basic physiology of water and sodium balance as well as the breadth of common and rarer causes. An approach to basic

Practical Pediatric Endocrinology in a Limited Resource Setting
http://dx.doi.org/10.1016/B978-0-12-407822-2.00008-6

investigations and initial management will be emphasised, but relevant specialised testing will also be described.

PATHOPHYSIOLOGY

The body fluid compartments are divided into two-thirds intracellular and one-third extracellular, with the latter subdivided into interstitial and intravascular. Control of fluid volume and sodium homeostasis is essential in protecting the integrity of these compartments.

Water Regulation

The regulation and the stability of plasma osmolality is an extremely important system and tightly regulated despite large variations in water consumption or water loss. Serum osmolality is controlled by receptors and organs of the hypothalamic-neurohypophyseal axis which includes organs responsible for sensing plasma osmolality and volume, and the synthesis and secretion of the antidiuretic hormone 'vasopressin (AVP)'. The osmoregulatory system also regulates thirst and drinking behaviour and is stimulated by osmotic changes in plasma. The kidney — the renal collecting duct — is responsive to vasopressin and varies urinary flow in order to maintain water balance.

Thus, three factors are involved in the regulation of water balance:

1. vasopressin synthesis and secretion
2. the kidney's response to vasopressin
3. thirst.

Vasopressin

The peptides arginine vasopressin (antidiuretic hormone, AVP) and oxytocin are synthesised in the supraoptic and paraventricular nuclei of the hypothalamus and transported via the supraopticohypophyseal tract through the pituitary stalk to the posterior pituitary. The secretion is then stimulated and regulated via osmo-receptors and volume (baro)-receptors.

The osmotically sensitive cells are located in the anterior hypothalamus whereas the volume receptors are situated in the atria of the heart and the great veins of the chest and the carotid body and the arch of the aorta.

Normal osmolality ranges from 280 to 300 mOsm/kg H_2O. The osmoreceptor is very sensitive and AVP secretion is stimulated by an increase of as little as 1% of serum osmolality.

Thirst

Thirst is sensed at a plasma osmolality of 295 mOsm/kg H_2O, which causes a maximal stimulation of AVP with a high urine osmolality.

Kidney and Water Regulation

The main physiologic function of vasopressin is the concentration of urine. Vasopressin binds to specific receptors (V2-receptor) along the basolateral membrane of the tubular cells of the distal collecting ducts of the nephron, which stimulate the insertion of water channels (aquaporin-2) into the luminal membrane, thereby promoting reabsorption of water.

Under the influence of AVP, urine is concentrated and urine flow decreases, causing urine osmolality to rise to a maximum of 800—1200 mOsm/kg in humans.

Alternatively, free water clearance is possible when AVP secretion is suppressed. This decreases water reabsorption in the collecting duct, resulting in a urine osmolality as low as 50—100 mOsm/kg.

Sodium Regulation

Sodium accounts for over 90% of the osmotically active solute. It is the main determinant of the extracellular fluid (ECF) and hence the water content of the body. The sodium level and the water content of the body are tightly regulated by a variety of control mechanisms and through these regulatory mechanisms the amount of sodium excreted equals the amount of sodium ingested. The excretion of sodium can vary from 1 mmol/day on a low-sodium diet to 400 mmol/day on a high-sodium diet.

- The most important regulatory system of sodium balance is the renin-angiotensin-aldosterone system. Aldosterone, the most potent naturally occurring mineralocorticoid, is synthesised in the zona glomerulosa of the adrenal gland and is regulated by the renin-angiotensin-system (RAS).
- Renin is produced by juxta-glomerular cells in the nephron, located at the junction of the afferent arteriole, efferent arteriole and distal convoluted tubule. This provides a tailored sensor to monitor glomerular perfusion and tubular flow, in turn establishing a rapid capacity to alter RAS activity in response to shifts in fluid state.
- The other potent stimulator of aldosterone is potassium, while ACTH and vasopressin transiently stimulate aldosterone secretion.

Mechanism of Aldosterone Action

As with other steroid hormones, the actions of aldosterone are mediated by an intracellular receptor. The aldosterone or mineralocorticoid receptor is closely related to the progesterone, androgen and glucocorticoid receptors, and more distantly to the oestrogen receptor within the nuclear receptor superfamily.

Aldosterone exerts its physiological action by binding to receptors that belong to the steroid/thyroid/retinoid receptor family of ligand-dependent transcription factors. Aldosterone regulates sodium homeostasis by stimulating sodium reabsorption in the distal nephron and the distal colon. The response in these epithelia is mediated via the amiloride-sensitive sodium channel in the apical membrane and the energy-dependent sodium pump (Na^+/K^+-ATPase) in the basolateral membrane. These receptors, channels and pumps are linked together and form a complex system that is regulated and controlled at various levels.

The molecular and genetic basis of the response is known for a number of the components. Mutations causing defects or overactivity of these pathways are the basis for a variety of inherited diseases whose clinical picture is either that of salt retention or salt loss.

In addition to aldosterone and cortisol, a number of steroids may act as agonists at the mineralocorticoid receptor including deoxycorticosterone (DOC) and the synthetic steroid 9-a-fludrocortisone (Florinef®). Other synthetic steroids such as 9-a-fluoroprednisolone also have unexpected mineralocorticoid activity. Their administration in nasal sprays has been associated with mineralocorticoid-like side effects. Several steroids in therapeutic use, able to act as antagonists of the mineralocorticoid receptor, are spironolactone and eplerenone.

While the most important organ system for sodium regulation is the kidney, sodium can also be lost via other organ systems — particularly the gastrointestinal tract. Acute diarrhoea is associated with salt and water loss, and depending upon the infective agent results either in hyponatraemic or hypernatraemic dehydration. The diagnosis can usually be made on clinical grounds.

CLINICAL FEATURES OF DISTURBED SALT AND WATER BALANCE

The reliable assessment of the fluid state of a child is essential in ensuring safe management and correct diagnosis of the underlying disorder. A history of excessive fluid losses (diarrhoea, vomiting, polyuria), lethargy, observed rapid weight loss, tachycardia, blood pressure, oedema, skin turgor and capillary refill time are a simple group of clinical features to assess, but are reliable and integral to subsequent management.

Estimation of dehydration (equivalent to percentage of body weight loss) allows calculation of targets for volume replenishment and are categorised as follows: Mild 3–5%; Moderate 6–10%; Severe/Shock 10–15%. The normal range for serum sodium is 135–145 mEq/L. Features of deranged sodium are largely neurological and can be subtle and insidious, even in extreme cases. Non-specific symptoms of headache, lethargy, irritability and confusion may progress to loss of consciousness and seizures.

AETIOLOGY AND INVESTIGATIONS FOR HYPONATRAEMIA

Hyponatraemia is diagnosed on the basis of the serum sodium, but can occur in association with reduced, normal or increased volume states, depending on the cause. A methodical approach depends on the assessment of these parameters and further information on the serum and urine osmolalities and electrolyte levels will direct the clinician to the diagnosis in the majority of cases.

Clinical assessment of volume state is the first step and assessment of urine sodium is the second step. Measurement of sodium excretion in other body fluids, like the faeces and the saliva, is tedious and usually does not help much in the clinical diagnosis. The sequence of investigations logically follows the steps taken after the clinical assessment and correlation with urine sodium. Basic initial investigations will include serum Na^+, K^+, Cl^-, HCO_3, osmolality and urine Na and osmolality. Appropriate tests are then conducted to distinguish the remaining differential diagnoses. Figure 8.1 outlines such an approach, incorporating the causes of hyponatraemia. Uncommonly, hyponatraemia may be fictitious, due to elevated impermeable solutes drawing water into the plasma (e.g. hyperglycaemia or mannitol) or decreased plasma water by soluble molecules (e.g. hyperlipidaemia, hyperproteinaemia).

The following section outlines the main causes of hyponatraemia and a practical approach to diagnosis and treatment. Greater detail is provided at the end of the section on endocrine disorders associated with hyponatraemia.

CLINICAL CONDITIONS WITH HYPERVOLAEMIC HYPONATRAEMIA

Organ Failure

Heart failure, liver failure and nephrotic syndrome are all characterised by **intravascular depletion**, despite the presence of generalised oedema. There is therefore a highly activated renin-angiotensin-aldosterone axis, leading to stimulation of thirst, AVP and maximal sodium and water retention from urine. This results in salt retention, but even greater fluid retention and loss of this fluid into subcutaneous and interstitial tissues due to decreased oncotic pressure in the blood.

Primary Renal Disease

Any oliguric acute or chronic kidney disease associated with damage to glomerular and tubular function can lead to **fluid overload** and hyponatraemia. This is largely dependent on the nature of fluid intake. In most situations humans consume hypotonic fluids. Therefore, excess water will result in dilution of serum sodium and expansion of the intravascular space, but the high renal perfusion pressure in concert with a damaged renal tubule will still allow sodium to leak out in the urine.

Diagnosis

- A simple initial test is to examine the urine: high levels of protein in isolation suggest nephrotic syndrome.

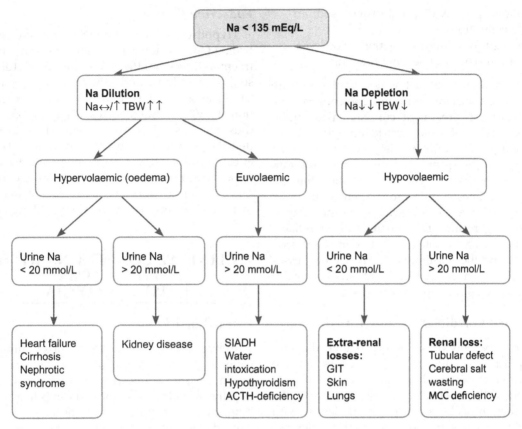

FIGURE 8.1 Causes of hyponatraemia.

Notes: TBW — total body water; GIT — gastrointestinal tract; MCC — mineralocorticoid. See text for details of individual causes.

- Urine microscopy as well as serum levels of urea, creatinine, albumin and liver enzymes can then be used to identify alternative causes.
- ECG, chest X-ray and echocardiography will be necessary for cardiac assessment.

CLINICAL CONDITIONS WITH EUVOLAEMIC HYPONATRAEMIA

Syndrome of Inappropriate Secretion of Antidiuretic Hormone (SIADH)

Inappropriate secretion of ADH occurs in adults usually as an ectopic secretion of AVP in lung cancer. In children it is associated most commonly with severe pulmonary or central nervous system infections (viral or bacterial). It is also seen following some neurosurgical procedures, particularly those around the area of the hypothalamus. The so-called 'triple response' of immediate post-operative diabetes insipidus is followed 3—10 days later by hyponatraemia and SIADH, with relapse of diabetes insipidus around 2 weeks after surgery. The cardinal features are as follows:

- hyponatremia and hypo-osmolality of the serum
- urine osmolality near or above plasma osmolality

- inappropriately elevated urinary sodium concentration
- no signs of volume depletion or oedema
- normal renal and adrenal function.

In children, the vast majority of cases are acute and transient, responding to conservative management. Treatment consists in the more severe cases of fluid restriction (50–75% of normal fluid requirements). In adults, some cases can be prolonged and may warrant specific treatments. The latter include the use of tetracyclines and, in more recent years, AVP antagonists such as tolvaptan have shown very promising results. Due to the lack of reliable paediatric data, potential for significant side effects and the self-limited nature of most cases in children, these agents should only be considered in exceptional paediatric cases.

Primary Polydipsia (Water Intoxication)

Primary polydipsia or dipsogenic diabetes insipidus in children often occurs for no apparent reason while in adults it is often associated with psychiatric illness or due to the destruction of the anterior hypothalamus with conditions like sarcoidosis or multiple sclerosis. Sometimes the child may have developed a drinking habit during an episode of stress or acute illness, with continued increased intake later becoming a habit. The problem is more commonly seen in bottle-fed children.

While vasopressin is low in primary polydipsia the renal action of vasopressin might also be impaired due to prolonged excessive fluid intake, which can reduce the kidney's concentration ability due to a 'wash out' effect on the osmotic gradient across the renal tubular cell.

In most cases the diagnosis can be made with a history of high fluid intake and polyuria, in association with a low serum osmolality and low urine osmolality. Correction occurs with restriction of fluid intake, but may take some days until the renal concentrating gradient is re-established.

Endocrine Causes

Hypothyroidism and deficiency of glucocorticoids (ACTH deficiency) can lead to hyponatraemia through effects on the distal tubule sodium handling and concentrating capacity as well as some inadvertent stimulation of secretion of AVP. Central diabetes insipidus (cDI) can thus be masked by unrecognised endocrine deficits of anterior pituitary hormones. These effects do not appear to be mediated through mineralocorticoid activity. Importantly, correction of thyroid hormone and cortisol deficits increases free water clearance, unmasking cDI.

CLINICAL CONDITIONS WITH HYPOVOLAEMIC HYPONATRAEMIA

Extra-Renal Losses

Dehydration due to an excess of sodium and water loss is most commonly due to enteric losses in gastroenteritis. Any non-renal loss will usually be evident on clinical findings (e.g. vomiting, diarrhoea, burns, cystic fibrosis, abdominal distension, heat stress) and can be confirmed by a low urine sodium concentration (usually less than 10 mmol/L).

- Acute diarrhoea is associated with salt and water loss and depending upon the infective agent results in either hyponatraemic or hypernatraemic dehydration.
- Chronic sodium loss can occur in chronic malabsorption; for example, due to short bowel syndrome.

In these patients urinary sodium excretion is extremely low and can be used as a measure of adequate replacement therapy. During adequate replacement therapy the kidneys start to excrete sodium again and an excretion of greater than 10 mmol/L of sodium is usually considered as an index of adequate replacement therapy.

Losses Due to a Renal Tubular Defect

Hyponatraemia in the context of a urine sodium greater than 20 mmol/L suggests an inappropriate natriuresis and the renal tubule is the source of sodium losses.

- This includes renal parenchymal disorder (sometimes called renal salt wasting); diuretics, nephrotoxins and inherited tubular channel defects; or mineralocorticoid resistance (see later).
- Developmental defects in the kidneys, including dysplasia, cystic kidneys, reflux nephropathy and obstructive uropathy, result in damage to the interstitium, which is critical to the concentrating capacity of the kidneys. Such children may fail to thrive and frequently present with polyuria, high urinary sodium and mild to moderate hyponatraemia. Serum electrolytes and creatinine as well as a renal ultrasound are essential for diagnosis, to exclude obstruction and to identify other structural defects.
- History of diuretic use may not always be forthcoming, but will usually present with dehydration, hyponatraemia, hypokalaemia and other electrolyte derangements and will improve with careful observation and fluid and electrolyte replacement. If there is no improvement, a primary tubular defect, such as Bartter syndrome or Gitelman syndrome will have identical findings to the chronic use of loop diuretics or thiazide diuretics, respectively. A detailed account of these disorders is beyond the scope of this chapter, but is available in a textbook of paediatric nephrology.

Cerebral Salt Wasting (CSW)

CSW results from a systemic mediator, thought to be a brain natriuretic peptide, driving a natriuresis. It occurs in a variety of intracranial disorders, including trauma, malignancy and haemorrhage. CSW is characterised by polyuria, in association with elevated urinary sodium and a low intravascular state. In some situations, the volume state can be difficult to assess without invasive monitoring and the biochemical findings can resemble SIADH.

CSW tends to occur later in the course of an interference to brain function, in contrast to acute onset of cDI which is usually manifest within hours of the insult.

One clue is the tendency for CSW to be associated with low serum uric acid levels. Serial monitoring of weight and urine output will allow the distinction to be made between CSW and SIADH. In contrast to SIADH, management requires maintenance of normal to high fluids and sodium supplementation with gradual tapering.

ENDOCRINE DISEASE

Defects of mineralocorticoid secretion or action are the major endocrine causes of sodium loss in the urine. In the absence of mineralocorticoids, primarily aldosterone, Na^+/water is lost and K^+/H^+ cannot be excreted in the distal tubule. The biochemical and clinical features are as follows.

1 Significant water loss, causing life-threatening dehydration, particularly in the neonatal period.
2 Sodium loss causing severe hyponatraemia.
3 Hyperkalaemia with a risk of life-threatening cardiac arrhythmias.
4 Acidosis.

Less severe salt loss results in failure-to-thrive and growth retardation.

Table 8.1 details the endocrine disorders associated with mineralocorticoid (MCC) deficiency and resistance. These include defects in the synthesis of mineralocorticoids as well as end-organ resistance to their action. *Details of the synthetic pathways for adrenal hormones and the*

TABLE 8.1 Summary of Endocrine Disorders Associated with Sodium Loss

Disorder	Mode of transmission	Defective protein	Gene	Sentinel findings for salt loss
Aldosterone and cortisol synthesis defects				
Congenital adrenal hypoplasia	XLR	DAX-1-protein	DAX-1 AHC/ NROB1	• Renin ↑ • Aldosterone ↓
	AD	SF-1 (Ad4BP)	FTZ-F1/SF1	
Congenital lipoid adrenal hyperplasia	AR	StAR protein	STAR	
Congenital adrenal hyperplasia (CAH)	AR	3β-hydroxysteroid dehydrogenase type II	HSD3B2	
	AR	21-hydroxylase [21OHD]	CYP21A2	
Isolated aldosterone deficiency				
Aldosterone synthase deficiency	AR	Aldosterone synthase	CYP11B2	• Renin ↑ • Aldosterone ↓
Aldosterone resistance syndromes				
PHA type I	AR	α,β γ-subunits of ENaC	βENaCGT-1 SCNN1 A,B,C	• Renin ↑ • Aldosterone ↑
PHA type I	AD	Mineralocorticoid (type I) Receptor	MLR/MCR/ WR3C2	• Renin ↑ • Aldosterone ↑
Transient PHA type I	Acquired	Not applicable	Not applicable	• Renin ↑ • Aldosterone ↑ • Urinary tract abnormality

clinical effects of glucocorticoid function (see 'Addisonian crisis') can be found in Chapter 4, Adrenal Disorders.

Congenital Adrenal Insufficiency

The most frequent causes of congenital adrenal insufficiency are associated with congenital adrenal hyperplasia (CAH), of which the most common is a defect in the 21-hydroxylase enzyme. This leads to a syndrome of androgen excess, causing virilisation of newborn female infants. The steroid pattern depends upon the enzymatic defect being both characteristic and diagnostic, but this does require some specialised laboratory facilities (*see Chapter 4 Adrenal Disorders*). However, in all cases plasma and urine aldosterone levels are low and plasma renin activity is high. In 21-hydroxylase deficient CAH, salt loss is present in 60% of affected patients. It can be confirmed when serum potassium levels are above 6 mmol/L and serum sodium falls below

130 mmol/L in association with urine sodium greater than 20 mmol/L.

Aldosterone Synthesis Defects

Defects in the final steps of aldosterone synthesis (not involving cortisol) result from autosomal recessive mutations in the aldosterone synthase gene. Sporadic cases are rare, but as with pseudohypoaldosteronism (below), in certain ethnic groups and consanguineous pedigrees these may present more commonly. Clinically, symptoms of salt loss tend to improve with age. As expected, aldosterone is very low and plasma renin high. Biochemical diagnosis is based on relative levels of 18-hydroxycorticosterone (19-OH-B), B (corticosterone), 18-OH-B and aldosterone:

- **Aldosterone synthase deficiency type I**: normal or low 19-OH-B, no aldosterone synthase activity. Ratio of B : 18-OH-B greater than 40; ratio of 18-OH-B : aldosterone less than 10.
- **Aldosterone synthase deficiency type II**: elevated 19-OH-B, aldosterone synthase retains 11-hydroxylase but not 18-oxidase activity. Ratio of B : 18-OH-B less than 10; ratio of plasma 18-OH-B : aldosterone greater than 100.

Pseudohypoaldosteronism (PHA)

Presenting a similar clinical picture to disorders of MCC synthesis, PHA is distinguished by the biochemical detection of very high levels of renin and aldosterone. Forgoing access to these investigations and the time taken to obtain results, a practical and more rapid diagnosis can be made on the basis of a lack of response to a therapeutic trial with 0.1 to 0.2 mg fludrocortisone for 2 to 3 days.

Maintenance therapy consists of an intake of high fluid, sodium chloride and sometimes sodium bicarbonate supplementation, but in severe cases, also potassium binding resins

(Na-resonium) may be required. During episodes of acute decompensation intravenous fluids and sodium are necessary. Specific treatment is curative for the transient/acquired form (see below).

PHA Type I

Autosomal recessive PHA type I is caused by an inactivating mutation in one of the three subunits of epithelial sodium channel (ENaC), located along the distal renal tubule and pulmonary epithelia. All patients reported so far are from consanguineous marriages. In addition to severe unremitting sodium loss, potassium and acid retention, these patients may exhibit pulmonary manifestations akin to those in cystic fibrosis. Most children succumb in early childhood, but even for the older child, a fatal crisis remains a risk.

Autosomal-dominant PHA type I is a mild disorder and affected family members who transmit the disorder to their offspring can often be detected biochemically, but not clinically. Although dangerous and life-threatening crises can occur during the neonatal period, in later childhood, salt loss tends to improve and a relatively mild disorder remains which does not require any therapy. Only in a minority of cases can a genetic basis be established and is found to be due to heterozygous inactivating mutations of the mineralocorticoid receptor.

Transient PHA Type I (Type IV Renal Tubular Acidosis)

Not surprisingly, any acute or chronic insult that damages the function of the renal ENaC leads to the renal phenotype of PHA. Most commonly, this reversible defect is due to a partially obstructed urinary tract, especially with superimposed pyelonephritis. Less common causes include sickle cell disease, lead nephropathy and amyloidosis. The transient form is commoner than the inherited forms of PHA or CAH. It is therefore sensible to perform urine microscopy and culture as well as a renal ultrasound in the diagnostic assessment of any child with these biochemical abnormalities. Appropriate treatment of obstruction and infection is curative.

Investigations for the Hyponatraemic Child Due to Endocrine Causes

For clinical purposes sodium loss due to hormonal deficiency can be readily diagnosed by measuring paired serum and urinary sodium, whereas resistance to the action of aldosterone can be evaluated by giving therapeutic doses of a synthetic aldosterone (fludrocortisone) which should have no effect upon the excretion of sodium. However, the initial approach requires the methodical approach outlined in Figure 8.1.

Basic Investigations for the Hyponatraemic Child

- Serum sodium, potassium, calcium, acid-base, urea, creatinine, albumin and osmolality
- Urine sodium, osmolality, dipstick for blood and protein
- Organ-specific according to the above: liver, kidney, heart, gastrointestinal.

Subsequent Investigations for the Hyponatraemic Child without a Cause Identified

- Thyroid function
- Urine microscopy and culture to exclude urosepsis and primary renal disease
- Renal ultrasound to identify parenchymal abnormalities or obstruction.

Investigations Available in Dedicated Specialised Laboratories

- Plasma renin activity, urine/plasma aldosterone, aldosterone metabolites and

precursors: all these tests require careful handling, often with critical care to maintain at 4°C immediately after collection and laboratories must have rigorous quality control to ensure reliable normal ranges. Therefore, clinicians planning to perform these tests are advised to liaise directly with the specialist laboratory for details about specimen collection, handling and transport, as well as subsequent interpretation of results.

- Urine steroid profile and short ACTH stimulation test (*see Chapter 4, Adrenal Disorders, section on laboratory investigations of CAH in the neonatal period*).
- Genetic mutational analysis (often only available on research basis in a handful of laboratories around the world and is not necessary for practical management).

MANAGEMENT OF HYPONATRAEMIA: FLUID AND SODIUM CORRECTION

Until a specific diagnosis can be made which allows a targeted treatment, the general approach to correction of hyponatraemia requires a correction of the volume state and then of any sodium deficit. In many circumstances, there will only be a need for volume correction, which will spontaneously correct the hyponatraemia. The initial management involves the following.

- **Hypovolaemic hyponatraemia**: administration of one or more boluses of 0.9% NaCl 20 mL/kg over 1 hour each to correct shock. Subsequent fluids as 0.45–0.9% NaCl according to serum sodium levels.
- **Euvolaemic hyponatraemia**: water restriction by 50–75% in SIADH or water intoxication is the key to therapy. If intravenous fluids are used, 0.9% NaCl is appropriate.

- **Hypervolaemic hyponatraemia:** fluid and salt restriction are the keys to therapy. Furosemide (0.5–1 mg/kg) can be used to promote fluid mobilisation, but only after restoration of intravascular volume in hypovolaemic cases.

Intravascular depletion associated with hypoalbuminaemia, as in cirrhosis and nephrotic syndrome, should be corrected with intravenous albumin (1 g/kg as 20% albumin over 4 hours) and the furosemide given halfway through the albumin infusion.

The major challenge is to ensure the rate of sodium rise is not too rapid as there is a conceivable risk of demyelination of the central nervous system (central pontine myelinolysis). This risk is greatest in states of chronic hyponatraemia, in which the intracellular adaptation exposes neurons to fluid shifts if extracellular sodium rises rapidly. Monitoring weight, fluid intake, urine output, urine sodium and serum sodium direct ongoing treatment.

- As a guide, the **serum sodium should rise by a maximum of 0.5 mmol/L hourly.** Any plan of treatment will require frequent revision, as the renal and endocrine responses to rehydration will themselves alter ongoing losses. Measurement of weight and serum sodium (2-hourly in severe cases) is therefore critical to ensuring safe correction.
- In cases of severe hyponatraemia, with serum sodium less than 120 mEq/L, associated with neurological disturbance, the risk of imminent seizures mandates that treatment is undertaken with extreme care. In the **life-threatening** situations of recurrent seizures, respiratory arrest or signs of brainstem herniation, 3 mmol/kg of sodium as hypertonic saline (3% NaCl) should be administered over 30 minutes to increase the serum sodium by approximately 5 mEq/L. In all other circumstances, irrespective of the level of serum sodium, the aim should remain a slow and steady rise in serum sodium by 10–12 mmol/L/24 hours.
- In moderate hyponatraemia, gradual correction of sodium should occur over 24–48 hours using 0.45–0.9% NaCl intravenously, according to successive serum sodium levels.
- Use of oral fluids for replacement is preferable to intravenous fluids as soon as the patient can tolerate these and is neurologically stable. Intestinal transport buffers against the risk of miscalculations leading to iatrogenic complications of therapy. Oral rehydration solutions may be suitable, but still require monitoring of serum sodium, potassium and fluid balance.
- Additional sodium can be supplemented orally as well. A usual starting supplemental dose is 0.5 mmol/kg twice per day. This can be done using commercial preparations of sodium chloride and sodium bicarbonate. Alternatively, these can be easily prepared in any setting by dissolving the substrate in cooled boiled water. The following directions produce a solution at the most concentrated level that can be tolerated orally by most children:
  - Sodium chloride: 1 standard imperial teaspoon of table salt is equivalent to 100 mmol of sodium. Dissolve in 100 mL to produce a 1 mmol/mL solution.
  - Sodium bicarbonate: 1 standard imperial teaspoon of table sodium bicarbonate (baking soda) is equivalent to 60 mmol of sodium. Dissolve in 60 mL to produce a 1 mmol/mL solution.

HYPERKALAEMIA

Hyperkalaemia is a frequent accompanying complication to hyponatraemia, dehydration and acidosis. Hyperkalaemia merits urgent treatment as it can lead to fatal cardiac arrhythmias. Neonates are more tolerant of higher potassium levels and rarely require treatment for potassium levels up to 6.5 mmol/L, but for older children potassium levels over 6.0 mmol/L require monitoring and treatment if they do not improve with initial fluid resuscitation.

Please note: children with high potassium levels due to endocrine disease are often used to high levels and may tolerate them without need for intervention. For endocrine disorders, as opposed to renal disorders, treatment of the underlying condition usually resolves the accompanying potassium problem.

Specific medical management of hyperkalaemia includes the following:

- Administer 10% calcium gluconate 0.5 mL/kg over 15 minutes through a reliable intravenous line (beware extravasation burns) if any of the following are present:
  - Serum potassium greater than 6.5
  - ECG shows prolonged PR interval, depressed ST, QRS widening or peaked T waves
  - Ionised calcium less than 1.10 mmol/L.

Note: this stabilises the myocardium, but does *not* affect the potassium level. Additional measures are also required. Flush line well if infusing sodium bicarbonate as well.

- Shift potassium intracellularly:
  - Sodium bicarbonate over 30 minutes: 0.3 mmol x weight x base deficit. This is usually the first line of treatment as it addresses hyperkalaemia, hyponatraemia and acidosis. Caution: it can cause hypocalcaemia and hypertension in the hypervolaemic patient.
  - Salbutamol nebulised 2.5 −5 mg per dose
  - Insulin and glucose can be used, but require careful monitoring for hypoglycaemia, especially in the neonate and is therefore not the first line.
- Increase potassium excretion:
  - Sodium-resonium exchange resin oral or rectally: 0.5−1 g/kg up to 6-hourly

- Furosemide 1−2 mg/kg IV over 30 minutes only if fluid replete.

AETIOLOGIES AND INVESTIGATIONS FOR HYPERNATRAEMIA

Clinical features of hypernatraemia are also mainly neurological including headaches, nausea and lethargy in mild cases, progressing to impaired conscious state and seizures in severe cases. Two further unusual findings are as follows.

1. Fever, which resolves with correction of hypernatraemia.
2. Dehydration associated with a doughy texture to the skin. The latter is an unusual form of decreased skin turgor, resulting from the loss of fluid from the intracellular space into the interstitial space. This can mask the severity of dehydration if one relies on the more typical wrinkled skin appearance of dehydration. Most cases of hypernatraemia are associated with dehydration, but occasionally patients will present well-perfused and hypertensive, reflecting hypervolaemic hypernatraemia.

Figure 8.2 provides a diagnostic approach to hypernatraemia. As outlined for hyponatraemia, a methodical approach to hypernatraemia depends on a reliable clinical assessment of fluid state and serum and urine sodium and osmolality. Causes associated with dehydration can then be divided into those due to pure water loss or those due to both water and sodium loss.

Causes of Pure Water Loss Leading to Hypernatraemia

Polyuria or diabetes insipidus can be defined by the excretion of large amounts of dilute urine more than 2.5 L/24 hours (40 mL/kg/24 hours) in adults or more than 100 mL/kg/24 hours in

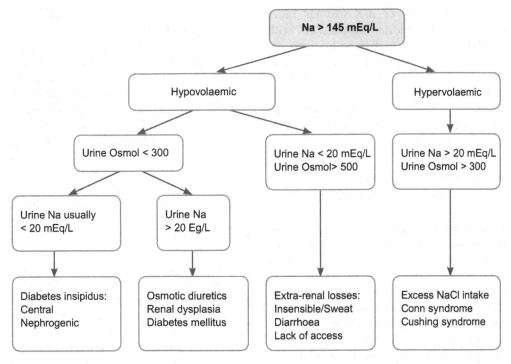

FIGURE 8.2 Diagnostic approach to hypernatraemia.

infants. This is accompanied by increased thirst and polydipsia. In the child a common presentation is for enuresis or nocturia. Although primary polydipsia leads to polyuria, it results in dilutional hyponatraemia (see section on hyponatraemia). There are two basic aetiologies of polyuria associated with hypernatraemia: nephrogenic diabetes insipidus and central diabetes insipidus.

Nephrogenic Diabetes Insipidus (nDI)

nDI is an example of end-organ resistance, with lack of AVP responsiveness in the renal collecting duct. The kidney is unable to concentrate urine, making the child vulnerable to severe dehydration, hypernatraemia and failure to thrive. While the polyuria is expected to be severe from birth, this may be delayed in the breast-fed infant. Because the urine cannot be concentrated, any increase in solute load placed on the kidneys

must be met by a greater urine volume in order to ensure excretion of solutes. Human breast milk is relatively low in sodium and protein, in comparison to cow's milk. For this reason, infants with inherited forms of nDI may thrive for several weeks or even until they are weaned off breast milk onto cow's milk or solids.

There are two inherited forms of nDI, both of which are rare:

- V2-receptor (AVP receptor) gene mutations: responsible for 90% of inherited cases and follows an X-linked recessive inheritance (mapped to Xq28). Males are severely affected, but female carriers often exhibit impaired concentrating capacity.
- AQP-2 (aquaporin) gene mutations: responsible for 10% of inherited cases and follows either autosomal-recessive or autosomal-dominant inheritance.

The acquired forms of nDI are far more common than the hereditary forms. As with transient PHA type I (see section on hyponatrae-mia) an insult to the distal nephron can lead to this tubular defect. Recognised causes include chronic kidney disease (obstruction, dysplasia, pyelonephritis, nephrocalcinosis), hypercalcae-mia, hypokalaemia, drugs (tetracyclines, lithium) and sarcoidosis.

Central Diabetes Insipidus (cDI)

Congenital, familial diabetes insipidus is a rare disorder with an autosomal-dominant inheritance pattern. Diagnosis is often delayed until the second year of life, particularly if the vasopressin deficiency is mild or where there is a strong family history and the chronic poly-dipsia is an accepted feature of life. In these cases, the child may simply present with failure to thrive and a careful history and family history are required to establish the cause. In some countries genetic testing may be available to confirm the heritable nature of the disorder and thus to obviate the need for repeated imaging surveillance when a diagnosis is made in later childhood.

Acquired forms of DI are more common.

- cDI may occur acutely, following a head injury. This can occur even in the absence of loss of consciousness, and is due to a contra-coup injury to the pituitary stalk. It may be short-lived or permanent, when stalk transaction occurs.
- Tumour in the hypothalamic pituitary region in childhood not uncommonly presents with diabetes insipidus. Large tumours such as glioma or astrocytoma are more likely to present with symptoms of visual loss or of raised intracranial pressure. Small lesions are often associated with cDI, such as germinoma. The onset of cDI may precede the diagnosis of a germinoma by up to 7 years, making it mandatory to repeat imaging studies, preferably with MRI, at 3—6-month

intervals, when sudden onset cDI is diagnosed beyond late infancy.
- Langerhans histiocytosis is the major differential diagnosis to be considered, with childhood onset DI. In very young children granulomatous rash, mouth granuloma or skeletal defects may immediately indicate the correct diagnosis, with confirmatory biopsy. However, isolated pituitary stalk thickening is more common in the older child. This is not usually amenable to safe biopsy, so a presumptive diagnosis must include the possibility of early germinoma, with suitable ongoing surveillance, as outlined above.
- Craniopharyngioma may rarely present with DI as a primary complaint but onset of DI is more frequently seen after surgery to the hypothalamic area in this condition.
- Septo-optic dysplasia or other major midline defects may be associated with DI but it is relatively rare. It is more common to see a raised set point in the hypothalamus for thirst, with chronic serum sodium levels around 155 mmol/L. Acute illness can precipitate acute onset DI which seems to settle after recovery but which recurs.
- Radiation treatment of tumours does not induce cDI except as a rare late phenomenon, with radiation fibrosis of the area. cDI in the context of midline tumour is related to position and/or size of tumour or to its surgical treatment.

Sarcoidosis is a very rare cause of cDI in children or adolescents, although more common in adults.

DIAGNOSIS

The simplest and most important diagnostic tool is measurement of weight, urine volume, as well as paired serum and urine osmolarity and sodium levels. Healthy children can maintain serum osmolality over a 14-hour period. As the condition of DI is due to excess water loss, serum sodium and osmolality will rise, but the urine will remain inappropriately dilute with low sodium and osmolality. Although plasma AVP will distinguish between nDI (high) and cDI (low), the measurement of AVP is not readily available and problematic due to lack of normative data.

A more practical approach is to confirm DI on formal water deprivation and then assess the response to a therapeutic trial of desmopressin.

If the condition is mild, it is possible to undertake an overnight fast with early morning paired samples.

However, if there is any suspicion of a severe condition, exemplified by more than 3–4 L/day fluid intake, this should be avoided due to the chance of producing severe dehydration. A formal water deprivation test should be performed, with admission of the child to hospital early in the day and the test only commenced once staff are available for frequent observation.

PROCEDURE FOR WATER DEPRIVATION TEST

The test is started at 6 pm and ends at 8 am in patients without frank polyuria. In very young infants or in patients with polyuria (urine volume above 4 L/24 hours) the test should be started in the early morning. No food or drink is allowed during the test, blood pressure and weight is taken every 1–2 hours, and the test terminated at any time if 5% of the body weight is lost.

At the end of the 6–8-hour fast or after 5% weight loss, or a serum sodium level rising above 155 mmol/L with serum osmolarity greater than 300 mOsm/kg, whichever is sooner, a spot urine and a blood specimen are taken to measure urine and plasma osmolality.

A test dose of desmopressin 5–10 µg is then administered, with a further paired sample for serum and urine osmolality after 1 hour. This allows the differentiation between nDI and cDI: cDI, being due to lack of vasopressin, will respond by immediate urine concentration and a fall in serum sodium, whereas there will be no response if the problem is nephrogenic. Table 8.2 details the diagnoses derived from different levels of urine osmolality after dehydration and desmopressin.

TREATMENT OF DI

Fluids for DI should be as close to pure water as possible. Five per cent dextrose is the ideal solution as it generally matches the composition of the urine. However, in partial DI, fluids with some sodium content will be necessary and this will be determined based on serial urine and plasma sodium levels. The administration of common intravenous fluids, such as 0.45% or 0.9% NaCl, will usually lead to worsening hypernatraemia as they provide a net sodium load, due to the lack of sodium excretion in the urine. Enteral intake of water orally or via nasogastric tube is suitable if the child is neurologically stable.

Once the diagnosis is confirmed, cDI is treated with desmopressin (DDAVP®) orally 0.1–1 mg/day or intranasally 2–40 µg/day.

TABLE 8.2 Interpretation of the Water Deprivation Test

Urine osmolality (mOsm/kg) after dehydration	Urine osmolality (mOsm/kg) after desmopressin	Diagnosis
> 750	> 750	normal
< 300	> 750	cDI
< 300	< 300	nDI
300–750	< 750	Partial cDI or Partial nDI or Primary polydipsia

Each child will require dose titration, in association with knowledge of an ideal target fluid intake, and is best arranged under close supervision in hospital. This is especially the case for infants soon after diagnosis.

On the contrary, there is no specific treatment for nDI. The crux of treatment is provision of high volumes of fluid to match the polyuria. However, some measures may help reduce the polyuria to more manageable levels. These include:

- low salt intake to reduce the renal solute load
- diuretics (hydrochlorothiazide or amiloride), which act to increase reabsorption in more proximal segments of the nephron
- indomethacin, which decreases renal perfusion, but may also have a direct tubular effect.

Causes of Combined Water and Sodium Loss Leading to Hypernatraemia

Loss of water and sodium through the kidneys will be reflected by a high urine output, high urine sodium and low urine osmolality. Osmotic diuretics and hyperglycaemia lead to an osmotic diuresis, whereas renal parenchymal pathology such as renal dysplasia can impair the concentrating ability of the kidneys. A good history, urinalysis, blood/urine glucose level, serum creatinine and renal ultrasound will provide the additional information for diagnosis.

Where the urine sodium is extremely low and the urine osmolality high, the primary losses are extra-renal. As with hyponatraemia, this is usually due to gastroenteritis, but can occasionally occur with skin loss in severe exertion or lack of access to water in victims of major disasters.

Causes of Sodium Retention Leading to Hypernatraemia

Uncommonly, hypernatraemia results from a net excess of body sodium. This can be induced by exogenous or endogenous mineralocorticoid (e.g. Conn syndrome) or glucocorticoid (e.g. Cushing syndrome) over-activity. There will usually be a number of additional findings in patients with Cushing syndrome (see Chapter 4, Adrenal Disorders), but the patient with Conn syndrome will have manifestations resulting from hypertension, hypernatraemia, hypokalaemia and alkalosis. Often these produce minimal complaints, but can lead to headaches, muscle weakness, constipation and polyuria. Diagnostic tests include the following:

- sodium, potassium, calcium, acid-base, blood glucose
- ECG: ST depression or U wave
- endocrine testing includes plasma renin activity, aldosterone, urine steroids, ACTH stimulation, but require specialised laboratory testing (see section on hyponatraemia and Chapter 4, Adrenal Disorders).

Rarely, hypernatraemia is due to salt poisoning through excess sodium consumption, salt water drowning or, most commonly, iatrogenically induced (e.g. excess sodium bicarbonate during cardiac resuscitation). There have been cases in infants reported as a result of incorrect preparation of formula milk.

TREATMENT OF HYPERNATRAEMIA

Specific treatment of DI is described under the section on DI earlier in this chapter. This section describes the general approach to management of hypernatraemia.

Severe hypernatraemia needs to be extremely cautiously corrected. While rapid shifts in sodium can be dangerous in hyponatraemia, this problem is more acute when treating hypernatraemia due to the risk of inducing sudden cerebral oedema. It is therefore essential that the neurological state is carefully monitored during sodium correction and if conscious state alters, management is modified to maintain the sodium level. Only if life-threatening neurological signs emerge as sodium falls should hypertonic saline be administered to acutely raise the serum sodium by 5 mEq/L (see above for treatment of hyponatraemia). As a rule, the maximum rate of change should be 0.5 mEq/L/hour and the **correction of sodium to the upper limit of normal should occur over 48–72 hours**.

Use of intravenous fluid to manage hypernatraemia will depend on the underlying cause. The urine sodium and osmolality are therefore critical.

- Shock should be corrected with 0.9% NaCl 20 mL/kg boluses every 30–60 minutes until perfusion is adequate.
- Subsequent fluid will depend on the net sodium and fluid deficit, ongoing losses and maintenance requirements. Body fluid deficit is calculated according to the clinical assessment of percentage dehydration. In order to rehydrate carefully, calculate the total volume of the water deficit and the 48-hour maintenance requirement for that child. Administer this total volume as constant rate divided over 48 hours. Additional fluid will need to be added for extra losses such as vomiting and diarrhoea.
- There are formulae to calculate total sodium deficit and rate of replacement, but from a practical perspective, once perfusion is satisfactory, 0.45% NaCl is usually the fluid of choice.
- Monitoring of weight, fluid balance and serum sodium will then direct any increase or decrease in fluid rate and sodium composition.
- Often the accompanying acidosis requires NaHCO3 and this can be used to increase serum sodium if the intravenous fluid is insufficient.
- Potassium should be administered once urine output is documented and serum potassium is known to be in the normal range.

HIV AND DERANGEMENTS OF FLUID AND SODIUM

Patients infected with HIV can have a number of disease-related complications resulting in hyponatraemia or hypernatraemia. The investigation of such children therefore follows the steps detailed in this chapter to first determine the source of fluid and salt loss/retention and then treat accordingly.

The important point is to consider HIV as the underlying cause in areas of high HIV prevalence and after stabilisation of fluid and electrolytes to address treatment of the HIV infection. Examples of some of these HIV-associated complications are listed in Table 8.3.

CONCLUSION

Deranged sodium and fluid states are a common clinical problem and can lead to life-threatening complications, as can the inappropriate and over-enthusiastic therapeutic attempts to correct these abnormalities. A logical approach to these patients involves a simple clinical assessment, followed by measurement of urine and serum sodium and osmolality. Armed with these basic data and an understanding of targeted rates of correction of these abnormalities, the clinician can ascertain the source of these derangements and thereby allow a tailored course of management. This alone is sufficient to successfully treat the patient in the acute setting and to diagnose many of the acquired causes. For other acquired causes and especially for inherited disorders, a panel of sophisticated laboratory investigations and imaging may then be necessary.

TABLE 8.3   The Spectrum of Sodium and Water Disturbances in HIV/AIDS

HIV-related complication	Sodium/fluid disturbance
HIV nephropathy	Hypervolaemic hyponatraemia (nephrotic syndrome)
Cryptosporidium gastroenteritis	Hypernatraemic dehydration (non-renal loss)
Tenofovir	Hypernatraemic dehydration (nDI)
Tenofovir	Hyponatraemic dehydration (renal tubular loss)
CMV colitis	Hyponatraemic dehydration (non-renal loss)
Toxoplasmosis/ cerebral lymphoma	Hypernatraemic dehydration (cDI)
Cryptococcal meningitis	Euvolaemic hyponatraemia (SIADH)

References and Further Reading

Ackermann MJ, Clapham DE. Ion channels: basic science and clinical disease. *N Engl J Med* 1997; **336**: 1575–1600.

Adrogue HJ, Madias NE. Hyponatremia. *N Engl J Med* 2000; **342**: 1581–89.

Beattie TJ. Disorders of fluid and electrolyte balance. In: Webb N, Postlethwaite R (eds). *Clinical Paediatric Nephrology,* 3rd ed, Oxford: Oxford University Press, 2003.

Hughes I. Disorders of sex differentiation. In: Melmed S (ed). *Williams Textbook of Endocrinology,* 11th ed, New York: WB Saunders, 2008.

Kuhnle U, Lewicka S, Fuller PJ. Endocrine disorders of sodium regulation. *Horm Res* 2004; **61**: 68–83.

Lifton RP, Gharavi AG, Geller DS. Molecular mechanisms of human hypertension. *Cell* 2001; **104**: 545–66.

Rogerson FM, Fuller PJ. Mineralocorticoid action. *Steroids* 2000; **65**: 61–73.

Scheinmann SJ, Guay-Woodford LM, Thakker RV, Warnock DG. Genetic disorders of renal electrolyte transport. *N Engl J Med* 1999; **340**: 1177–87.

Stewart P. The adrenal cortex. In: Melmed S (ed). *Williams Textbook of Endocrinology,* 11th ed, New York: WB Saunders, 2008.

Trachtman H. Sodium and water. In: Avner ED, Harmon WE, Niaudet P (eds). *Pediatric Nephrology,* 5th ed, Baltimore: Lippincott Williams and Wilkins, 2004.

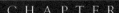

CHAPTER

9

Bone Health

Craig F. Munns, Annemieke M. Boot

OUTLINE

INTRODUCTION

This chapter provides the paediatrician/physician charged with the care of children with a background to disorders affecting bone health. It outlines a strategy for the investigation and management of disorders of low bone mass, high bone mass, skeletal dysplasia and metabolic disorders associated with a skeletal phenotype. With this information, the clinician will be able to formulate treatment tailored to their available resources.

It is hoped that this chapter will also help the healthcare provider avoid misdiagnosis such as non-accidental injury in cases of bone fragility and the instigation of inappropriate treatments such as growth hormone in skeletal dysplasia.

However, it is not meant to be a definitive text on this complex and ever-progressing field of paediatric medicine and the reader is directed to the references at the end of this chapter for further reading.

BACKGROUND

Approximately 30% of children sustain a long bone fracture before the age of 18 years. A small proportion of these will have an underlying bone fragility disorder, either of primary bone origin or secondary to an underlying medical condition. As practitioners involved in the care of children, it is important to be able to identify those with bone fragility and

Practical Pediatric Endocrinology in a Limited Resource Setting
http://dx.doi.org/10.1016/B978-0-12-407822-2.00009-8

develop treatment strategies to improve bone strength.

As children grow, their bones not only get longer but also wider and thicker, through a process known as modelling. The strength of the bone is governed by its size, shape, mineral density and material properties. Genetics are responsible for determining approximately 80% of bone mass (strength). Of the remaining 20%, 15% is determined by muscle mass. The remaining 5% is determined by factors such as pubertal hormones, calcium intake and serum vitamin D concentration. As such, the child health professional can help maximise bone health in all children by:

- encouraging physical activity
- ensuring adequate and timely pubertal progression
- providing adequate dietary calcium intake
- maintaining serum vitamin D concentrations within the normal range.

TOOLS FOR ASSESSMENT

DXA

Osteoporosis in children is defined as a bone mineral content (BMC) or areal bone mineral density (aBMD) age adjusted z-score of less than −2.0 plus a clinically significant fracture (lower extremity long fracture, vertebral compression fracture or two or more upper extremity long bone fracture).[1] It is the authors' experience that children with bone fragility conditions such as osteogenesis imperfecta may also present with ill-defined bone pain, in the absence of overt fracture.

To diagnose osteoporosis in children as per the above definition, it is necessary to have access to a dual-energy X-ray absorptiometry (DXA, previously DEXA) machine. Although this type of test may not currently be available in some countries, its use is becoming widespread throughout the world and there is a vast body of medical literature on the subject. As this is an increasingly important adjunct to good clinical care of many patients with chronic diseases as well as those who have primary bone disorders, we feel it is important to understand the use and interpretation of this methodology.

Bone mineral density (BMD) as accessed by DXA is not a true volumetric density but, rather, it is the mass of bone mineral per projection area (grams/cm^2) and is given the term 'areal BMD' (aBMD). Areal BMD is a size-dependent measure. Shorter children therefore have a reduced aBMD compared to aged-matched controls. Children with chronic illness frequently have short stature resulting from their primary disease or its treatment, and may have a reduction in aBMD, not because there is anything abnormal with the composition or structure of their bones, but simply because the bones are small. It is therefore important to correct for height when interpreting aBMD.

Despite these issues with DXA it is the preferred method of assessing for reduced bone mass and density as it is estimated that a child will have to have a 30% reduction in bone mass before it can be appreciated on plain radiographs.

However, if BMD is not available, second metacarpal cortical thickness is a recognised method of assessing for reduction of cortical long bone thickness and can be easily attained from a bone age X-ray.[2] A lateral thoracolumbar spine X-ray is also useful for the assessment of bone mass as well as the detection of vertebral crush fractures.[3]

Mineral Homeostasis

In children with a suspected abnormality of bone health, as well as an assessment of bone mass/density, evaluation of mineral homeostasis and secondary causes of osteoporosis should be undertaken where possible.[3]

Mineral homeostasis: Serum calcium, magnesium, phosphorus, alkaline phosphatase,

25-hydroxy vitamin D and parathyroid hormone. Urinary calcium: creatinine ratio.

Secondary causes of osteoporosis: Full blood count, coeliac screen, renal function, thyroid function, gonadotropins and sex hormones (if pubertal delay).

Note: Bone turnover markers in children are more a reflection of growth and are of little clinical use outside the research setting.

PRIMARY BONE DISORDERS

Primary Osteoporosis

Clinical Setting

This large group of heterogeneous genetic disorders of the skeleton consists of diseases that are characterised by decreased bone density, abnormal biomechanical properties of bone (e.g. bone fragility) and reduced longitudinal growth. The most common disorder is osteogenesis imperfecta (OI) with an incidence of approximately 1 : 20,000. Within the Caucasian population OI is most often the result of a mutation in the type I collagen gene (COL1).[4] Recent reports from families of African descent have described severe forms of OI that arise from mutations in non-COL1 genes. This has resulted in an expansion of the nomenclature of OI from the original four groups described by Sillence in 1973, to upwards of eight. For practical purposes it is reasonable to use an abridged classification of five groups as described below (Table 9.1).

At present, treatment options for OI do not rely on the presence or otherwise of a COL1 mutation, but rather on the phenotype of the child. Response to treatment has been shown to be similarly effective for all groups.

Treatment of Children with Osteogenesis Imperfecta

The aim of treatment in OI is to maximise mobility and other functional capacities.[5] The

TABLE 9.1 Types of Osteogenesis Imperfecta

Type	Clinical severity	Sclerae	Hearing loss	Gene
I	Mild-non deforming	blue	in about 50%	COL1A1/2 related
II	Perinatal lethal	dark blue		COL1A1/2
III	Severely deforming	blue	frequent	CRTAP-related LEPRE1-related PPIB-related
IV	Moderately deforming	grey	some	CRTAP-related LEPRE1-related PPIB-related
V	Moderately to severely deforming	normal	no	unknown

Notes:

COL1A1/2: collagen 1 alpha 1 or 2

CRTAP: cartilage associated protein

LEPRE1: leucine and proline enriched proteoglycan 1

PPIB: peptidylprolyl isomerase B

optimal treatment approach involves an interdisciplinary team consisting of physicians, orthopaedic surgeons, rehabilitation specialists and physiotherapists.[6]

Despite optimal surgical and rehabilitative care, extreme bone fragility and deformity persists in many patients. The major medical advance in the past 10 years has come from the introduction of bisphosphonate therapy, and cyclic intravenous pamidronate is now viewed as the 'gold standard' for the treatment of children and adults with moderate to severe OI and its Cole-Carpenter and Bruck variants. To date, little data are available on the treatment of mild OI (two or fewer fractures per year, no verte-bral crush fractures, and no long-bone defor-mities) or the use of oral bisphosphonates in OI.

Although the availability of bisphosphonates is extremely limited in many countries, the use of the Internet is not! Thus, most parents who have a child with OI now are aware of this treat-ment option and, even in surprisingly difficult circumstances, have sought, obtained and successfully used it. We therefore believe it is appropriate to include detailed information on this management option and when it should be considered.

Bisphosphonates

Most published experience has used pamidr-onate. Zoledronic acid as a third-generation bisphosphonate is currently also being used in research studies

EFFICACY

Bisphosphonates are potent antiresorptive agents that disrupt osteoclastic activity by inter-fering with the mevalonate pathway of choles-terol biosynthesis.

Intravenous pamidronate in children with OI has been reported to decrease bone pain, enhance well-being, improve mobility and muscle strength, reduce fracture incidence, increase long bone cortical thickness, increase vertebral size with vertebral reshaping, and increase bone mass and bone mineral density.[5]

Even in settings where optimal orthopaedic and allied therapies are not available, the improvement in bone pain and reduction in vertebral fracture makes treatment worthwhile.

In an attempt to prevent growth disturbance and spine and limb deformity, cyclical intrave-nous pamidronate has also been used in babies and infants with OI.[7] The treatment was safe in infants (see 'Safety' below) and response more pronounced than in the older cohort. It is reasonable therefore to commence treatment in babies with severe forms of OI before 6 months of age.

SAFETY

The safety of bisphosphonate therapy continues to be of concern to many clinicians. Pamidronate lowers serum calcium concentra-tions and this is most marked following the first infusion cycle. In vitamin D-replete indi-viduals receiving the recommended calcium intake, the hypocalcaemia is self-remitting. The majority of children have an acute phase reaction (fever, muscle pain, headache and vomiting) 12—36 hours following initial expo-sure to pamidronate.[3] These side effects can be minimised by the administration of acet-aminophen (paracetamol) or anti-inflamma-tory medication. Transient uveitis occurs in approximately 1% of children who receive pamidronate.[5]

Pamidronate has been shown to significantly improve the growth of children and adolescents with moderate to severe OI compared to histor-ical controls, over a 4-year treatment period, by preventing limb and spine deformity.

CONTRAINDICATIONS TO USE

Bisphosphonates are contraindicated during pregnancy, and all females of reproductive age should have a negative pregnancy test before each pamidronate treatment cycle or before commencing oral bisphosphonates. Because bisphosphonates persist in mineralised bone for many years, concern has also been expressed that bisphosphonates administered before conception could be released from the maternal skeleton during the pregnancy and affect the fetus. To date there has been no evidence to support this concern.

MONITORING OF BISPHOSPHONATE TREATMENT

Ideally, bone mineral density 6—12 monthly should be performed to assess efficiency of treatment. This should be accompanied by assessment of mineral homeostasis (serum calcium, 25(OH)D and PTH). The dose of pamidronate can be reduced once bone density has normalised and vertebral shape improved. This is usually possible within 3–4 years of start of treatment. Treatment should not be continued long-term without a defined form of assessment of bone response (BMD). Continued use without assessment will inevitably result in production of hard, brittle bone and ultimately a type of osteopetrosis.

IN SUMMARY

- Cyclic intravenous pamidronate (9 mg/kg/ year, with a dose and treatment interval that varies with age)[5] should be offered to children with moderate to severe OI as defined by: two or more long-bone fractures per year, and/or vertebral crush fractures, and/or long-bone deformities, and/or children with OI type III or IV.
- Following normalisation of bone density and improvement in vertebral shape the dose of pamidronate can be reduced to 3–4 mg/kg/ year.
- Pamidronate therapy has good short-term safety and efficacy in children and adolescents with moderate to severe osteogenesis imperfecta and related disorders.
- In severe cases, treatment can be started during infancy, but these children need to be monitored very closely, especially during the first infusion cycle.
- Treatment continues to be effective in older teenagers and the upper age limit of responsiveness still remains to be defined.
- All children treated with a bisphosphonate should be monitored closely as the long-term safety and efficacy of these compounds can be adequately evaluated.
- Further study is required before bisphosphonates can be administered to all patients with OI on the basis of low BMD alone.

Osteogenesis Imperfecta Type I

OI type I is an autosomal dominant disorder of COL1, characterised by excessive bone fragility, which is usually associated with low bone mass, distinctly blue sclerae, and susceptibility to conductive hearing loss. This is the most common form of OI and has a birth frequency in the order of 1/30,000 and a similar population frequency.[4]

Dentinogenesis imperfecta (DI) is observed in some families and requires specialised dental care. Type I collagen is the predominant structural component of dentin. Abnormalities in dentin development are present in all children with OI who have a COL1 mutation, but is only clinically significant in those with DI where it results in opalescent teeth that are predisposed to dental caries and chipping of teeth. Children should be encouraged to clean teeth regularly and avoid eating hard foodstuffs. Some institutions place metal caps on the molars of children with DI to preserve their integrity and capping of permanent teeth is also undertaken. Primary dentition is often more severely affected than secondary dentition.

When fractures occur at birth, these are usually only a few in number. Individuals with fractures at birth subsequently have no more deformity, handicap, or number of fractures than other individuals who have their first fracture after 1 year of age. Deformities of the limbs in this group are usually the result of fractures, but bowing, particularly of the lower limbs, is common in children with moderate disease not treated with bisphosphonates. Although rare in children, some adults have progressive kyphoscoliosis, which may be of a severe degree. There is usually excessive hypermobility in the small joints of the hands and feet, but this feature is less marked in adults.

Hearing impairment and vestibular dysfunction are rare before the end of the second decade of life.

Patients with OI type I frequently have easy bruising, which in children may be mistaken for child abuse, particularly when associated with unexplained fractures. It is not uncommon for families to have repeated adversity and repeated experience of accusations of non-accidental injury levelled against them, prior to a diagnosis of OI being made.

Bone densitometry determined by dual energy X-ray absorptiometry falls into the low normal range in many children with OI type I. However, in late childhood, bone density in the long bone and spine frequently falls to two standard deviations below the mean.

Radiographic studies in most patients in this group have the following indications.

- They show generalised osteopaenia, evidence of previous fractures, and normal callus formation at the site of recent fractures.
- Severe osteoporosis of the spine with codfish vertebrae is occasionally seen in these patients, but most have normally formed vertebral bodies with some wedging and flattening.
- Wormian bones are not necessarily present in the skull and are found in no more than 70% of subjects. However, their finding provides immediate evidence of the underlying condition and acts as a deterrent to making a diagnosis of non-accidental injury.

Natural history: spontaneous improvement is observed during adolescence, with a marked reduction in the frequency of fractures. This may represent an increase in bone strength secondary to the osteogenic effects of the sex hormones or a reduction in risk-taking behaviour, as the young person appreciates their limitations. There is exaggerated postmenopausal bone loss, and adults who have not had fractures for many years may commence having fractures again in their late 40s to 50s.

Treatment of OI Type I

Children and adults with OI type I have less tendency to progressive skeletal deformity than in other types of OI and thus they maintain better mobility. If there are recurrent long-bone fractures or vertebral crush fractures in children and adults, cyclic intravenous pamidronate (see above) can be used with a very favourable response to therapy. Oral bisphosphonates are yet to be proven beneficial in those requiring treatment.

Practice Points

- There is currently no evidence to recommend bisphosphonate therapy in children with mild OI type I.
- It may be valuable to monitor the clinical state and bone density in adult women planning a pregnancy before and immediately after the pregnancy.
- Given the caveats discussed above, it may be advisable to institute therapy with a bisphosphonate for those women whose pregnancy-related bone loss has resulted in symptomatic osteopaenia and/or reduced bone mineral density into the symptomatic/fracture range.
- Where dentinogenesis imperfecta is present, regular (6–12 monthly) dental reviews should be undertaken.
- Joint hypermobility may require specific therapy input with assistance at school for hand writing.

Genetic Counselling and Prenatal Diagnosis

For an affected adult marrying a normal partner, there is a 50% chance of an affected child. Where two adults with OI type I marry, there is a 25% chance for a homozygous-affected infant, which is likely to be perinatally lethal or severely affected. Prenatal detection is possible as is pre-implantation diagnosis. Ultrasound and radiographic studies prenatally will occasionally differentiate a normal from an affected fetus.

Osteogenesis Imperfecta Type II

OI type II is characterised by extreme bone fragility, leading to intrauterine or early infant death. The group is clinically and biochemically heterogeneous with a recurrence rate of approximately 6%, although most cases of OI type II are caused by fresh constitutional dominant mutations. Collagen and DNA studies show that within each subgroup there is further biochemical and molecular heterogeneity. Treatment with pamidronate is not recommended in this OI type.[4]

Osteogenesis Imperfecta Type III

OI type III is the most severe form of OI that is compatible with life. It is characterised by progressive deformity of the spine and long bones. OI type III shows molecular heterogeneity with identification of a number of non-COL1 gene mutations over recent years (Table 9.1). OI type III can be inherited as either autosomal dominant or recessive. Although there are subtle phenotypic differences between those with COL1 and non-COL1 OI type III their management is similar.[4]

Clinical Features

These individuals have newborn or infant presentation with severe bone fragility and multiple fractures leading to progressive deformity of the skeleton. They are generally born at or near term and have normal birth weight and often normal birth length, although this may be reduced because of deformities of the lower limbs at birth. Fractures are present in most cases at birth and occur frequently during childhood even if treated with pamidronate.

Although the sclerae may be blue at birth, observation of many patients with this syndrome reveals that the sclerae become progressively less blue with age.

The childhood phenotype of OI type III has been altered by the use of intravenous pamidronate coupled with timely intramedullary rodding of long bones. Because of these changes in practice, the phenotype described below may vary considerably, dependent on the level of care available to these children.

At birth, there is usually over-modelling of the shafts of the long bones, with widening of the femoral metaphyses and angulation of the tibiae. There is generalised osteopaenia and multiple fractures. Within weeks to months, in most infants, the shafts of the long bones show under-modelling, producing a 'broad-bone' appearance.

Progressive disruption and repair of metaphyseal trabeculae may produce a 'popcorn' appearance. There is poor longitudinal growth well below the third percentile in height for age and sex. The ribs are thin, osteopaenic, and progressively crowded as platyspondyly increases.

The skull shows multiple Wormian bones, although these may not be evident until several weeks to months of age. Progressive kyphoscoliosis develops during childhood and adolescence. Hearing loss is rare during childhood, but reported in 16–80% of adults.

In the past, approximately one-third of the patients survived long-term, reflecting not only the severity of the disorder but also the heterogeneity within the group. Death usually resulted from the complications of severe bone fragility, skeletal deformity including kyphoscoliosis, pulmonary hypertension, and cardio-respiratory failure. Given the present therapeutic options, specifically treatment with cyclic intravenous pamidronate commenced in infancy, it can be expected that the majority of patients with OI type III will survive into adult life.

Treatment

Cyclic intravenous pamidronate has been used in children with OI type III, resulting in decreased fracture frequency, increased mobility and improved quality of life, and it should be offered from infancy.

Rehabilitation and orthopaedic care should be instituted as able to prevent progressive deformity and provide for as normal a development as possible.

Intramedullary rodding may improve mobility and prevent fractures and is also used to correct and prevent progressive deformity.

Various orthoses can be provided or designed which assist in the rehabilitation of these children; these orthoses improve mobility and normalise activities of daily living.

Where dentinogenesis imperfecta is present, 6—12-monthly dental reviews should be undertaken.

Most cases of OI type III are caused by fresh constitutional dominant mutations. Due to rare recessive forms of OI type III as well as germline mosaicism for heterozygous mutations, however, the quoted recurrence risk of OI type III is approximately 6%.

Osteogenesis Imperfecta Type IV

OI type IV is an autosomal dominant disorder of COL1 characterised by osteoporosis leading to bone fragility without the characteristic features of the OI type I syndrome (i.e. blue sclerae and early onset deafness).[4]

Clinical Findings

The sclerae may be bluish at birth but become progressively less blue as the patient matures. These individuals have variable ages of onset of fractures, which may be present at birth (approximately 25%) or may not occur until adult life. Significant bowing of the lower limbs has been present at birth as the only feature of this syndrome. Some patients improve with age in that bowing lessens.

Just as in OI type I, these patients appeared to show a spontaneous improvement at the time of puberty, and generally fewer fractures are encountered in adolescents and adults. However, the majority of patients have short stature and measurement

of bone density by DXA reveals persistent osteopaenia.

A small proportion of affected children have severe progressive deformity of long bones and spine that is out of proportion to their severity as judged by fracture frequency.

Wormian bones are absent in 30—50% of subjects.

Dentinogenesis imperfecta has been observed in some families and not others.

Hearing impairment and vestibular dysfunction are reported and get more common with age.

Radiographically, this group is defined by generalised osteopaenia, although multiple fractures may be observed in the skeleton at birth and throughout life.

Treatment is as for OI in general.

Where there are recurrent long bone fractures, vertebral crush fractures or skeletal deformity, cyclic intravenous pamidronate should be offered as the first line of treatment. The response in OI type IV is particularly good. In the osteopaenic but asymptomatic child, one can make the case to treat before the first vertebral or femoral fracture occurs as the immobilisation following a fracture in an osteopaenic OI child is usually worsened and can rarely be reversed by physical activity alone.

Rehabilitation and orthopaedic care should be instituted as able to prevent progressive deformity and provide for as normal a development as possible.

Intramedullary rodding may improve mobility and prevent fractures and is also used to correct and prevent progressive deformity.

Various orthoses can be provided or designed which assist in the rehabilitation of these children; these orthoses improve mobility and normalise activities of daily living.

Where dentinogenesis imperfecta is present, 6-monthly dental reviews should be undertaken.

Genetic counselling and prenatal diagnosis. For an affected adult marrying a normal partner, there is a 50% chance of an affected child. Where two adults with OI type IV marry, there is a 25% chance for a homozygous-affected infant, which is likely to be perinatally lethal or severely affected. Prenatal genetic and pre-implantation diagnosis is possible. Ultrasound and radiographic studies prenatally will occasionally differentiate a normal from an affected fetus.

Differential Diagnosis

Juvenile idiopathic osteoporosis (IJO). IJO is a rare and self-limiting disorder that may be difficult to distinguish from mildly affected cases of OI type IV (with normal teeth). Features of IJO not associated with OI are: onset of symptoms 2 to 3 years prior to the onset of puberty and usually self-remitting. In addition, there is a negative family history, metaphyseal fracture, neo-osseous ossification, straight long bones with normal cortical thickness, no extra-skeletal manifestations as in OI and decreased bone turnover.[8] Osteopaenia in IJO is most marked in the axial skeleton.

Osteogenesis Imperfecta Type V

OI type V is an autosomal dominant disorder characterised by moderate to severe bone fragility, and accounts for approximately 5% of individuals with OI seen in the hospital setting.[5]

Clinical Features

From early in life, calcification of the interosseous membrane in the forearms is observed, which leads to restriction of pronation and supination, and eventual dislocation of the radial heads.

- The sclerae are white.
- Opalescent dentine and Wormian bones are not present.
- There is an increased risk of developing hyperplastic callus following a fracture or orthopaedic surgery.

This disorder has a distinct pattern of bone histomorphometry with coarse mesh-like lamellation.[4] Hyperplastic callus describes a massive callus with swelling and pain at the site of the fracture, which can mimic osteosarcoma, but may be distinguished from it on MRI and CT.

Its progress may be prevented by the prompt use of indomethacin, an anti-inflammatory prostaglandin inhibitor, following fracture.

Management

Treatment is as for OI in general. Where there are recurrent long bone fractures, vertebral crush fractures or skeletal deformity, cyclic intravenous pamidronate should be offered as the first line of treatment.

As with OI types III and IV, OI type V responds well to cyclical intravenous pamidronate.

Anti-inflammatory medication is of benefit to reduce the severity of hypertrophic callus development.

Forearm/hand orthoses may decrease the pain and improve the function associated with intraosseous membrane calcification.

FIBROUS DYSPLASIA

Clinical Features

Fibrous dysplasia (FD) of bone is a congenital, non-heritable skeletal disorder. FD affects both sexes equally and usually is diagnosed in childhood or adolescence. FD occurs when bone marrow cells are affected by somatic activating mutations of the gene encoding the a- subunit of the stimulatory G-protein, Gsa. The mutation has a mosaic distribution and results in locally increased stimulation of adenylyl cyclase and over production of cAMP. In bone mesenchymal cells, the downstream effects of the mutation include increased production of c-fos protein and IL-6.[7] At the bone tissue level, FD is characterised by dysplastic lesions that consist of abnormal fibrous tissue in the marrow space intertwined with poorly oriented, irregular trabeculae of woven bone.[7]

Radiologic Appearance

On X-rays, dysplastic lesions have a lytic or cystic appearance with surrounding bone cortex reduced in thickness. Occasionally, the entire bone is widened. Radioisotopic bone scans usually disclose increased uptake in affected areas and bone turnover markers are often elevated, especially if lesions are widespread. Production of FGF23 by the dysplastic lesions may result in hypophosphataemia.

Associations

FD may be part of the McCune–Albright syndrome, a rare disorder that combines polyostotic fibrous dysplasia, skin pigmentation (café-au-lait spots) and one or several endocrinopathies like gonadotropin independent precocious puberty.

The natural evolution of the disorder is variable. Lesions may remain stable for decades, but can also progress relentlessly, leading to multiple fractures and severe bone deformities. The disease progress appears to be more rapid in the growing skeleton. Skull lesions can result in visual impairment and/or facial asymmetry. Lesions may be localised on one bone (monostotic) or widespread (polyostotic or panostotic).

Investigations

In the lesion the normal bone is replaced by tissue that is more radiolucent with a ground-glass appearance on X-ray. Bone scintigraphy is useful for assessing the extent of the disease.

Alkaline phosphatase is often high and can be used to assess response to treatment.

Serum phosphate should be assessed at diagnosis as lesions will worsen if a deficit is not corrected.

If **McCune–Albright syndrome** is suspected, examination for signs of associated endocrinopathy should be undertaken, including signs of the following.

- Precocious puberty in both females and males. Macroorchidism is common in males without progressive pubertal changes.
- Growth hormone excess (acromegaly). This is common in late childhood or early adolescence but can be delayed until adulthood.
- Thyrotoxicosis is usually due to a thyroid adenoma but Tx3 toxicosis has been reported. Seventy percent of affected individuals will have this problem at some time.
- Cortisol excess (Cushing syndrome) can occur at any age, even infancy.
- All the endocrinopathies adversely affect bone health.

Treatment

The mainstay of treatment for FD remains orthopaedic surgery, consisting of preventive measures (curettage, bone grafting, internal fixation of long bones) and management of fractures. Intravenous pamidronate in children is effective in reducing bone pain but does not appear to influence the natural history.[7] In severe hypophosphataemia, phosphate replacement may be indicated.

In the case of severe fibrous dysplasia of the skull, where the optic foramina are affected with resulting visual pathway compromise, every attempt should be made to use bisphosphonate, if at all possible. It will usually halt progress and often resolves field defects. Decompression surgery must be reserved only for progressive visual loss. When surgery is used in the absence of progressive visual loss, there is a 50% chance of a worse visual outcome and very low chance of improvement.

If asymptomatic, no treatment of bone lesions is required. If bone pain, intravenous bisphosphonates may be of benefit.[7] The optimal treatment regimen remains to be defined, but one approach found useful is to treat as per treatment of moderate-to-severe OI with regular infusions of bisphosphonate, if available, for the first 2 years then on an as-needs basis to control bone pain.

SECONDARY OSTEOPOROSIS

A chronically ill child will usually have multiple factors influencing bone health and strength, with the number increasing as does the severity of the illness.[9] These factors are outlined in Table 9.2 and discussed below.

Reduced Mobility

Bones develop to withstand the mechanical forces applied to them in everyday life. The magnitude of these forces and the skeleton's ability to sense and respond to them have a major influence on the mineral content and architectural design of bone, and therefore its strength.[3] In the normally ambulatory child, the major bone strains result from muscle pull and growth. These fare of paramount importance to chronically ill children, in whom reduced mobility and thus muscle load is a major cause of reduced bone mass and strength. This is most notable in children with neuromuscular disorders such as cerebral palsy, Duchenne muscular dystrophy and spinal muscular atrophy, and children with congenital or acquired spinal cord lesions. Transiliac bone biopsies from children with various neurological disorders and immobility have shown that the reduced mass results from small bone size, thin cortices and a reduced trabecular bone volume.

The most common site of fracture in children with immobility is the distal femur. This is because their long bones tend to be slender with thin cortices and reduced trabecular density, and the lower extremities are subject to trauma from accidents or handling. Vertebral

TABLE 9.2   Causes of Secondary Osteoporosis

Endocrine	• glucocorticoid excess
	• hypogonadism
	• hyperthyroidism
	• hyperparathyroidism
Deficiencies	• calcium
	• vitamin D
	• malnutrition
Inflammation	• juvenile idiopathic arthritis,
	• inflammatory bowel disease
Immobilisation	• paraplegia
	• cerebral palsy
	• Duchenne muscular dystrophy
Neoplasia	• leukaemia
Medication	• glucocorticosteroids
	• methotrexate
	• anticonvulsants
Inborn errors of metabolism	• glycogen storage disease, Gaucher disease
Haematological disorders	• thalassaemia, sickle cell disease
Renal	• chronic renal failure
	• chronic metabolic acidosis
Malabsorption	• coeliac disease
	• chronic liver failure
	• pancreatic insufficiency

crush fractures are less frequent, but can be complicated by the development of scoliosis.

To prevent immobilisation bone loss in children with chronic illness, weight-bearing activity should be maximised, which in healthy children and adolescents and those with cerebral palsy has been shown to increase bone mineral accrual and bone size. For children with extreme bone fragility, swimming and hydrotherapy may be beneficial. In ambulant and non-ambulant children with spastic cerebral palsy, weight-bearing activity has been shown to significantly improve femoral neck bone mineral content and volumetric BMD compared to controls.

Pubertal Delay

Delayed or arrested pubertal development may occur as a result of an underlying chronic illness and/or its treatment, and unless assessed prospectively may be easily overlooked in the care of the chronically ill child.[3] Pubertal hormones (oestradiol in females and testosterone in males) influence longitudinal bone growth and bone mineral accrual, with their appropriate timing being important for normal skeletal development and the attainment of peak bone mass. Pubertal hormones may also help provide children with the emotional maturity required to cope with chronic illness.[3]

It is unclear if the induction of puberty in otherwise normal children with constitutional delay (CD) positively influences bone mass at final height. The situation is even less clear for children with a chronic illness, where osteoporosis is associated with low bone turnover and small bone size.

Short-term (6-month) androgen therapy has been demonstrated to progress puberty without adversely affecting final height in males with CD. Androgen therapy does not, however, positively affect bone mass.

No data on sex steroid 'priming' is available in females. Here, if there is no pubertal development by age 13.5 years, it is recommended to introduce low dose oestrogen with a gradual increase in dose over 2–3 years. Once pubertal development has been achieved, it may be possible to withdraw therapy to see if puberty can be maintained spontaneously.

In the chronically ill or disabled child, pubertal induction may exacerbate behavioural difficulties and raise concerns about hygiene. These are important issues and need to be addressed appropriately.

(See Chapter 2, Puberty: Normal and Abnormal, for detailed information.)

Nutrition and Low Body Weight

Adequate nutrition is essential for normal growth and development. It is not surprising, therefore, that osteoporosis is associated with nutritional and low body weight disorders such as anorexia nervosa, inflammatory bowel disease, malignancy and cystic fibrosis.[3] The aetiology of the osteoporosis in such disorders is multifactorial with interplay between low body weight, low calcium, vitamin D and protein intake, gonadal deficiency, growth hormone resistance and malabsorption.

An adequate intake of calcium and vitamin D is essential for skeletal mineralisation. In adolescents, a dietary intake of approximately 1100 mg/day is associated with peak calcium accretion rates of 350 mg/day in boys and 300 mg/day in girls.[10] In healthy adolescents, short-term gains in BMD have been achieved through calcium supplementation.[8] It is unclear, however, whether such gains are sustainable, improve peak bone mass or, most importantly, increase bone strength. Given this, the recommended daily intake of calcium for healthy children is summarised in Table 9.3. Further studies are required to assess if the calcium needs are similar for children with a chronic illness. Until then, children during both health and illness should receive the recommended daily requirement of calcium.

Without adequate sun exposure, as is often the case in the chronically ill, even children living in sunny climates can become vitamin D deficient.[11] Because of this, the vitamin D status

TABLE 9.3 Recommended Daily Intake of Calcium for Healthy Children[3]

	0–6 months	6–12 months	1–3 years	4–8 years	9–18 years
Adequate intake of calcium (mg/day)	210	270	500	800	1300

of chronically ill children should be evaluated on an annual basis and, if necessary, vitamin D supplementation commenced at 400 IU to 800 IU/day (10–20 μg/day).

Iatrogenic Factors Affecting Bone Health

Glucocorticoids

Glucocorticoids are commonly prescribed to children with chronic inflammatory and autoimmune disorders. Even at low doses, glucocorticoids may result in osteopaenia by decreasing bone formation and increasing bone resorption.[11] In the majority of situations there will be multiple factors responsible for the deterioration in bone health of children receiving glucocorticoid therapy including the medication itself, inflammatory cytokines, decreased mobility, poor nutrition and hormonal disturbance.

Vertebral crush fractures are the most prevalent fractures associated with glucocorticoid use in children. A prednisolone dose of 0.62 mg/kg/day in children with juvenile idiopathic arthritis is associated with a mean time to vertebral collapse of 2.6 years. Intermittent steroid use may also predispose to fracture, with a recent study reporting an increased fracture incidence in children who received over four courses of glucocorticoids. It is, however, difficult to differentiate between glucocorticoid-induced bone loss and that associated with the primary disorder and its associated increase in inflammatory cytokines, malnutrition and decrease in weight bearing.[12]

It is unclear if there is a safe, yet therapeutic, dose below which glucocorticoids do not adversely influence bone in children. Until this data is available, it is essential that children be prescribed the smallest effective dose of glucocorticoid and be withdrawn from these drugs and commenced on steroid-sparing medication as rapidly as possible. Alternate day dosing may prevent bone loss secondary to glucocorticoid use while maintaining the therapeutic benefits.

The role of calcium and vitamin D supplementation in the prevention of glucocorticoid-induced osteoporosis remains controversial. Paediatric data are lacking, with conflicting results on the effectiveness of calcium and vitamin D supplementation on improving BMD. There is no data on the use of calcium and vitamin D supplementation and fracture incidence in children on glucocorticoid therapy. Until further data are available, children on glucocorticoid therapy should receive the recommended daily intake of calcium (Table 9.3) and vitamin D supplementation, 400–800 IU/day, if their serum vitamin D concentrations are low.

Inflammatory Cytokines and Growth Factors

Systemic inflammatory disorders are frequently associated with osteopaenia and osteoporosis.[3] The aetiology of the bone loss is multifactorial, but increased circulating and focal concentrations of inflammatory cytokines (IL-1, IL-6, IL-7, TNF-α and β, and RANKL) and growth factors (PDGF) are likely to play an important role. Cytokines have been shown to stimulate osteoclastogenesis, suppress osteoblast recruitment and induce resistance to 1,25-dihydroxyvitamin D_3, thus increasing bone resorption and decreasing bone formation.

Treatment of Osteopaenia/Osteoporosis

Treatment aims to optimise weight-bearing activity, vitamin D and calcium status, together with inducing and maintaining puberty if required, in a window of opportunity when health is relatively good and corticosteroid needs are low.

These measures are frequently inadequate in preventing the development of osteoporosis with chronic bone pain or fragility fractures. In these situations, specific anti-osteoporosis therapy should be considered, where available.

Bisphosphonates are the most widely used medications for the treatment of paediatric osteoporosis.[13] Similar clinical and densitometric results have been demonstrated in small numbers of children with osteoporosis associated with various chronic illness including glucocorticoid-induced osteoporosis, cystic fibrosis, cerebral palsy, Duchenne muscular dystrophy, spina bifida and Gaucher disease. Oral bisphosphonates have been shown to be well tolerated and increase BMD in children with diffuse connective tissue diseases.

Specific Disorders

Cerebral Palsy

Cerebral palsy (CP) is a non-progressive encephalopathy with disordered posture and movement, and a prevalence of between 2 and 4/1000. It results from an abnormality in brain development, although the precise aetiology remains unclear in the majority of cases.[17]

Orthopaedic complications of CP include scoliosis, joint subluxation and dislocation and fracture of long bones and vertebrae.[3] Fracture incidence in children with CP is variously reported between 5 and 30%, with the majority of fractures occurring in the femoral shaft and supracondylar region.[3]

Reduced mobility is the major aetiological factor for bone fragility in children with CP. Reduced mobility results in bone with a low bone mass and abnormal architectural design, which is unable to withstand the occasional mechanical challenges placed upon it, such as forceful muscle contractures associated with a seizure or unusual weight bearing or transfer.[3]

Other factors include vitamin D deficiency from reduced sunlight exposure and possibly anticonvulsant therapy, disorders of puberty and nutritional disorders.

Lumbar spine BMD is often normal in children with CP who sustain a pathological fracture. Specialised DXA examination of the distal femur has been helpful to provide a reproducible measure of bone quality in this group.

To prevent osteoporosis in children with CP a concerted effort must be made to maintain ambulation and weight bearing. To this end, a multidisciplinary team consisting of rehabilitation specialists, physiotherapists, orthopaedic surgeons and bone and mineral physicians provides the optimal treatment approach. As outlined above, biomechanical stimulation of bone requires further investigation as it holds great promise. Other general measures such as ensuring adequate calcium and vitamin D intake and general nutrition, minimising iatrogenic causes of bone loss and ensuring timely pubertal development are also important to the child with CP.

Once osteoporosis is established, the use of bisphosphonate therapy is justified. Because the majority of children with CP have difficulty swallowing, intravenous therapy is preferable. Although bone density has been shown to increase, further trials are required to investigate if bisphosphonates reduce fracture incidence in this cohort of children.

BONE DYSPLASIAS

Skeletal dysplasias are a heterogeneous group of over 370 disorders of bone and/or cartilage with varied clinical phenotypes and genetic aetiologies. The skeletal dysplasias can be divided into three main groups — osteodysplasias (abnormalities of bone density and mineralisation), chondrodysplasias (abnormalities of cartilage with associated short stature) and dysostoses (malformation of single bones alone or in combination). The majority of skeletal dysplasias are defined by their clinical and radiological appearance. More and more, however, the molecular basis and causative genetic defect are also being recognised.[14]

Resources for Diagnosis

In countries where expert radiologic diagnosis may not be readily available, the advent of the Internet has permitted major advances in accurate diagnosis of these disorders. Radiographs of a skeletal survey can now be sent to a specialised unit for early diagnosis.

Clinical Setting

Errors of diagnosis and confusion with other disorders still abound. Attention to basic techniques of examination and the recognition of skeletal disproportion will avoid many errors, such as short stature being considered to be due to growth hormone deficiency. Conversely, the relative skeletal disproportion of early androgen excess may be misinterpreted as a skeletal dysplasia if adequate clinical examination is omitted.

In countries where consanguinity is common, rare disorders such as mucopolysaccharidoses and lipoidoses are seen more frequently. While many of these present with developmental delay or acute ill health and organomegaly, short stature with abnormalities of skeletal proportions, together with a relatively large head, may be the first clinical presentation.

Diagnostic Approach

The diagnosis of skeletal dysplasia often requires a multidisciplinary approach incorporating clinical geneticists, radiologists and molecular biologists. The cornerstone of diagnosis remains a detailed clinical and radiological evaluation.

In the history, birth length and previous growth data are important as is family history.

On examination attention should be paid to height and body proportions (arm span, sitting height and leg length). Serial radiographs (skeletal survey) are often required as the radiological phenotype may develop over time.

The key to diagnosis is comparison of radiographs to age-matched controls. Small and irregular epiphyseal ossification suggest an epiphyseal dysplasia; widened, flared and irregular metaphyses suggest a metaphyseal dysplasia, and osteodysplasias are characterised by cortical thickening or marrow expansion. When these changes are associated with spinal flattening or irregularity, spondylo is added to describe the dysplasia, e.g. spondylo-epiphyseal dysplasia (SED).[14]

Management

With such a huge range of disorders encompassed within skeletal dysplasia it is not possible to discuss their detailed management in this chapter. Osteogenesis imperfecta and fibrous dysplasia have been discussed above and a few specific disorders will be briefly mentioned below.

Osteopetrosis

Osteopetrosis (marble bone disease) is the most common sclerosing bone disorder and is due to abnormal number and or function of the osteoclasts (bone-resorbing cells). There are two major clinical forms of osteopetrosis, the autosomal recessive infantile (malignant) type and the autosomal dominant juvenile (benign) type.[15]

INFANTILE OSTEOPETROSIS

The infantile type is uniformly lethal without bone marrow transplant and presents in the first year of life. Neonatal hypocalcaemic seizure with rickets (osteopetro-rickets) is well recognised. Due to lack of widening of cranial foramina, there is compression of cranial nerves resulting in optic, ocular motor and facial nerve compression. Hearing impairment and visual impairment are common as is raised intracranial pressure due to communicating hydrocephalus. Although dense, bones are fragile and fracture with delayed healing is seen. There is delayed tooth eruption with dental abscess. Due to narrowing of the medullary canal, anaemia with hypersplenism is observed. On physical examination children are short, with macrocephaly and frontal bossing, nystagmus and hepatosplenomegaly. Without treatment, children die within the first decade from haemorrhage, pneumonia, anaemia, sepsis or raised intracranial pressure. The most common cause of infantile osteopetrosis is a mutation in TCIRG1, which encodes the α3 subunit of the vascular proton pump.[15]

JUVENILE OSTEOPETROSIS

Radiological features appear in childhood and there is phenotypic heterogeneity within kindreds with both symptomatic infants to asymptomatic carriers within the same family. Features include long-bone fracture, cranial nerve palsy, motor delay, abnormal dental development and dental abscess.

Treatment is supportive, e.g. surgical decompression of cranial nerves, fracture management, good dental hygiene and avoidance of activities associated with increased risk of trauma. The molecular basis for juvenile osteopetrosis includes mutations in CLCN7 and LRP5.[15]

Achondroplasia

Achondroplasia is the most common form of rhizomelic short stature and is due to dominant mutations in FGFR3. Approximately 75% of cases are due to new mutations with no family history. Children with achondroplasia show *in utero* growth restriction that is maintained throughout childhood, with a final adult height of approximately 120 cm in both males and females.

The diagnosis is based on radiographic features, including contracted base of skull, a square shape to the pelvis with a small sacroiliac notch, short vertebral pedicles, rhizomelic (proximal) shortening of the long bones, trident hands, normal trunk length, proximal femoral radiolucency and by mid-childhood chevron shape of the distal femoral epiphysis. The differential diagnosis includes the two other FGFR3-related disorders, hypochondroplasia (milder) and thanatophoric dysplasia (more severe).[16]

Children with achondroplasia commonly have delayed motor milestones, recurrent middle ear infections and lower limb bowing. Other complications in early childhood include airways obstruction, thoracolumbar kyphosis, hydrocephalus and upper spinal cord compression. Intellect and life expectancy are normal.

Management is supportive and anticipatory with frequent review for assessment of potential complications.

SHOX Related Disorders

The short stature homeobox gene (SHOX) is an important growth gene located on the X and Y chromosomes. SHOX haploinsufficiency is associated with the short stature seen in Turner syndrome, Leri–Weill syndrome (LWS) and a percentage of idiopathic short stature.

The skeletal abnormalities associated with SHOX haploinsufficiency include mesomelic short stature, scoliosis, high arched palate, Madelung deformity of the wrist, short fourth metacarpals and exostoses. Those with LWS also tend to have a muscular body habitus. Unlike other skeletal dysplasias, there is good evidence that the short stature of SHOX-related disorders responds well to growth hormone therapy, with gains in final height of approximately 8 cm. It should be noted that the non-skeletal features of Turner syndrome, namely lymphoedema, cardiac abnormalities, gonadal failure and renal abnormalities, are not related to SHOX haploinsufficiency.[17]

Mucopolysaccharidoses and Lipoidoses

The mucopolysaccharidoses comprise disorders such as Hunter, Hurler and Morquio disease that are caused by reduced activity of the lysosomal enzymes that break down glycosaminoglycans. Accumulation of glycosaminoglycans within the marrow cells results in a pattern of skeletal abnormalities collectively referred to as 'dysostosis multiplex'. The phenotype can vary widely between and within disorders depending on the specific enzymopathy and mutation. Features of the skeletal phenotype include macrocephaly, dyscephaly, a J-shaped sella turcica, osteoporosis, abnormal ribs and clavicles, ova/hook-shaped vertebral bodies, dysplasia of the capital femoral epiphyses, coxa valga, epiphyseal and metaphyseal dysplasia and proximal tapering of the metacarpals. Joint contractures are also seen. Due to the variability of phenotype that clinical picture can be similar to that of growth hormone deficiency. Treatment is largely supportive, although in some centres bone marrow transplant and enzyme replacement therapy are being used.

References

1. Rauch F, Plotkin H, DiMeglio L, Engelbert RH, et al. Fracture prediction and the definition of osteoporosis in children and adolescents: the ISCD 2007 Pediatric Official Positions. *J Clin Densitom* 2008; **11**:22–8.

2. Garn SM, Poznanski AK, Nagt JM. Bone measurements in the differential diagnosis of osteopenia and osteoporosis. *Diagnostic Radiology* 1971;**100**: 509–18.

3. Munns CF, Cowell CT. Prevention and treatment of osteoporosis in chronically ill children. *J Musculoskelet Neuronal Interact* 2005;**5**:262–72.

4. Munns CFJ, Sillence DO. Disorders predisposing to bone fragility and decreased bone density. In: Rimoin DL, Connor JM, Pyeritz RE, Korf BR, editors. *Principles and Practice of Medical Genetics*. Philadelphia: Churchill Livingstone Elsevier; 2007. p. 3671–91.

5. Rauch F, Glorieux FH. Osteogenesis imperfecta. *Lancet* 2004;**363**:1377–85.

6. Chaisson R, Munns C, Zeitlin L. *Interdisciplinary Treatment of Osteogenesis Imperfecta*. Montreal: Shriners Hospital for Children (Canada); 2004.

7. Plotkin H, Rauch F, Zeitlin L, et al. Effect of pamidronate treatment in children with polyostotic fibrous dysplasia of bone. *J Clin Endocrinol Metab* 2003;**88**: 4569–75.

8. Ward LM, Glorieux FH. The spectrum of pediatric osteoporosis. In: Glorieux FH, Pettifor J, Jueppner H, editors. *Pediatric Bone: biology and disease*, San Diego: Academic Press; 2003. p. 401–42.

9. Zacharin M. Current advances in bone health of disabled children. *Curr Opin Pediatr* 2004;**16**:545–51.

10. Bailey DA, Martin AD, McKay HA, et al. Calcium accretion in girls and boys during puberty: a longitudinal analysis. *J Bone Miner Res* 2000;**15**:2245–50.

11. Greenway A, Zacharin M. Vitamin D status of chronically ill or disabled children in Victoria. *J Paediatr Child Health* 2003;**39**:543–7.

12. Leonard MB, Feldman HI, Shults J, Zemel BS, et al. Long-term, high-dose glucocorticoids and bone mineral content in childhood glucocorticoid-sensitive nephrotic syndrome. *N Engl J Med* 2004;**351**:868–75.

13. Batch JA, Couper JJ, Rodda C, et al. Use of bisphosphonate therapy for osteoporosis in childhood and adolescence. *J Paediatr Child Health* 2003;**39**: 88–92.

14. Alanay Y, Rimoin DL. Chondrodysplasias. In: Rosen CJ, editor. *Primer on the Metabolic Bone Diseases and Disorders of Mineral Metabolism*. 7th ed. Washington: The American Society for Bone and Mineral Research; 2008. p. 428–9.

15. Whyte MP. Sclerosing bone disorders. In: Rosen CJ, editor. *Primer on the Metabolic Bone Diseases and Disorders of Mineral Metabolism*. 7th ed. Washington: The American Society for Bone and Mineral Research; 2008. p. 412–23.

16. American Academy of Pediatrics Committee on Genetics. Health supervision for children with achondroplasia. *Pediatrics* 1995;**95**:443–51.

17. Munns CF, Glass IA, Flanagan S, et al. Familial growth and skeletal features associated with SHOX haploinsufficiency. *J Pediatr Endocrinol Metab* 2003;**16**: 987–96.

Paediatric and Adolescent Gynaecology

Sonia Grover

PAEDIATRIC GYNAECOLOGY

Although childhood is a period when reproductive hormones are relatively inactive, nevertheless there are a few problems that do present under the guise of possible paediatric endocrinology.

Concerns regarding the genitalia of young girls do occasionally present to the paediatric endocrinologist.

Abnormal Genital Appearance with No Visible Vagina

The commonest problem with this presentation is labial adhesions/fusion/agglutination. This is not present at birth when maternal oestrogen levels are transmitted to the infant (sometimes accompanied by the presence of a breast bud), but when the oestrogen levels fall (and the breast bud disappears), thinning and irritation of the labial skin can result in labial adhesions occurring. These are relatively common, with reported rates of up to 50%.

Vulval examination reveals a midline stripe, where the fusion has occurred.

Management

As labial adhesions never persist after puberty, there is usually no reason to undertake any intervention. It is very rare for complete occlusion of the introitus and vulva to occur, in which situation the young girl will present with acute urinary retention.

Occasionally, toilet-trained girls will complain of urine loss after voiding. This can usually be managed with simple advice of sitting on the toilet for longer, to allow the urine that is behind the labial adhesions to drain.

Practical Pediatric Endocrinology in a Limited Resource Setting
http://dx.doi.org/10.1016/B978-0-12-407822-2.00010-4

Other treatment options that have been used in the past include lateral traction to separate the adhesions, but there is a greater than 50% recurrence rate and the approach can be traumatic for the girl. An alternative that has been used is topical oestrogen cream. This is effective in about 50% of cases, but also has a greater than 50% recurrence rate. Topical oestrogen can result in systemic oestrogenisation and consequent breast development.

Pressure to investigate and to prove that a vagina and uterus are present should be resisted. In this age group, the uterus may be very small and ultrasound and other imaging techniques can have great difficulty identifying these structures.

(An alternative explanation for apparent labial adhesions may be female genital mutilation [FGM]. See later section on FGM.)

Vulvovaginitis

Vulvovaginitis occurs as a consequence of the low-oestrogen state, which is normal in prepubescent girls. The usual clinical presentation is one of smelly vaginal discharge, burning with micturition and perineal soreness. Other diagnoses such as child sexual abuse need to be considered and excluded.

In the low-oestrogen state, the vaginal and introital skin is relatively atrophic, and thus is easily irritated, with a resultant vaginal discharge. The moisture from the discharge then irritates the external skin.

Management

Investigations are rarely required (once child sexual abuse has been excluded). Microscopy and culture from the introital area will reveal only mixed bowel flora, which is normal. Barrier cream to the irritated skin reduces the burning and stinging sensation. Bathing will reduce the discharge. The natural history of this is for intermittent recurrences to occur until puberty, when oestrogens change the vaginal flora and thicken the vaginal and introital skin.

In the presence of a bloodstained discharge, other diagnoses need consideration, including foreign body and the rare childhood vaginal and urethral tumour (sarcoma botryoides). Referral to a specialist gynaecologist is required. Examination under anaesthetic of the vagina requires the use of an appropriate paediatric-size speculum (often a nasal speculum will suffice when a small size is required).

ADOLESCENT GYNAECOLOGY

Disorders of pubertal development, including precocious puberty and delayed puberty, are discussed at length in Chapter 2. As the age of puberty and menarche are influenced by parental age of puberty, weight, general health, altitude and level of physical activity, some care needs to be taken in deciding when to investigate.

Primary Amenorrhoea

Presentation with primary amenorrhoea can be quite late, with some older teenage girls presenting with primary infertility. The usual interval between the onset of breast development and menarche is about 2 years. When the delay is greater than 4 years, then investigation is warranted.

Additionally, features that suggest the progression through puberty may be atypical also warrant investigation. Development of excess hirsutism, clitoromegaly or voice changes, or an unexplained regression of previous changes with a reduction in size of breasts, would also provoke the need for investigation.

Settings in which Primary Amenorrhoea may Occur

NORMAL PUBERTAL PROGRESSION, NORMAL PUBIC AND AXILLARY HAIR

In the presence of apparently normal completion of pubertal development, with normal pubic and axillary hair development, if menarche is delayed for many months, a structural anomaly is most likely.

- **In the presence of cyclic pain**, imperforate hymen is most likely. Palpation of the lower abdomen will reveal some suprapubic fullness or a mass. With visualisation of the perineal area, and gentle pressure on the suprapubic area, the hymen can be seen to bulge. No imaging is required to clarify the diagnosis. A simple hymenectomy will resolve the problem. If gentle pressure on the suprapubic area does not result in distension of the perineal area, it is likely that a transverse septum is present. The management of this is more complex and further investigation and expertise will be required. Suppression of menses with medroxyprogesterone acetate (MPA) or continuous oral contraceptive pill can be administered while access to further specialist surgical care is organised.
- **In the absence of cyclic pain,** the commonest diagnosis is vaginal agenesis. Young women with vaginal agenesis often have associated anomalies, including renal agenesis, and spinal and/or cardiac anomalies. Examination of the genital area will enable some assessment of whether a hymen is present or not. Where a normal hymen is visible, gentle insertion of a cotton wool stick will allow measurement of the length of the vagina. Dilatation (with either dilators or with sexual activity) is likely to be successful in these young women. Where a hymen is visible there are likely to be two kidneys present and no other anomalies. In the absence of a hymen, there is a higher likelihood of an absent kidney and other anomalies. Although dilatation can be successful in this group as well, there is a suggestion that it may be more difficult.

A further diagnosis for primary amenorrhoea, to consider in the setting of normal pubertal development and normal hymen visible on genital examination, is tuberculous endometritis. Examination under anaesthetic will allow the identification of a cervix. The endometrial cavity may be obliterated by tuberculosis (TB).

NORMAL PUBERTAL PROGRESSION, LESS THAN NORMAL PUBIC AND AXILLARY HAIR

Where pubertal changes have occurred but there is less pubic and axillary hair than expected, a diagnosis of androgen insensitivity syndrome (AIS) needs to be considered. Careful examination and palpation of the inguinal region and labia may allow identification of testes. *(See Chapter 5 on DSD for management)*. Removal of intra-abdominal testes is recommended due to the increased malignancy risk of about 15%. This is in contrast to complete androgen insensitivity where cancer risk is very low. Extra-abdominal testes may be left, although they may be the source of pain with sexual activity.

Although leaving the testes means that there is a source of endogenous oestrogens due to the conversion of testosterone to oestrogen, this is often inadequate for bone mineral density protection. Alternatively, the need for ongoing compliance with oestrogen therapy following removal of testes is always an issue of concern.

The vaginal length in women with AIS does not usually require any intervention, with improvement in length readily occurring with sexual activity or dilatation.

NORMAL PUBERTAL PROGRESSION, INCREASED PUBIC AND AXILLARY HAIR

Where excess hair has occurred as pubertal changes progress, other diagnoses need consideration.

- **Polycystic ovarian disease.** Although the description of polycystic ovary syndrome (PCOS) is often one of oligomenorrhoea, it can present as primary amenorrhoea. This is most likely in the presence of significant weight gain or obesity, often with other markers of the metabolic syndrome – with acanthosis nigricans, hyperlipidaemia and sometimes elevated blood glucose. There is usually no evidence of clitoromegaly.

A progesterone challenge test (7 days of oral progestogen – either norethisterone acetate or medroxyprogesterone acetate) will often provoke a withdrawal bleed, thus enabling confirmation that a functional uterus and oestrogenisation are present. (See below for further discussion regarding management of PCOS.)

- **Congenital Adrenal Hyperplasia.** The hirsutism associated with congenital adrenal hyperplasia will often begin in childhood rather than after puberty. Associated clinical findings may be evidence of clitoromegaly and posterior labial fusion. If androgen levels are high enough there will be suppression of ovarian function with subsequent low oestrogens. This may manifest as relatively poor breast development with otherwise normal linear pubertal growth or as early growth cessation after tall stature and rapid childhood growth. A progesterone challenge test will thus be negative – despite the presence of a uterus. Abnormal or increased pigmentation compared to other family members may assist in making a clinical diagnosis. (*See Chapter 4, Adrenal Disorders.*)
- **Partial AIS and other XY conditions.** Some clitoromegaly and posterior labial fusion is usually present in these conditions – as well as hirsutism. Karyotype may allow confirmation of a diagnosis of mixed gonadal dysgenesis. Complex testing is usually required to clarify other diagnoses. (*See Chapter 4, Adrenal Disorders, and Chapter 5, Disorders of Sexual Development.*)

Testes need to be removed if they are intra-abdominal due to the risk of malignancy of these structures. The urgency to remove the testes if they are extra-abdominal is not so great as the malignancy risk is not as high, and palpation is possible. Nevertheless, removal should be considered due to the need for follow-up and the likelihood of pain associated with sexual activity if the gonads are sited externally. Following removal of the testes, oestrogen replacement therapy is required. Correction of the posterior labial fusion may be necessary to allow sexual intercourse. Vaginal length may be amenable to dilatation and may not require surgical intervention.

Polycystic Ovarian Syndrome

The internationally agreed criteria for this entity have been changed a number of times, and they were developed primarily to reach a consensus for the diagnosis for adult women.

The application of these criteria to teenagers is thus problematic. Teenagers have irregular menses for the first 1 to 3 years post menarche, thus oligomenorrhoea is of no assistance in making the diagnosis within the first 3 years post menarche. Another diagnostic criterion relates to evidence of excess androgens, which includes acne. As teenagers get acne as part of the pubertal adrenarche, this criteria can provoke unnecessary concern. Although the international criteria do include the possibility of measuring serum androgens, interpretation may be misleading. Laboratory variations in measured androgen levels are such that many young women are inappropriately labelled as having excess androgens on blood results. If there is clinical concern regarding the possibility of excess androgens – as demonstrated by excess hirsutism, voice changes, or clitoromegaly – androgen levels should be measured to ensure exclusion of androgen-producing tumours and 17-OH progesterone should be performed, to exclude non-classical congenital adrenal hyperplasia. Otherwise, measurement of androgens rarely contributes to management in this condition.

The clinical findings of a young woman who is overweight, with oligomenorrhoea (not within the first 3 years post menarche) and evidence of acanthosis is likely to fulfil the criteria for PCOS, without any laboratory investigations having been performed. A pelvic ultrasound to clarify the number of follicles on the ovaries is not likely to be of any assistance. In young teenagers, the ovaries are a little disorganised due to the relative immaturity of the hypothalamic-pituitary-ovarian axis, with consequent anovulatory cycles. The normal number of follicles in an adolescent ovary is between 10 and 20 follicles. A teenage ovary is thus normally multicystic. A polycystic ovary by definition is larger with more than 20 peripherally located follicles. Around 22% of the female population have the ultrasound appearance of PCOS whereas only around 8% have PCOS.

The most important aspect of PCOS is the risk for diabetes, metabolic syndrome and the complications relating to obesity. Concerns regarding oligomenorrhoea (and ovulation) are largely corrected by increased exercise and weight reduction which result in a return of ovulation. There is evidence that fertility will return with regular exercise of 30–40 minutes four times a week within 6 months.

Management

HIRSUTISM

Interventions relating to reduction in hirsutism (spironolactone 100–200 mg daily, acting as an androgen receptor blocker; or cyproterone acetate 50–100 mg daily, from day 1–10 of the menstrual cycle) should be provided at the same time as measures to increase exercise and decrease weight. Both types of medication often cause either polymenorrhoea or oligomenorrhoea. Concomitant use of the oral contraceptive pill is usually given for this reason and also because it may have an additive effect on suppression of ovarian androgen production.

FERTILITY INDUCTION

Regular exercise and weight reduction should be the major focus. This has the additional benefit of reducing the risks to the woman during pregnancy and to the fetus, associated with maternal obesity and gestational diabetes. Other approaches that have been advocated in the past include diathermy (known as 'golf balling') to the ovary. This practice should be avoided as ovarian failure has been reported as a consequence and the pregnancy-associated risks of excess maternal weight are not addressed by this approach.

Clomiphene citrate can be used as an alternative to metformin for ovulation induction. Care needs to be taken with the doses due to the risk of multiple pregnancy. In the first two cycles of clomiphene use, it is appropriate to commence with clomiphene 25 mg from day 5–9 of cycle, where day 1 is the first day of the menses. When there has been amenorrhoea or significant oligomenorrhoea, the menses may be provoked with the use of oral progestogen – either medroxyprogesterone acetate 10 mg daily or norethisterone acetate 5 mg daily for 10–14 days, with the first day of bleeding again being considered day 1).

Ideally, tests for ovulation should occur – usually on about day 24 (testing for both serum progesterone and oestrogen). In the first cycle ovulation often does not occur, as there is a significant lag time to adequately stimulate the follicles. Dose change should not occur after the first cycle, but can be adjusted after the second cycle if ovulation does not occur. As ovulation occurs, the cycle length shortens down to 30–35 days. This means that ovulation is still occurring at about day 16–20 rather than day 14. Hence it is important that couples know that regular intercourse needs to be occurring, preferably every day or alternate days from around day 12 till day 22.

Metformin is used as an alternative approach to induce regular menses and ovulation, at a dose of 500–100 mg twice a day and is particularly useful in the context of evidence of elevated glucose and insulin (which will be apparent with the presence of acanthosis nigricans). Concomitant efforts to increase exercise and reduce weight should be encouraged.

Heavy Menses

Normal Menstruation

Normal periods last between 3 to 7 or 8 days. Measuring heaviness of menses is fraught with difficulty due to the variations in interpretation of what is heavy. This is particularly the case in families where several of the women experience heavy menses – and thus consider this to be normal. Additionally, the variation in the types of menstrual hygiene products and their respective absorptive capacity, as well as the comfort of the young women in terms of desire to change these (i.e. when the menstrual pad may be only partly stained with blood versus one where it is completely soaked), will all influence the frequency of pad changes or the number of pads used per day.

In general, if menstrual hygiene pads require changing under 2-hourly because they are soaked, or overnight changes are necessary, or flooding is occurring (when menstrual loss cannot be constrained by menstrual hygiene pads or tampons), concern needs to be present that the loss is excessive. Prolonged moderate loss can also be an important problem. The presence of clots is usually not very helpful – unless the clots are large (greater than 6 cm diameter).

Abnormal Menstruation

Although bleeding disorders may be responsible for heavy periods, in the girl presenting within a few cycles of menarche, the most likely explanation will be anovulatory bleeding. Bleeding disorders can often be recognised by the presence of other bleeding symptoms or by the presence of other family members with bleeding problems. Prolonged epistaxes, bleeding post tonsillectomy, maternal postpartum haemorrhage, and recurrent significant ovulation pain are all helpful features in trying to identify those with bleeding disorders. Testing for bleeding disorders is difficult, with false normal results frequently seen if testing is undertaken at the time of an acute bleed or when the girl is stressed.

The main benefit in knowing that a bleeding disorder is present is being aware of the risks of significant bleeding in future at the time of surgery, and also the recognition that the problems will not settle with time (unlike anovulatory bleeding in the girl who is just post menarchal).

As pregnancy and stress result in improved coagulation factors, girls with mild bleeding disorders may not experience major problems at the time of delivery. Nevertheless it should be noted that studies suggest their risk of a postpartum haemorrhage is approximately 25%, which is higher than the usual background rate of 5%.

Acute and Short-Term Management of Menorrhagia

There is only limited evidence regarding the various management options.

TRANEXAMIC ACID

In the first instance, the use of tranexamic acid (500 mg 4 times daily if less than 50 kg, 1 g 4 times daily if greater than 50 kg) on days of heavy bleeding may be adequate to reduce heavy bleeding to lighter bleeding (studies suggest a reduction in menstrual loss of 50% with this medication).

PROGESTOGEN

In the context of a prolonged period, the first option would be the use of a progestogen – either medroxyprogesterone acetate 10 mg or norethisterone acetate (NEA) 5 mg tablets. Either of these can be used acutely, as 2 tablets administered 2-hourly till the bleeding settles, then maintaining three times daily doses for a week, before a very gradual reduction over the subsequent 3 weeks. On ceasing the progestogen, a bleed is expected to occur. It is desirable to delay a period, particularly if the girl is anaemic.

(An alternative may be to use the combined oral contraceptive pill instead of a progestogen.)

Occasionally, despite progestogen and/or the combined oral contraceptive pill, bleeding does not settle. In these contexts, it is presumed that the endometrium has been completely shed and there is no endometrium on which the progestogen can work.

OESTROGEN

In this setting the use of oestrogens (either IV combined equine oestrogens [Premarin®] 25 mg if this is available, or oral Premarin 0.625, 2 tablets twice or three times a day) will provoke the development of endometrium and 36 hours later progestogen or the oral contraceptive pill can then be commenced. The bleeding may not completely settle during the use of the oestrogen, but the subsequent addition of progestogen will then be effective. The dose of progestogen required in this setting is not usually as high — and 1 tablet twice a day of either NEA 5 mg or medroxyprogesterone acetate 10 mg will suffice.

Long-Term Management of Menorrhagia

AIMING TO REDUCE MENSTRUAL FLOW BUT TO MAINTAIN CURRENT FERTILITY

On a long-term basis, heavy menses can be managed with tranexamic acid (50% reduction in menstrual loss) or non-steroidal anti-inflammatory agents (30% reduction in menstrual loss) if fertility is desired.

AIMING TO REDUCE MENSTRUAL FLOW BUT IMPAIR CURRENT FERTILITY

All these hormonal options could be used with tranexamic acid.

Cyclic progestogen used for 21 out of 28 days will reduce menstrual loss (MPA10 mg or NEA 5 mg daily) but may reduce fertility, although it would not be considered reliable as contraception.

The combined oral contraceptive pill, or the levonorgestrel intrauterine system (IUS), will also both reduce menstrual loss but they are both contraceptive.

AIMING FOR AMENORRHOEA

Achievement of amenorrhoea is likely with the use of depot medroxyprogesterone acetate, oral MPA 10 mg twice a day, NEA 5 mg twice a day, or continuous combined oral contraceptive pill (i.e. skipping all sugar pills). These options are particularly useful if the young woman has been experiencing significant ovulation-related pains or has had a recognised haemoperitoneum in association with ovulation, because these approaches will suppress ovulation.

Menstrual Management for Girls who Have a Disability

Physical and/or intellectual disability can be associated with significant practical difficulties for menstrual management in an affected adolescent or young adult. While menstruation may be regular and otherwise normal, the need for care by a variety of people may put an extra burden on families and can lead to social isolation for part of each month.

Various management options exist, although financial constraint may reduce access.

- Use of the continuous contraceptive pill (cutting off the sugar pills) often results in minimisation of endometrial thickness and oligomenorrhoea.
- A progesterone-bearing intrauterine device provides 5 years of amenorrhoea and 5 years of contraception. It is thus often seen as a major advantage to families. Insertion requires that the uterus is of adult dimensions and insertion is limited only by the ability to negotiate a tight nulliparous

cervix. A light general anaesthetic is required for these girls.

• Depot progestogen is undesirable as it switches off the hypothalamic-pituitary-ovarian axis and causes ongoing bone loss with increased osteoporosis risk in an already compromised situation of reduced weight bearing and immobility. If used it must be in combination with oestrogen.

Contraception

Sexual activity carries the risk of both pregnancy and sexually transmitted infections (STI). Condoms are important for STI protection and have limited value for contraception. Alternative more reliable contraception using oral contraceptives and longer acting alternative such as depot medroxyprogesterone acetate (3 months), etonogestrel (3 years), copper intrauterine devices (IUDs) (5 years) and levo-norgestrel IUDs are all options. See web sites for further information on contraception (www.ippf.org/en/Resources/Contraception/Myths+WholeData.htm), for young people about sex, relationships and STIs (www.likeitis.org); for organisation and international perspectives on approaches to managing reproductive health problems in developing countries (http://www.mariestopes.org/Publication.aspx?Frid=1).

Ovarian Cysts

Normal ovarian function is dependent on the production of hormones, which occurs in follicles — which are physiological cysts. In childhood it is common to see a small number (2—5) of ovarian follicles of 2—3 mm diameter in each ovary on an ultrasound. With the onset of puberty the number and size of the follicles increases. Thus, in 20-year-old women, 25% of young women will have 20 follicles visible on each ovary. This is normal and should not be considered part of or diagnostic of PCOS. Other

features are required to make this diagnosis (see earlier section on PCOS). With the maturation of the hypothalamic-pituitary-ovarian axis, ovulation begins to occur. For those girls who have their menarche earlier, regular ovulatory cycles are established sooner, often within a year. For those who reach menarche at 15 years or older, it may take 3 or 4 years before ovulatory cycles occur.

With ovulation, the ovary produces a 3—4 cm ovulation follicle. This is completely normal, and may at times be associated with pain. At the time of ovulation the egg is released and is attracted to the fimbria by chemotaxis. Fertilisation occurs within the fallopian tube. The process of the egg leaving the ovulation follicle can result in rupture of the follicle, or haemorrhage within the ovulation follicle resulting in a haemorrhagic corpus luteum. This can be quite painful, and on ultrasound can give a complex appearance. Resolution of this haemorrhagic cyst can take a few weeks. If undertaking a follow-up ultrasound, it is worth waiting 6 weeks.

Teen Pregnancy

The socially acceptable age for pregnancy and marriage varies significantly in different cultures and communities. For many countries, marriage and pregnancy tends to occur at younger ages where there are other contributing factors such as poverty and lower levels of education. There is an interaction here, as girls who are not achieving within an educational environment may then chose to discontinue their study and prefer to have children. Unfortunately, in most parts of the world, lower levels of education are associated with ongoing poverty and poorer options and outcomes for children. Not surprisingly, education of women is seen as a critical factor in improving the survival and welfare of their children.

For young teenagers who are pregnant there are common themes throughout the world. Their ability to continue with their education is often limited, and their capacity to return to education once they have had children is equally difficult. Thus they and their children are likely to remain in poverty.

Teenagers who are pregnant are usually living in circumstances associated with financial hardship.

- Their ability to access healthcare is thus limited, placing them at increased risk for pregnancy-related complications which may have been amenable to intervention if they had been able to attend for antenatal care.
- Due to poverty as well as lack of support, the teenagers' knowledge and access to adequate nutrition may be limited. In some communities this may be associated with malnutrition, in others this may be obesity with a poor diet, and for others this may be associated with eating disorders.
- Endemic problems of vitamin D deficiency are frequent in these circumstances, particularly in cultures where covering clothing is worn. In turn this puts an infant at high risk of early, severe vitamin D deficiency and its complications.
- Housing and community support and social isolation or exclusion may also be consequences of teenage pregnancy.
- Other health-risk behaviours also need to be considered. They are often at increased risk of sexually transmitted infections (human immunodeficiency virus [HIV], chlamydia, *Neisseria gonorrhoeae*, *Herpes simplex*, syphilis) and they should be screened for these infections. The use of drugs, tobacco and alcohol are also increased in some communities — and as these have significant impact on the health of the young woman as well as the pregnancy, careful questions regarding these need to occur.

Female Genital Mutilation/Cutting

There has been considerable discussion and debate about this expression, with the suggestion that the alternative expression of female genital cutting (FGC) may be more respectful to the women who have undergone this procedure. In recognition of this the expression female genital mutilation/cutting (FGM/C) will be used in this chapter. When talking to women and their families it may be appropriate to use the expressions 'traditional cutting' or 'female circumcision'.

FGM/C covers a spectrum of genital procedures, from very minor cutting, where in some cases the women may be unaware that anything has been done to their genitalia, to more significant procedures. These procedures are undertaken for cultural reasons, are not specifically linked to any religious group and occur in many parts of Africa but also in parts of Asia. With the substantial migration that has occurred in the last two decades, women and girls with FGM/C are now seen and cared for in all parts of the world.

There is an international classification of FGM/C, although the classification is not without problems. For example, the external appearance of the genitalia of a young woman who has had FGM/C performed may result in the labia majora being joined in the midline, suggestive of a more significant or severe procedure (e.g. a 'type 3', implying that the clitoris and labia minora have been completely removed), but underneath the labial adhesions both the clitoris and labia minora may in fact be untouched. The age at which the procedure is performed varies in different communities, but can be undertaken in the neonate through to the teenager. With international and national efforts to ban these procedures, there is evidence that the number of procedures as well as the severity of the procedures are reducing. In the past, all such procedures were carried out in the local communities without analgesia, but today an increasing number are being done in hospitals, partly as a harm-minimisation tactic, although clearly completely discontinuing the practice is the aim.

Complications associated with FGM/C include acute complications of haemorrhage and infection. Inclusion cysts occur with the accumulation of skin secretions, with the child presenting with a 'genital anomaly' which may be periclitoral in position. The presence of the midline fusion of either the labia minor or labia majora, combined with the history of FGM/C, will confirm the diagnosis.

Urinary symptoms are not usually reported. However, it should be recognised that with voiding, the urine flow is not usually direct but instead is associated with dribbling. Most often the FGM/C was undertaken in childhood. A girl/adolescent or young woman seeking reversal of the procedure will not remember a more normal urine flow pattern. She should be warned of this difference prior to 'undoing' the labial adhesions of the FGM/C.

Although dysmenorrhoea has been reported, the single opening for both urine and menses is usually at least 1 cm — and thus is very unlikely to be responsible for any obstruction to the menstrual loss (compared to the cervical canal which is only 2 or 3 mm in diameter). An inability to have sexual intercourse and dyspareunia are both important issues for most women who have had a FGM/C, and they will often require surgical division of the FGM/C labial adhesions. This should be done with adequate analgesia to avoid any further trauma to the young woman.

Pregnancy can occur in the presence of persistent labial adhesions of FGM/C (despite the inability for penetration to occur). The FGM/C may then be responsible for obstructed labour during childbirth, with the risk of bladder and bowel fistulae if assistance is not available.

Further Reading

Knight R, Hotchin A, Bayly C, Grover S. Female Genital Mutilation: experience of the Royal Women's Hospital, Melbourne. *Aust N Z J Obstet Gynaecol* 1999;**39**:5054.

Moran LJ, Hutchison SK, Norman RJ, Teede HJ. Lifestyle changes in women with polycystic ovary syndrome. *Cochrane Database Syst Rev* 2011;7:CD007506.

United Nations Children's Fund, The Strategic Information Section and Child Protection Section. *Female Genital Mutilation/Cutting: a statistical exploration*. New York: UNICEF, 2005.

World Health Organization, Department of Reproductive Health and Research. *Eliminating Female Genital Mutilation: an interagency statement*, Geneva: WHO, 2008.

Endocrine Dysfunction and Disease in the Neonatal Period

Amanda L. Ogilvy-Stuart, Paula Midgley

INTRODUCTION

While endocrine disease in the newborn is uncommon, it may be life-threatening or have profound long-term sequelae if not diagnosed and treated promptly. Endocrine dysfunction, however, is common, particularly in the preterm and sick newborn baby.

The hormonal milieu is influenced by the mother and the placenta. Maternal nutritional deficiencies such as iodine or vitamin D may have lasting effects on the fetus and infant.

Severe malnutrition in pregnancy and lactation may result not only in long-term metabolic consequences for the baby but lasting effects into subsequent generations.

Abrupt hormonal changes occur at parturition, and interpretation of results needs to take this into account. In the preterm baby, the situation can be more complex as there are no truly normative data, because the baby should still be *in utero*.

The symptoms and signs of endocrine disease or dysfunction in the newborn are

Practical Pediatric Endocrinology in a Limited Resource Setting
http://dx.doi.org/10.1016/B978-0-12-407822-2.00011-6

non-specific, so they need to be thought of in the differential diagnosis of babies who present with these symptoms. This chapter explores some of the endocrine pathologies which are unique to the newborn or which may have a different presentation or management from older children.

FETAL AND NEONATAL GLUCOSE PHYSIOLOGY

Fetal glucose levels are determined by the placenta and reflect maternal levels. There is no endogenous glucose production. Glycogen stores are laid down in the last month of gestation and adipose tissue in the last trimester. Sugar levels fall over the first 2 hours of life. In healthy term babies this activates the counter-regulatory hormones, resulting in high levels of adrenaline, glucagon and growth hormone levels and a fall in insulin levels. Glycogenolysis, gluconeogenesis and lipolysis are induced, causing a rapid rise in fatty acids and ketone bodies providing alternative metabolic fuels. Glycogen levels are rapidly depleted, but glucose levels stabilise by 4—6 hours of age.

HYPOGLYCAEMIA

The healthy term baby of normal birth weight does not need blood sugar levels to be measured — if sugar levels were to be measured in the first 4 hours of life, they would like to be low. In contrast *symptomatic* hypoglycaemia (see Box 11.1) in a term baby is always pathological until proved otherwise.

Hypoglycaemia Should be Anticipated in the Following Babies

- **Small for gestational age (SGA) babies.** Many will be normal, healthy,

---

> ### BOX 11.1
> ### SYMPTOMS OF HYPOGLYCAEMIA
>
> Neuroglycopaenic symptoms: Jittering, irritability, lethargy, apnoea, hypotonia, feeding problems, convulsions, coma.
>
> (Autonomic symptoms, e.g. pallor, sweating, tachypnoea, are not prominent in the newborn.)

---

constitutionally small babies. Those that have been growth restricted *in utero* fail to lay down adipose tissue and glycogen stores and are vulnerable to hypoglycaemia. Generally, they will have asymmetrical growth restriction, with relative sparing of head growth and length. Babies with symmetrical growth retardation are more likely to have an underlying chromosomal problem or congenital infection. These babies often have defective counter-regulatory responses, resulting in a poor ketogenic response, enhanced glycolysis and high insulin levels.

- **Large for gestational age babies.** Some will be healthy, constitutionally large babies while others will be exposed to excessive insulin or insulin-like growth factors *in utero* (such as infants of diabetic mothers and babies with Beckwith—Wiedemann syndrome).
- **Preterm babies.** Like SGA babies, these babies have a lack of glycogen stores, immature enzymes involved in glucose homeostasis and often inappropriately high insulin levels.
- **Babies with a history of birth depression** (who utilised glycogen stores during delivery).
- **Polycythaemic babies** in whom the erythrocytes utilise glucose.
- **Maternal or neonatal β-blocker use.**

Management Plan

As hypoglycaemia is anticipated, these babies require diligent review of sugar measurements after birth until stable. Blood sugar should be measured using a method which is accurate at low levels.

For sick, small or premature babies glucose level may be measured on admission to the neonatal unit.

If able to feed, milk should be given 1—3-hourly depending on gestation, size and well-being, usually via a nasogastric tube. The baby usually requires at least 60 mL/kg/day to maintain normoglycaemia.

Vulnerable babies, who remain with their mothers, should be encouraged to feed within an hour of birth, establishing normal hormonal regulation of glucose. Breast milk results in better ketogenic responses than formula milk. Skin-to-skin contact keeps baby warm and supports breast feeding. If the baby does not breastfeed, give expressed breast milk, or formula feed (7.5 mL/kg, i.e. 3-hourly amount of 60 mL/kg/day). Check blood sugar levels and observe temperature, respiratory rate, heart rate, work of breathing, colour and behaviour pre-feed starting before the second feed (after the physiological dip in blood sugar). If the blood sugars are maintained at or above 2.6 mmol/L, for three consecutive readings, discontinue monitoring but ensure at least eight feeds in 24 hours. If there is concern about clinical condition or nutritional intake, another blood sugar reading should be taken.

If enteral feeding is not possible, commence an intravenous 10% dextrose infusion (at least 5 mg/kg/minute, i.e. 72 mL/kg/day). Increase the infusion rate if hypoglycaemia is not controlled. Care should be taken with large volumes, which can result in hyponatraemia. If hypoglycaemia is difficult to control on reasonable volumes, or fluid restriction is required, a central line and higher glucose concentrations will be needed. Enteral feeds should be introduced as soon as possible. Once sugar levels are stable, intravenous (IV) fluids should be reduced and oral feeds increased.

If the baby is unexpectedly hypoglycaemic investigate as outlined in *Chapter 13, Hypoglycaemia*.

In the majority of cases, hypoglycaemia is transient and outcome would be expected to be normal and no follow-up required. If hypoglycaemia is severe or prolonged, brain injury may occur and long-term neurodevelopmental outcome guarded.

HYPERGLYCAEMIA

Blood sugar levels greater than 7 mmol/L are unusual in healthy term babies. Most neonatologists would treat by reducing sugar intake or with insulin if the blood sugar was greater than 10—12 mmol/L, especially with significant glycosuria causing an osmotic diuresis, particularly in sick preterm babies.

Hyperglycaemia is usually picked up incidentally on routine blood glucose assessment or in response to finding glycosuria or it may be noted in the work-up of a sick baby.

Hyperglycaemia is common in very preterm or SGA babies due to impaired insulin secretion and/or insulin resistance and immaturity of liver enzymes involved in glucose metabolism. If hyperglycaemia occurs out of context (such as a previously healthy, appropriate for gestational age, enterally fed infant), the cause needs to be identified. Other common causes of hyperglycaemia include sepsis, stress, iatrogenic (excessive intravenous glucose), or drugs, particularly corticosteroids. Rare causes include transient or permanent neonatal diabetes or pancreatic agenesis.

To confirm the diagnosis, measure the true blood glucose and calculate the glucose infusion rate to exclude excessive glucose delivery.

To exclude neonatal diabetes if hyperglycaemia is persistent measure concomitant:

glucose, insulin, C-peptide and ketone bodies and urine for ketones. Genetic investigations are possible but are expensive and not readily available.

Management

- Treat underlying cause (sepsis etc.).
- Reduce glucose infusion rate (if high) and/or calorie intake to 5 mg/kg/minute (equivalent to 3 mL/kg/hour of 10% dextrose, fetal glucose production rate) but not below 3 mg/kg/minute of glucose or 45 kcal/kg/day.
- Some very premature babies develop hyperglycaemia and an osmotic diuresis with normal infusions of glucose. This can be treated by reducing the glucose input or giving an insulin infusion.
- Treatment with insulin should be considered when the blood sugar is greater than 10 mmol/L or there is an osmotic diuresis. The suggested starting treatment dose of insulin is 0.05 unit/kg/hour. This may need to be altered depending on response. When using insulin it is *essential* to have accurate blood sugar measurements to identify and avoid hypoglycaemia. Insulin therapy can usually be discontinued after a few days once hormonal maturation and maturation of the liver has occurred, but hyperglycaemia secondary to dysregulation in preterm babies resulting from delayed maturation of hepatic enzymes may persist beyond time of discharge.
- If hyperglycaemia persists, consider neonatal diabetes (this is rare — incidence 1 in 400,000). Treatment with insulin may be temporary (months) or permanent. This may be given as subcutaneous intermittent injections.
- Babies diagnosed with neonatal diabetes will require referral to a paediatric diabetologist and geneticist.
  - Permanent neonatal diabetes will require lifelong insulin therapy.

- Transient neonatal diabetes may re-emerge as type 2 diabetes in adolescence.

THE ADRENAL GLAND IN THE PERINATAL PERIOD

The adrenal gland *in utero* primarily produces androgens (DHEA, DHEAS) that are essential as substrate for placental oestrogen synthesis. Thus, fetal adrenal cortical enzyme activity (high 3BHSD activity) favours androgen production rather than cortisol production. Fetal plasma cortisol levels are low, partly due to low production, and partly due to inactivation of maternal and fetal cortisol by 11BHSD2 in the placenta and fetus. After birth there is a sudden rise in cortisol. Adrenal androgen production, which is high at birth, falls rapidly in the first few weeks of life. In preterm infants this fetal adrenal androgen production persists and declines around term. These fetal androgens do not appear to produce clinical effects, but can interfere with steroid assays. Diurnal variation in cortisol levels develops at 8–12 weeks of age in term infants, and in preterm infants less than 31 weeks' gestation, but is delayed in less mature preterm infants.

Infants exposed to high levels of maternal glucocorticoids (dexamethasone, prednisolone, maternal Cushing syndrome) can have transient adrenal insufficiency in the first few days of life — monitor blood glucose levels and blood pressure for 48 hours.

Preterm infants given antenatal steroids have subtle changes in cortisol production, but this does not appear to be of clinical significance.

Although preterm infants are capable of producing high levels of cortisol in response to severe stress, there is debate as to whether these infants produce or sustain appropriate levels for the ongoing stresses of intensive care. However, high doses of postnatal dexamethasone are known to be harmful to the preterm infant brain, and so steroid use in this population is usually restricted to infants showing possible signs of adrenal insufficiency — such as hypotension refractory to inotropes.

The symptoms and signs of adrenal failure/abnormal adrenal function in the newborn include:

- hypoglycaemia (glucocorticoid deficiency),
- hyponatraemia combined with hyperkalaemia (mineralocorticoid deficiency)
- collapse
- hypotension
- genital anomalies/disorders of sex development or micropenis
- excessive adrenocorticotrophic hormone (ACTH) can lead to skin pigmentation (commonly, but not exclusively, scrotal) — but this clinical sign is only discernable in white infants.

Adrenal failure secondary to pituitary insufficiency commonly presents with hypoglycaemia and prolonged jaundice, but can present as an adrenal crisis at any stage in the presence of intercurrent illness.

Stimulation tests: In preterm infants, neither the appropriate dose of Synacthen®, nor the cortisol response, has been established. Most clinicians would use the same dose (adjusted for birth weight) and response as described for term infants. (*See Chapter 4, Adrenal Disorders.*)

THYROID PHYSIOLOGY IN THE FETUS AND NEWBORN

Maternal thyroxine (T4) crosses the placenta in limited amounts throughout gestation and is important for early central nervous system development which is crucial in hypothyroid fetuses. In conditions of severe maternal and fetal hypothyroidism, particularly in areas of endemic iodine deficiency, significant neurological impairment will occur unless iodine supplementation is provided before the third trimester.

After delivery at term, there is an abrupt increase in thyroid stimulating hormone (TSH) peaking at about 30 minutes of age to about 70 mU/L, before decreasing to normal infant levels by 3—5 days of age. This is accompanied by a two to six-fold increase in both T4 and triiodothyronine (T3) levels, peaking at 2—3 days. Thyroxine levels remain elevated for several weeks. Results of thyroid function taken in the neonatal period must be interpreted in the light of expected values during this period.

Preterm infants born after 30 weeks' gestation have a similar but attenuated surge in TSH, T4 and T3 after birth. T4 peaks between 12 and 72 hours and declines in a similar pattern to that in term babies. T4 levels increase over the next 4—8 weeks to levels found in term babies. Babies born before 30 weeks' gestation and very low birth weight babies (less than 1500 g), have a limited or absent TSH and T4 surge.

Although the more preterm the baby the more marked the hypothyroxinaemia, T4 levels also reflect the severity of the neonatal illness, with the sickest babies having the lowest T4 levels. Contributing factors include loss of maternal transplacental T4 contribution, immaturity of the hypothalamic-pituitary-thyroid axis, immaturity of peripheral tissue deiodination and negative iodine balance, the use of drugs which reduce the pituitary secretion of TSH (such as dopamine and glucocorticoids), the use of iodine-containing antiseptic and contrast media, and iodine deficiency in areas of the world with low environmental iodine.

Low T4 levels are associated with morbidity and mortality in preterm babies; however, data do not support benefit from thyroid hormone supplementation either to prevent or to treat hypothyroxinaemia and cannot be recommended.

(*For hyperthyroidism and hypothyroidism, see Chapter 3, Thyroid Disorders.*)

PROBLEMS WITH SALT AND WATER BALANCE

Hyponatraemia

Hyponatraemia (plasma sodium less than 130 mmol/L) may be due to water overload (excessive IV fluids, inappropriate antidiuretic hormone [ADH] secretion, renal failure) or salt depletion (vomiting, diarrhoea, excessive urinary sodium loss, excessive sweating).

Hyponatraemia is common in preterm infants. In the first 5–7 days of life plasma sodium primarily reflects water balance (i.e. hyponatraemia suggests water overload), but thereafter urinary sodium loss by the immature kidney is the usual cause of hyponatraemia in preterm infants.

In sick term and preterm infants, particularly those with intracranial or lung pathology, there may be inappropriate secretion of ADH (syndrome of inappropriate ADH, SIADH), i.e. ADH is produced in response to illness which causes inappropriate retention of water by the kidney. This results in low plasma osmolality, and an inappropriately high urine osmolality (i.e. concentrated urine, when dilute urine would be expected).

The treatment of fluid overload, either iatrogenic or SIADH, is reduction in fluid intake. With severe hyponatraemia in SIADH, it may be necessary to provide a small amount of salt in addition.

Salt loss can be due to vomiting or diarrhoea. In the absence of these symptoms urinary salt loss should be suspected. The plasma potassium measurement may be helpful in interpretation of the cause. When hyponatraemia occurs together with hyperkalaemia this suggests either aldosterone deficiency (or resistance) or renal impairment. The commonest cause of aldosterone deficiency presenting in the neonatal period is salt losing congenital adrenal hyperplasia (CAH). In this condition

salt loss starts from about day 4, but infants usually present in the second week of life, by which time salt loss can be severe and life-threatening. Salt (and fluid) replacement is the most important aspect of management, together with steroid replacement (glucocorticoid and mineralocorticoid) once the diagnosis has been made (see Chapter 4, Adrenal Disorders). Occasionally, hyperkalaemia is so severe that it requires specific management (e.g. calcium resonium). Rarer causes of aldosterone deficiency include congenital adrenal hypoplasia (also causing glucocorticoid deficiency), aldosterone biosynthetic defects, and aldosterone resistance (also known as pseudo-hypoaldosteronism) (see Chapter 4, Adrenal Disorders).

To investigate hyponatraemia, make an assessment of fluid intake, and current body weight in relation to birth or previous weight(s). Lack of normal postnatal weight loss or weight gain suggests fluid retention whereas weight loss suggests sodium (and water) loss.

Measure urine output and make serial measurements of blood sodium, blood osmolality (estimated by $2[Na + K] + [urea] + [glucose]$), blood potassium, urea and creatinine. Assess urinary sodium, potassium, osmolality, creatinine (paired with plasma osmolality, creatinine). (Infants with CAH have inappropriately high urinary sodium levels.)

Hypernatraemia

Hypernatraemia (plasma sodium greater than 145 mmol/L) may be due to water depletion (inadequate intake or excessive loss) or sodium excess (excessive salt intake, sodium bicarbonate infusions, IV saline including flushes, malicious salt poisoning).

The commonest cause of hypernatraemia in the newborn is dehydration secondary to inadequate milk intake. The infant has usually lost weight, and the urine is concentrated.

Clinical Approach

Identify those causes which have urgent implications in terms of management, e.g. septo-optic dysplasia, diabetes insipidus (DI), renal concentrating defect.

Rarely, hypernatraemia is secondary to a renal concentration defect or to diabetes insipidus. In DI, urine is inappropriately dilute for the plasma sodium level, i.e. there is a failure to concentrate the urine. Clinical pointers to this diagnosis include midline defects (suggestive of septo-optic dysplasia: hypo or hypertelorism, central cleft palate, absent corpus callosum or holoprosencephaly on head ultrasound scan, micropenis, hypoplastic optic discs).

Presentation is with polydipsia and polyuria. In infants with an intact sense of thirst, drinking may compensate for urine output, leading to a relatively normal (or only slightly elevated) plasma sodium and osmolality, until the infant is stressed by illness, or fluid intake is limited.

Excessive fluid intake can affect the kidneys chronically due to high solute load, and can lead to high plasma calcium levels.

A water deprivation test is not safe in the newborn, and diagnosis rests on documenting fluid intake and output (both will be excessive), and paired plasma and urine osmolality. Where urine osmolality is inappropriately low, a small test dose of DDAVP® is used to distinguish central (pituitary) DI from renal DI. Available preparations of DDAVP make it difficult to administer sufficiently low doses for infants, particularly by the intranasal route (more potent that oral administration).

However, the intranasal solution can be given orally, and the solution can be diluted to 10 μg/mL, which gives more flexibility for administering small doses. (See Chapter 8, Disturbances of Sodium and Water.)

Other pituitary hormone insufficiencies should be suspected and sought, and in infants deficient in ACTH, DI may not be manifest until hydrocortisone replacement is started (cortisol is required to excrete a water load). In this situation DI may develop 1–2 days after starting hydrocortisone.

HYPERCALCAEMIA AND HYPOCALCAEMIA IN THE NEWBORN

The fetus is dependent on the mother for calcium, which is actively transported across the placenta, with the most rapid accretion occurring in the third trimester. Parathyroid hormone (PTH) levels are low but secreted from fetal parathyroid glands in response to hypocalcaemia, and suppressed in response to hypercalcaemia.

After birth, physiological hypocalcaemia occurs within the first 48 hours because of interrupted transplacental calcium supply, insufficient supply from the gastrointestinal tract and insufficient release of PTH. Total calcium levels drop to about 2 mmol/L and ionised to about 1 mmol/L. The newborn baby is dependent on parathyroid PTH secretion, dietary calcium, renal calcium reabsorption, skeletal calcium stores and vitamin D. PTH levels increase on the first day of life in response to the fall in serum calcium levels, peaking at 48 hours. In the first 2–4 weeks after birth, there is increased efficiency of intestinal absorption of calcium and maturation of renal tubular handling.

The fetus appears to be protected from the adverse effects of vitamin D deficiency during pregnancy. Even those with severe vitamin D deficiency are generally born with normal serum calcium levels and skeletal morphology. However, after birth, pregnancy and lactation vitamin D deficiency in the mother may lead to profound hypocalcaemia and rickets in the baby.

Hypocalcaemia

Hypocalcaemia is defined as a total calcium less than 2.2 mmol/L or ionised calcium less than 1.2 mmol/L. Ideally, ionised calcium level should be measured in the preterm baby as the normal relationship with total calcium is atypical.

Hypocalcaemia is common in the newborn, is usually physiological, or an exaggeration of the normal physiological response, or iatrogenic and short lasting. Other causes of hypocalcaemia are rare. Aetiologies are conventionally grouped according to the time of onset: early hypocalcaemia (occurring within 72 hours from birth) and late hypocalcaemia (after 72 hours of age).

The usual presentation is incidental asymptomatic hypocalcaemia on 'routine' blood samples. Symptoms include neuromuscular irritability (myoclonic jerks, jitteriness, exaggerated startle responses, seizures), apnoea, cyanosis, tachypnoea, vomiting, laryngospasm, or cardiac symptoms and signs (tachycardia, heart failure, prolonged Q-T interval on electrocardiogram, decreased contractility). Severe vitamin D deficiency may present with cardiomyopathy.

Other differential diagnoses of these common non-specific symptoms (sepsis, meningitis, hypoglycaemia, hypomagnesaemia, intracranial haemorrhage) must be excluded.

EARLY ONSET (FIRST 72 HOURS)

- Common causes include prematurity, delivery following pre-eclampsia, birth asphyxia, and infants of diabetic mothers.
- Maternal hyperparathyroidism (where intrauterine hypercalcaemia suppresses fetal parathyroid activity resulting in impaired parathyroid responsiveness to hypocalcaemia after birth). Hypocalcaemia may be severe and prolonged.

LATE ONSET (AFTER 72 HOURS)

- This is usually iatrogenic and caused by excessive phosphate intake, the use of citrated blood products, lipid infusions, bicarbonate therapy, loop and thiazide

diuretics, glucocorticoids and high phosphate-containing milk feeds, e.g. cow's milk.
- Other causes include vitamin D deficiency (usually secondary to maternal vitamin D deficiency). This may be associated with maternal anticonvulsant use (phenobarbitone or phenytoin), malabsorption of calcium or vitamin D, hypomagnesaemia, transient hypoparathyroidism, transient PTH resistance, renal failure, alkalosis, and congenital hypoparathyroidism.
  - Congenital hypoparathyroidism:
    - May be part of DiGeorge sequence/CATCH 22/velocardiofacial syndrome and may be transient, with resolution during infancy
    - May rarely be caused by activating mutations in calcium sensing receptor, agenesis of parathyroid glands or part of a number of metabolic syndromes.

Investigation of Hypocalcaemia

Blood samples should be taken for (ionised) calcium level, phosphate, creatinine, electrolytes, pH, alkaline phosphatase, magnesium and albumin.

A urine sample collected for calcium, phosphate, creatinine, glucose, and amino acids is helpful. The urinary calcium to creatinine ratio, and urinary PO4 excretion (tubular reabsorption of phosphate) should be determined.

Other investigations include an X-ray of the wrist for evidence of rickets or osteopenia.

Other helpful samples include: PTH level, vitamin D level and a sample for mutational analysis, but they may not be available.

For diagnosis and management see *Chapter 7, Disorders of Mineral and Bone Metabolism*.

Hypercalcaemia in the Newborn

Hypercalcaemia is defined as a total calcium greater than 2.82 mmol/L, or ionised calcium greater than 1.4 mmol/L. It may be picked up incidentally on 'routine' blood tests. Mild hypercalcaemia (2.74–3.2 mmol/L) is usually asymptomatic. Moderate-to-severe hypercalcaemia (greater than 3.2 mmol/L) may present with anorexia, gastro-oesophageal reflux, vomiting, or constipation (rarely diarrhoea).

Other symptoms and signs include polyuria (with dehydration), hypertension (secondary to vasoconstrictive effect of hypercalcaemia), shortened ST segment and heart block (secondary to direct effect on cardiac conduction) and central nervous system symptoms: irritability, hypotonia, drowsiness, seizures, stupor and coma. Chronic hypercalcaemia usually presents with failure to thrive.

Hyperparathyroidism may be associated with bone deformities or fractures, respiratory difficulties, hepatosplenomegaly and anaemia.

An assessment of calcium and phosphate intake should be made, especially in preterm infants receiving breast milk without phosphate supplementation and infants on prolonged low phosphate-containing intravenous infusions/parenteral nutrition. The vitamin D intake should be assessed (by checking the milk formulation and vitamin D supplementation).

Hypercalcaemia may be iatrogenic (hypophosphataemia, vitamin A or D excess, excessive calcium supplements and thiazide diuretics), or the result of functional hyperparathyroidism, or non-parathyroid hypercalcaemia (see Table 11.1 and Chapter 7, Disorders of Mineral and Bone Metabolism).

In functional hyperparathyroidism (raised serum calcium levels, low phosphate levels and normal or raised alkaline phosphatase levels), PTH levels would be raised (Table 11.1).

Investigation of Hypercalcaemia

- Blood samples for (ionised) calcium levels, phosphate, albumin, alkaline phosphatase, creatinine, electrolytes and magnesium.
- A urine sample for urinary calcium, phosphate and creatinine.
- A skeletal survey may be helpful.

TABLE 11.1 Causes of Functional Hyperparathyroidism and Non-Parathyroid Hypercalcaemia

Causes of functional hyperparathyroidism	Causes of non-parathyroid hypercalcaemia
• Maternal hypocalcaemia (secondary to pseudohypoparathyroidism, renal tubular acidosis)	• Disorders of vitamin D metabolism
• Congenital parathyroid hyperplasia	• Williams' syndrome
• Inactivating mutations in the calcium-sensing receptor gene: either familial hypocalciuric hypercalcaemia (heterozygous manifestation) or neonatal severe hyperparathyroidism (homozygous manifestation)	• Idiopathic infantile hypercalcaemia
	• Subcutaneous fat necrosis
	• Inborn errors of metabolism (lactase deficiency, disaccharidase deficiency, infantile hypophosphatasia, blue diaper syndrome)
• Jansen's metaphyseal chondrodysplasia (caused by constitutive mutation in the PTH/PTH- related peptide (PTHrP) receptor)	• Endocrine disorders (congenital hypothyroidism, thyrotoxicosis, adrenal insufficiency)
• Persistent parathyroid hormone-related peptide.	• Down syndrome
	• IMAGe syndrome
	• Malignancy

- Other helpful investigations include PTH level, vitamin D level (25(OH)D), and a sample for DNA (mutational analysis of calcium sensing receptor [CaSR] or Williams [elastin] gene, $1,25(OH)_2D$) but may not be available.

As the maternal calcium concentration and vitamin D status during pregnancy influences vitamin D levels and parathyroid function in the fetus, investigation of hypercalcaemia and unexplained hypocalcaemia should include an analysis of calcium metabolism in the mother (calcium, phosphate and, if possible, PTH). If defects in the calcium-sensing receptor are suspected, calcium levels in the father and siblings should be assessed. *(See Chapter 7, Disorders of Mineral and Bone Metabolism.)*

EPIGENETICS

In the developing world, there is a risk of maternal undernutrition during pregnancy and lactation. Epidemiological data in humans and studies in animals indicate that during critical periods of prenatal and postnatal development, nutrition and other environmental stimuli influence developmental pathways, inducing permanent changes in metabolism and chronic disease susceptibility, via epigenetic programming. Adverse consequences of altered intrauterine environments can be passed from first-generation to second-generation offspring. Transient environmental influences can have permanent effects on the developmental establishment of epigenetic gene regulation. A baby who has been subjected to an adverse *in utero* environment, who postnatally has an increased nutrient supply and postnatal weight gain, is at future risk of developing the metabolic syndrome (cardiovascular disease, insulin resistant diabetes and hypertension).

Preventing or treating the adverse pregnancy conditions will help to minimise the risk of transmission of metabolic diseases to future generations.

Maternal nutrition in early pregnancy and placental function both have major effects on developmental programming. Thus, the development of planning for improved medical and educational services for prospective mothers will in turn have profound consequences, in terms of reduced infant, child and future adult morbidity.

CONCLUSIONS

Endocrine dysfunction is common in the neonatal period, although endocrine disease is rare. Both may be picked up incidentally by abnormalities found on newborn examination or 'routine' blood samples or non-specific symptoms exhibited by the baby. Endocrine disease may also be picked up before symptoms are obvious on screening tests.

Because of the hormonal changes that occur with parturition, results need to be interpreted accordingly. In the preterm baby, there are no truly normative hormonal levels, and often treatment (particularly for adrenal dysfunction) needs to be given empirically if dysfunction is suspected.

References and Further Reading

References specific to management of individual disorders are included with each detailed chapter on a subject.

Gluckman P, Hanson M, Cooper C, Thornberg K. Effects of in utero and early life conditions on adult health and disease. *N Engl J Med* 2008;359:61–73.

Hall JG. Review and hypothesis: syndromes with severe intrauterine growth restriction and very short stature - are they related to the epigenetic mechanism(s) of fetal survival involved in the developmental origins of adult health and disease? *Am J Med Genet* 2010;152A:512–27.

12

Diabetes in Children and Adolescents: Basic Training for Healthcare Professionals in Developing Countries*

Stuart Brink, Warren Lee, Kubendran Pillay

INTRODUCTION

Diabetes can be a disease that kills in many parts of the developing world and particularly

so when it strikes children and adolescents. Compared to so many serious infectious diseases, diabetes is relatively rare so that those afflicted, their parents and family members as

---

* Based on the Changing Diabetes in Children (CDiC) Sub-Saharan African collaborative initiative of NovoNordisk, Roche Diagnostics and ISPAD

Practical Pediatric Endocrinology in a Limited Resource Setting
http://dx.doi.org/10.1016/B978-0-12-407822-2.00012-8

well as friends do not recognise its subtle symptoms even when the symptoms build and serious morbidity occurs. The subtleness of new enuresis, excess thirst, excess urination and unexplained weight loss should not be confused with AIDS wasting or parasitic bowel diseases nor with numerous bacterial infections, yet this happens all around the world. The key to understanding new diabetes is awareness that urination is increased in the face of unexplained dehydration — just the opposite of all the other lethal diseases which occur more commonly in the developing emergency care facilities around the world. Healthcare workers must learn to ask such questions that separate out newly diagnosed diabetic ketoacidosis (DKA) and type 1 diabetes mellitus (T1DM) from these other killer illnesses in severely ill children. Unfortunately, in the richer countries of the world, new diabetes and DKA are also misdiagnosed and often missed and the differential diagnosis almost never has diabetes considered.

If all emergency medical personnel were trained specifically to always ask about thirst and urination, enuresis or even whether there were ants near the toilet, missed diagnoses may be decreased and deaths from DKA, cerebral oedema and coma would similarly decrease dramatically in all the developed country emergency rooms and hospitals. Simple poster campaigns that highlight such facts with pictographs help save children's lives without any need for reading literacy, with postings at the town hall, religious institutions, schools and local stores.

This initiative sponsored by NovoNordisk's CDiC:[1] Changing Diabetes® in Children programme, co-sponsored with Roche Diagnostics and developed in collaboration with the International Society for Pediatric and Adolescent Diabetes (ISPAD), hopes to focus such attention, create partnerships and mentors, working with local paediatric and adult diabetologists interested in not only learning about paediatric and adolescent diabetes but setting up clinics and multidisciplinary teams to form the nucleus of future diabetes and paediatric endocrine services. Nevertheless, ISPAD's Declaration of Kos presented by ISPAD officers in 1984 remains unfulfilled (see Appendix).[2]

The only effective treatment for T1DM is injection of insulin. If insulin is unavailable, children and teenagers with T1DM die of ketoacidosis, dehydration and coma. If the diagnosis or treatment is delayed, DKA often progresses to coma and death within days of insulin deficiency becoming critical. If properly treated all around the world, even where resources are often not present, DKA can be recognised and prevented with appropriate education of healthcare personnel to consider and recognise this possible diagnosis. Short-term as well as long-term complications associated with chronic hyperglycaemia can be ameliorated or modified. T1DM can be enormously expensive with the costs of insulin, syringes, blood glucose meters, blood glucose test strips as well as provision of adequate nutrition on a regular basis all being necessary components of care. Trained healthcare professionals dedicated to knowing about diabetes and knowing about its treatment will make this happen with improved worldwide communication focusing on these efforts.

Why is Childhood Diabetes Different from Adult Diabetes?

Childhood and adolescent diabetes is different from adult diabetes.[3] Most youngsters with diabetes have type 1 or insulin-dependent diabetes compared to most adults with diabetes who have non-insulin dependent diabetes (diabetes mellitus type 2).[1] Children and adolescents grow and their insulin requirements change frequently, due to growth in size, puberty and the demands of school, sport and work. Insulin dosage is based on weight and insulin sensitivity. As children grow rapidly during childhood, their insulin doses need to be adjusted at each clinic visit, at a minimum every few months. During the pubertal growth spurt, insulin requirements increase even more rapidly, and then decrease back to normal adult levels as growth is completed. Children and teens with diabetes (and their families) need constant re-education as the child becomes older, more aware of their own needs and more able to make their own health-related decisions. The danger, of course, is that too-quick release of parental authorisation leaves children and adolescents too free to make too many mistakes, while too little transition to self-care also poses problems. The key to success reflects some personal balance between parental care and adult self-care, with appropriate transitioning and individual attention to needs based on clinical results.

Long-term complications of hyperlipidaemia, hypertension, diabetic retinopathy, nephropathy and neuropathy all begin in childhood and often accelerate in adolescence, especially if years of poor glucose control have occurred. These can be subtle and often subclinical. Assessment of daily glycaemia by home monitoring as well as by periodic haemoglobin A1c assessment provides an objective evaluation of those doing well and those needing further intervention from the healthcare team. Assessment of baseline function also needs to be done periodically and with standardised appropriate follow-up to determine who needs more intensified management and/or medical intervention (i.e. lipid-lowering agents, renal protective medications, antihypertensive treatment etc.). Standards of care proposed by ISPAD[4] and also by IDF[5] as well as those in numerous paediatric diabetes and endocrinology textbooks[3,6,7] around the world all suggest ongoing assessment and reassessment of specific diabetes issues as well as diabetes associated problems such as thyroid and coeliac disease. Treating a child or adolescent with diabetes requires more effort than treating an adult with diabetes. A multidisciplinary team approach is essential. Where manpower is limited, team members may have to take on more than one role, but the task must still be done. Childhood and adolescent diabetes needs a support system that includes the patient, his or her parents and sometimes grandparents, friends and neighbours, school personnel and the entire healthcare team all working together to provide practical, emotional and moral support where needed.

Type 1 Diabetes

Type 1 diabetes mellitus (T1DM) is the commonest type of diabetes in childhood and adolescence. In T1DM the pancreatic islets are 'attacked' through a non-infectious process called autoimmunity. Antibodies often can be measured in the blood. The β cells are damaged and stop being able to make insulin. Because there is not enough insulin, glucose in the blood is unable to move into the cells and a system of body 'starvation' occurs. Blood glucose levels rise. The person with T1DM feels tired and lethargic, sleeps excessively and does not want to work or play. The blood glucose levels as they rise get filtered by the normally working kidneys and drag water and salt with them as the kidneys try to get rid of the excess sugar in the blood. Sugar starts to appear in the urine (glycosuria) where more sodium and potassium salt and water continue to be lost. Another question that healthcare workers should consider asking anyone who is dehydrated (or their family members) is whether or not there are **ants** near the toilet or where urination occurs outdoors; ants are attracted to sugar and the sugar in urine may provide the clue to the diagnosis of T1DM in many parts of the developing world! Excess urination (**polyuria**), night-time urination (**nocturia**) and bedwetting (**enuresis**) then occur and this explains the classic symptom presentation of new onset T1DM. Asking these three specific questions (four questions if one counts the 'ants') in any dehydrated child would immediately force healthcare professionals to consider T1DM in the differential diagnosis in any emergency room or triage facility, clinic or medical office around the world and these questions must become a near universal and central tenet of healthcare education if we are to successfully make the diagnosis of T1DM in children and adolescents. The same symptoms, of course, occur in anyone already diagnosed with diabetes who, when ill or facing several kinds of physiologic stress (i.e. surgery) or even relative lack of insulin (insulin unaffordability, insulin unavailability), continue to have hyperglycaemia.

Type 2 Diabetes Mellitus

Type 2 diabetes mellitus (T2DM) is the more common form of diabetes and usually seen in older people. As youngsters become more obese around the world, T2DM is also becoming more common at earlier ages. It is important not to mix up T1DM and T2DM since many healthcare workers and most people do not quite understand the differences between T1DM and T2DM aetiology, pathophysiology or treatment. Unlike T1DM, people with T2DM are usually older and usually overweight or obese rather than emaciated and thin. There are usually no antibodies present (although there is a T2DM variant called latent autoimmune diabetes in adults [LADA] where older and thinner adults present with diabetes). The biochemical abnormality in most with T2DM is related to insulin resistance concomitant with a demand for more insulin because of excess body fat. Such insulin resistance can be present for many years before symptomatic T2DM is diagnosed. T2DM ideally is treated by recognising the familial or genetic potential that exists, avoiding or correcting overweight and obesity and thus decreasing the underlying insulin resistance to some extent. Increasing physical activity helps enormously to do the same. Many pills are available for treating T2DM that also help to treat the insulin resistance and make more insulin available than is possible without such medication. In more than 50% of patients with T2DM,

ultimately insulin will be needed and only recently has this been sufficiently recognised in the natural history of T2DM.

With increasing obesity and overweight conditions occurring all around the world, more T2DM now is occurring in children and adolescents who are overweight. This occurs in the United States, Australia, Canada and in Western Europe in Caucasian populations but more so in so-called minority populations of Black, Latino, Asian and indigenous populations (American Indians, Canadian First Nation, Australian Aborigines) for presumed genetic reasons but driven by the obesity epidemic that is disproportionately present in such populations. As elsewhere, Japan, China, India, Southeast Asia, the Middle East, Africa and Latin America all have reported similar increases in T2DM not only in their adult populations as they become more prosperous, move from rural to urban environments and gain weight excessively with more money, less healthy and more caloric content of food and less daily physical activities. Family history of T2DM should serve as a warning signal of this potential that has been dubbed a true world epidemic by the WHO and the UN.

T2DM in childhood, adolescence and adults is closely associated with the **metabolic syndrome**. The metabolic syndrome includes (1) overweight, (2) obesity, (3) excess abdominal fat distribution, (4) elevated body mass index (BMI), (5) hypertension, (6) abnormal lipid levels (especially high triglycerides but also elevated LDL and total cholesterol and low HDL cholesterol, (7) hyperinsulinaemia, (8) fasting hyperglycaemia, (9) T2DM, (10) steatosis (fatty liver) with elevated liver enzymes (ALT, AST), (11) high uric acid levels with or without clinical gout, (12) acanthosis nigricans especially of the neck and the axillary region as well as the groin, (13) precocious adrenarche or (14) frank precocious puberty, (15) polycystic ovarian syndrome (PCOS). There is some debate as to which of these components of the metabolic syndrome are always required and which are highly associated but more variably present. However, clearly the metabolic syndrome and its central obesity and insulin-resistant states exist in many children and adolescents even before T2DM can be confirmed.

Other Forms of Diabetes

Other types of diabetes besides classical T1DM and T2DM also exist. A third form of diabetes often exists that has been called variably **T1.5 diabetes mellitus (T1.5DM), 'double diabetes' or LADA**, latent autoimmune diabetes in adults. This can also occur in adolescents. This is sometimes thought to be a combination of obesity-related T2DM but with more insulin deficiency and some β-cell autoimmunity (positive GAD antibodies or insulin antibodies, for instance). Such patients can present with incidental hyperglycaemia or insulin resistance or even in DKA. They seem to require insulin at diagnosis more like T1DM patients but are not as thin and emaciated, respond more quickly to DKA management and may come off insulin therapy and change to oral hypoglycaemic agents like metformin for quite some time if they can manage some weight loss with a balanced nutrition and increased activity each day. They also seem to eventually need insulin sooner than others with more classical, older-onset T2DM. In populations with larger African, Asian, Latino or indigenous ancestry (i.e. Australian Aborigines, American Indians, American, Canadian or Russian Eskimos) either in their countries or continents of origin or in whatever land they currently reside, T1.5DM (LADA) and T2DM are increasing in prevalence.

Diabetes associated with severe malnutrition also occurs (i.e. in India). This group includes fibrocalculous pancreatic diabetes.

Infants aged under 6 months may also develop a specific form of diabetes termed **neonatal diabetes**. This group of diabetes is extremely rare and occurs all around the world often with severe dehydration and hyperglycaemia at presentation and is now known to be caused by very specific and diagnosable genetic defects. Neonatal diabetes may be transient or permanent. Previously insulin was an absolute requirement and as difficult as the usual management of T1DM was, in such infants with neonatal diabetes, the management was even more problematic. Free genetic testing and treatment advice is available through a collaboration with special laboratories under the direction of Professor Andrew Hattersley in cooperation with ISPAD (see website www.ISPAD.org) and the rare diabetes initiative. Once the diagnosis is established with such genetic testing, many can be successfully changed to treatment with sulphonylurea oral tablets instead of insulin and not only can this be started at diagnosis in such infants, but transition from insulin even many years afterwards is successful with improved glycaemia, improved quality of life (no more injections!) and near-normalisation of haemoglobin A1c.

Maturity-onset diabetes of the young (MODY) is a group of several types of diabetes due to single gene abnormalities causing defects in insulin secretion. Children with MODY tend to have little insulin resistance and no ketones in urine. They often have a very autosomal-dominant family history usually affecting three or more generations of relatives and most often present before 25 years of age. Some may not need any insulin or oral hypoglycaemic treatment at all and there does *not* seem to be a steady progression towards insulin requirement as in many with classical T2DM.

DIAGNOSIS

Criteria for T1DM Diagnosis

Criteria include a high index of suspicion when reviewing a history, with classical symptoms as described above elicited from the adolescent, child or the parents/family members of those younger plus a casual glucose concentration equal to or greater than 11.1 mmol/L (equal to or greater than 200 mg/dL). Casual is defined as any time of day without regard to time since last eating or drinking or fasting plasma glucose equal to or greater than 7.0 mmol/L (equal to or greater than 126 mg/dL). If blood glucose measurement is not available, T1DM can be tentatively diagnosed by the finding of high levels of glucose and ketones in the urine. The date of onset of T1DM is estimated from the date of onset of symptoms reported whereas the date of diagnosis is the date of the urine or blood lab work and usually this coincides with the date of initiation of insulin treatment. There should be no delay in starting saline solutions for suspected T1DM-associated DKA or dehydration. There should be no delay in starting insulin or in transporting such a youngster to the nearest facility under emergency conditions where insulin can be started. Ideally, avoidance of DKA and coma should be a priority if appropriate awareness and questions from healthcare workers can be institutionalised. In parts of the world where incidence of T1DM is low, more DKA occurs (i.e. Africa vs Scandinavia). Similarly in parts of the world where access to medical care is problematic (urban ghettoes in the USA and Europe vs high-income suburbs) more DKA occurs.

Diagnosis of T1DM Without a Glucose Meter

- Ask the **key** questions of any ill infant, child or teenager **every time**: Polyuria? Polydipsia? Nocturia? Enuresis? Ants?
- Current weight and comparison with known prior weights.
- Slowed height velocity plotted on a standard growth chart.

- Complete physical examination including direct fundus examination if an ophthalmoscope is available.
- Use urine strips in those with suspicious history. Glycosuria and ketonuria are readily determined by urine test strips.

Diagnosis of T1DM Without a Glucose Meter and also Without any Urine Test Strips

- All the same history should be obtained and appropriate physical examination carried out according to the initial complaint and findings.
- The same **key** questions can be utilised to raise a high index of suspicion: Polyuria? Polydipsia? Nocturia? Enuresis? Ants? Remember that dehydration (i.e. less urination) is usually associated with less urination for almost all other causes except for diabetes!
- If the laboratory or hospital has Benedict's solution, this can also provide information about glycosuria, one of the reducing substances detected by such inexpensive Benedict's solution. Ants by the diaper disposal bin, ants where the worn underwear is kept before laundering or even a sample of urine left outdoors to be observed all can be a signal of sugar in the urine.

DIABETES EMERGENCY CARE: DKA, SEVERE HYPOGLYCAEMIA, MANAGING SURGICAL EMERGENCIES

Diabetic Ketoacidosis (DKA)

Diabetes is a chronic disease which needs to be well controlled. If it is not controlled because of lack of education facilities, lack of interested healthcare professionals, lack of priority given by the healthcare system, lack of insulin, poverty and lack of food and self-testing equipment, morbidity and mortality increase exponentially. Simple education about the symptoms of diabetes increases awareness in the community as well as in the healthcare professional community and has been shown in Italy, Canada and elsewhere to reduce the duration of symptoms of diabetes before diagnosis is made, reduce the severity of such symptoms and therefore reduce the need not only for emergency care and hospitalisation but also decrease death. DKA can occur if T1DM is not yet recognised and diagnosed. DKA can also occur in known patients with T1DM particularly during intercurrent illnesses and especially if self-monitoring is unavailable and/or insulin is not being provided correctly or is unaffordable.

Recognising DKA

Table 12.1 lists pathophysiologic effects and clinical features of DKA. DKA occurs when there is insufficient insulin. This obviously occurs at the time of diagnosis as the blood glucose levels increase. DKA refers to diabetic ketoacidosis, describing the decompensated metabolism. As ketones are produced, the fruity odour of acetone attempting to be excreted in the lungs/breath may be noted. If the diagnosis can be made earlier, the metabolic consequences are not so severe and DKA can be prevented at a level when there is only hyperglycaemia but not decompensated DKA. If nothing is recognised except that someone is ill, death may occur. At this late stage, severe dehydration and semi-coma or coma can readily be confused with overwhelming sepsis, cerebral malaria, severe dehydration from bacterial, viral or parasitic gastrointestinal disorders and numerous other kinds of severe infections (HIV/AIDS) that present to emergency room facilities around the world. It must be remembered, however, that new diagnoses of DKA do not start with coma or loss of consciousness but

TABLE 12.1 Diabetic Ketoacidosis

Pathophysiologic effects of DKA	Clinical features of DKA
Elevated blood glucose	Excess urination, excess thirst, night-time urination, enuresis, ants where urine is left
Dehydration when body unable to compensate and get sufficient fluid and electrolytes replaced	Weight loss, sunken eyes, dry mouth, decreased skin turgor, decreased circulatory perfusion, hypotension, shock and circulatory arrest
Decreased total body sodium: hyponatraemia	Irritability, change in level of consciousness, hypotension, shock and circulatory arrest
Decreased total body potassium: hypokalaemia	Irritability, change in level of consciousness, cardiac arrest, death
Metabolic acidosis; fat burning; diabetic ketoacidosis	Fruity odour (acetone breath), irritability, abdominal pain, nausea and vomiting, acidotic (Kussmaul) breathing, change in level of consciousness, cardiac arrest, death

Source: Adapted from ADA. http://www.diabetes.org/living-with-diabetes/treatment-and-care/blood-glucose-control/estimated-average-glucose.html

have usually had days if not weeks of **polyuria, nocturia, enuresis, polydipsia, weight loss and ants around sites of urination. These symptoms often have not been recognised for the early signals that they represent**: new insulin deficiency, rising hyperglycaemia and new T1DM.

DKA Management

Once DKA is diagnosed, treatment is aimed at correcting the biochemical and clinical abnormalities. This has to occur gradually and purposefully to prevent other potentially lethal complications, especially cerebral oedema. Fluid replacement with proper salt and water is probably more important than insulin treatment as early mortality is due to dehydration, electrolyte abnormalities and/or shock itself rather than hyperglycaemia per se. Of course, insulin therapy is part of DKA treatment to help correct the metabolic acidosis and underlying hyperglycaemia itself. Experience in recognition and treatment of DKA helps in making such decisions but initial treating facility should be expected to initiate slow saline and fluid management and then expedite transportation to the best facility to handle ongoing treatment and monitoring needs. DKA written guidelines should be available for review and strict adherence will save lives, decrease morbidity and also mortality associated with DKA. Not only is proper medical care needed but appropriate nursing expertise for such critically ill children and adolescents as well as laboratory support for monitoring are both key.

DKA Treatment

Treatment involves the following steps:

1. Correction of shock and provision of oxygen: airway, breathing, circulation (A, B, C).
2. Correction of salt and water deficits slowly and calculated to occur over 48 hours, not faster.
3. Decision about potassium treatment needs.
4. Slow reduction of insulin-deficiency-caused hyperglycaemia.
5. Slow correction of metabolic (keto)acidosis directly if at all.
6. Treatment of any infection if bacterial or parasitic.
7. Monitoring for and recognition and treatment of complications (i.e. cerebral oedema, inappropriate ADH).

Treatment of DKA often begins in an emergency room facility but sometimes this happens outside of an intensive care environment. Under such circumstances, telephone or other consultation should be available with appropriately trained DKA response teams to provide guidance and to facilitate initial treatment and stabilisation as well as transfer for ongoing management. If this is not possible for any

reason, the treating team should make all attempts to provide optimal medical, nursing and laboratory care as possible. A formal intensive care unit, while optimal, is also not always available but the DKA treatment team should be able to set up systems to maximise supervision and documentation of DKA.

For the effective treatment of DKA, one needs recognition and assessment of the problem including the following.

- A history and physical examination to include duration of symptoms, severity of dehydration. If uncertain about severity of dehydration, an assumption of a minimum of 10% dehydration can be used for replacement estimations.
- Ascertainment of level of consciousness is also critical since changes in neurologic status and sensorium can be subtle and must be checked hourly until stable and the dangers of cerebral oedema (sometimes not evident for 6–8 hours into therapy) are reduced.
- Initial weight should ideally be measured but if a scale is unavailable, an estimate should be used according to how much weight has been lost and last known actual weight.
- Ideally, blood glucose at the bedside should be obtained with confirmatory laboratory glucose measurement.
- Similarly either urine or blood ketone levels should be determined.
- Baseline sodium, chloride, potassium, bicarbonate, calcium and phosphate levels as well as blood urea nitrogen and creatinine levels should also be obtained if possible since these will help guide treatment decisions and also be invaluable for follow-up comparisons as treatment ensues. Most of these samples require a simple serum specimen. Blood for haemoglobin A1c requires collection in EDTA medium.
- If appropriate, samples for infection may also be needed. If there is no possibility of laboratory measurements, blood should still

be obtained for possible future measurement, after transportation to a higher level facility takes place. Appropriate microbiological samples if infection is suspected and laboratory support for such processing possible. If no laboratory is available, take the appropriate samples and send with patient to the next level of care.

The standard steps for emergency life support may be needed with initial DKA, depending upon the severity of presentation, degree of consciousness/coma and these are not different from any other emergency resuscitation process and *precede specific diabetes management.* The steps are as follows:

1. Resuscitation

- Ensure appropriate life support (**A**irway, **B**reathing, **C**irculation, etc.).
- Give oxygen to children with impaired circulation and/or shock; nasal oxygen low flow is usually adequate.
- Place a large IV cannula. If IV therapy not available at the site, set up intra-osseous access. If this is not available, place a nasogastric tube. Transfer child to a site with IV facilities as soon as possible.
- Treat shock (decreased perfusion) with fluid (intravenous, intraosseous) at ~10 cc/kg over 30 minutes. Use normal saline or Ringer's Lactate for initial resuscitation. Repeat boluses of 10 cc/kg until perfusion improves clinically.
- If the only access is by nasogastric tube, replace fluid over 60 minutes. Use normal saline, half-strength Darrow's solution with dextrose or oral rehydration solution until perfusion stabilises.

2. Fluid Replacement

- Rehydrate the child with normal saline. Aim to provide maintenance and 10% deficit over 48 hours with calculations designed to very slowly produce improvements. Too rapid correction of initial dehydration, salt and water

imbalance has been associated with cerebral oedema, morbidity and mortality in DKA. As a general rule, the sicker the child or teenager at presentation and the more comatose, the slower should be the initial rehydration.

- It is not necessary to add the urine output to the replacement volume calculations.
- Reassess clinical hydration regularly, i.e. hourly, and especially do not assume that your initial calculations were correct or are being followed without double checking these facts — particularly if your patient is not showing signs of improvement clinically. Make sure all tubes are connected, the electrolyte and fluid orders are being administered correctly and it is neither too fast nor too slow.
- Initial salt and water correction will help decrease the initial hyperglycaemia so a follow-up bedside blood glucose and/or laboratory glucose level in about 1 hour and then at 1—3-hour intervals will confirm response or need for treatment adjustment. Even before insulin effects are obvious, such rehydration efforts will reduce the initial hyperglycaemia and hyperosmolar state. When the blood glucose is less than 15 mmol/L, add dextrose to the saline (add 100 ml 50% dextrose to every litre of saline and use or create a ~5% dextrose-saline intravenous solution).
- If intravenous/osseous access is not available, rehydrate orally with oral rehydration solution (ORS). This can be done by nasogastric tube at a constant rate over 48 hours. If a nasogastric tube is not available, give ORS by oral sips at a rate of 1 mL/kg every 5 minutes. Arrange transfer of the child to a facility with resources to establish intravenous access as soon as possible.
- After the first 4—8 hours, consideration for changing from normal saline to

half-normal saline or similar intravenous solutions based upon clinical response and sequential sodium and other blood serum results.

3. Insulin Therapy

- Start insulin therapy only after circulation has been restored and the patient is haemodynamically stable.
- Start an insulin infusion of short-acting regular or analogue insulin (Actrapid®, NovoLog®, Humalog®, Apidra®) at 0.1 unit/kg/hour. This rate should be controlled with the best available technology (optimally an infusion pump) but piggyback intravenous infusions of insulin into the normal saline infusion work well. For example, a 14 kg child should receive 1.4 units/hour of Actrapid.
- In children under 3 years of age, consider using a lower rate on insulin delivery, e.g. 0.05 unit/kg/hour.
- If no suitable control of the rate of the insulin infusion is available or if intravenous access cannot be obtained or maintained, insulin can be given either subcutaneously or intramuscularly using a similar initial dose of 0.1 unit/kg of the same either short-acting regular insulin or rapid-acting insulins as above.
- Arrange transfer of the child to a facility with resources to establish intravenous access as soon as possible.
- Too rapid correction of hyperglycaemia, like too rapid correction of salt and water imbalance, is associated with cerebral oedema, morbidity and death during DKA treatment. A glucose lowering goal of ~5 mmol/litre/hour is a reasonable therapeutic goal.
- Ketones will classically rise for several hours after initial electrolyte, fluid and insulin treatment as the body metabolism changes and responds to the treatment itself and the metabolic acidosis begins to clear. Total ketones are, in fact, usually

decreasing but what is easily measured is often just a portion of the total ketones and falsely seems to be increasing as a result of the measurement being utilised (i.e. only acetone or acetoacetate instead of also the totality of ketones).

4. Potassium Replacement is needed for **every** child in DKA.

- Obtain a blood sample for determination of potassium as part of the initial assessment.
- If there is no suitable laboratory service (if not available or if results will be delayed beyond 4 hours), changes of hypokalaemia may be observed on an ECG where available. Flattening of the T wave, widening of the QT interval, and the appearance of U waves indicate **hypo**kalaemia. Tall, peaked, symmetrical T waves and shortening of the QT interval are signs of **hyper**kalaemia.
- Ideally, start replacing potassium once the serum potassium value is known or urine output has been documented.
- If the serum potassium values cannot be obtained within 4 hours, start potassium replacement within 4 hours of starting insulin therapy.
- Replace potassium by adding potassium chloride to the IV fluids at a concentration of 40 mmol/L (20 cc of a 15% KCl solution per litre of saline).
- It is not mandatory to utilise potassium phosphate even though total body phosphate is also almost always quite low in DKA. Excess or prolonged phosphate replacement has been linked to abnormalities of calcium and especially without sequential calcium and phosphate blood levels, this may pose additional problems.
- If intravenous potassium chloride is not available, potassium could be replaced by giving the child fruit juice or bananas since these are natural sources of potassium.

- For a child being rehydrated with ORS, no added potassium is needed as ORS contains potassium.
- Serum potassium ideally should be monitored every 4–6 hours, or as often as is possible, and cardiac monitoring should be considered to further document normal T waves without U waves being present.
- In sites where potassium cannot be measured, consider transfer of the child to a facility with resources to monitor potassium and electrolytes.

5. Correction of Acidosis

- Bicarbonate administration is not routinely recommended unless the acidosis is so profound that it is likely to affect cardiac function or resuscitative efforts.
- If bicarbonate is considered necessary, cautiously and slowly give 1–2 mmol/kg over 60 minutes intravenously.

6. Treatment of Infection

- Infection can be a precipitating event for the development of DKA, although most often such infections are viral and do not require antibiotics.
- It is often difficult to exclude infection in DKA, as the white cell count is elevated because of the severity of the metabolic distress and acidosis.
- If bacterial infection is suspected, treat with the most appropriate antibacterial antibiotics as indicated, i.e. treat bacterial pneumonia based upon gram staining, treat bacterial urinary tract infection based upon urinalysis and gram staining etc.
- While severe cerebral malaria and HIV/AIDS can be confused with severe DKA-producing coma, efforts should be considered to differentiate these possibilities. Similarly for common gastrointestinal parasites that can produce severe diarrhoea and dehydration.

7. Monitoring of Management must be ongoing and at least hourly for the first 8–12 hours

depending upon severity of presentation and clinical response to DKA treatment protocols. Specifically, attention to cardiovascular as well as neurologic clinical signs is imperative. One physician must be responsible for such supervision and one nurse similarly must take primary responsibility for such documentation in an appropriate DKA flow sheet.

- *Hourly* clinical parameters; heart rate, BP, respiratory rate, level of consciousness, neurologic status (i.e. pupillary response, gag reflex, reflexes) and glucose meter reading.
- Monitor urine ketones with every sample of urine passed.
- Record fluid intake parenterally as well as orally.
- Record all insulin therapy.
- Record urine output.
- Repeat urea and electrolytes every 4–6 hours.
- Once the blood glucose is less than 15 mmol/L, add dextrose to the saline (add 100 mL 50% dextrose to every litre of saline or use 5% dextrose saline). If replacing fluid orally, ensure that the child has ORS or fruit juice once the glucose gets is below 15 mmol/L.
- Remember that most ketone measurements will show a rise in ketones over the first several hours as these only measure some of the ketones present in DKA. Therefore, this should not require an automatic increase in insulin since it is an expected outcome of initial DKA treatment. Once the urine ketones are clear and oral intake is re-established, follow DKA protocols for transition to subcutaneous insulin.
- Acidosis should slowly but steadily improve with restoration of salt and water balance as well as reduction of ketoacids and lowering of glucose levels.

8. Transitioning to Subcutaneous Insulin

- Once the DKA has been adequately treated, i.e. hydration has been corrected, glucose controlled and ketones reduced (may not be entirely absent depending upon baseline values) and reasonable oral intake has taken place, the child or adolescent can be changed to subcutaneous insulin instead of intravenous insulin.
- The first subcutaneous dose of insulin should be given 30 minutes before stopping the insulin infusion.
- The treatment team should establish their treatment philosophy based on insulin availability and any financial restraints, i.e. twice-a-day insulins, multidose insulin regimens (MDI) and/or resumption of previous daily subcutaneous insulin regimens.

9. Cerebral Oedema

- Cerebral oedema is a rare but frequently fatal complication of DKA so all efforts should be focused on preventing cerebral oedema or at least recognising when it is more likely to occur as well as its earlier manifestations.
- Cerebral oedema is often idiosyncratic but its occurrence may be related to prior duration of DKA symptoms, severity of metabolic (keto)acidosis, too quick or excessive rate and treatment of rehydration, severity of electrolyte disturbance, exact replacement provided with sodium, potassium and bicarbonate errors all potentially contributory factors, degree of initial glucose elevation and too fast rate of decline of blood glucose.
- The rapidly rising intracranial pressure may manifest as a change in neurological state (restlessness, irritability, increased drowsiness or seizures), headache, increased blood pressure and slowing heart rate, decreasing respiratory effort or specific and/or focal neurological signs as

well as inappropriate antidiuretic hormone (unexplained excess urination). Worse neurologic signs or excessive urination — or both — are key to document and all staff should be aware of these possibilities. Hypoglycaemia, of course, can also be confused with such neurologic changes and so a blood glucose level must be obtained to be sure that this is not the case.

- Suspected cerebral oedema or diagnosed cerebral oedema is a true medical emergency so that treatment should not be delayed once diagnosis occurs.
- Reduce the rate of fluid administration by one-third.
- Elevate the head of the bed.
- Give mannitol 0.5–1 g/kg IV over 20 minutes and repeat if there is no initial response in 30 minutes to 2 hours.
- Hypertonic saline (3%), 5 mL/kg over 30 minutes, may be an alternative to mannitol, especially if there is no initial response to mannitol or if mannitol is not available.
- Intubation may be necessary for the patient with impending respiratory failure.
- Neurosurgical consultation should be obtained if available and CT scan or MRI may confirm dilated ventricles associated with cerebral oedema but treatment should not be delayed waiting for a neurosurgeon or for imaging studies.
- Intravenous prednisone or other corticosteroids should be considered if there is clinical worsening, uncontrolled seizures, respiratory arrest or other signs of ongoing cerebral compromise.

After treatment for cerebral oedema has been started, a cranial CT scan or MRI should be obtained to rule out other possible intracerebral causes of neurologic deterioration (approximately 10% of cases) including cerebral thrombosis or haemorrhage since other specific therapy may be available and needed under such circumstances. Cerebral oedema is an unpredictable complication of DKA and can occur even if all steps in DKA treatment are done correctly. Cerebral oedema has a high morbidity and mortality rate and patients who have experienced cerebral oedema are often left with significant lifelong neurologic deficits.

10. Renal Failure and Cardiac Arrest
While extremely rare, both can occur during treatment of severe cases of DKA. Ongoing cardiac monitoring and ongoing monitoring of renal function should allow appropriate recognition and consultation with cardiac and/or nephrology staff.

Hypoglycaemia

Hypoglycaemia means 'low blood glucose levels' and can be defined by symptoms and signs of hypoglycaemia but more recently by symptoms and signs of hypoglycaemia in association with actual blood glucose levels at the same time. The Diabetes Control and Complications Trial (DCCT) helped standardise these definitions that are now used around the world. Hypoglycaemia is said to occur with simultaneous symptoms when the blood glucose levels are less than 4.0 mmol/L (less than 70 mg/dL). There is some mild correlation of symptoms and signs with degree of hypoglycaemia but this is extremely variable, not necessarily reproducible from one episode to the next and may also depend upon rate of decline of blood glucose levels as much as absolute blood glucose level. There is an additional difficulty in that brain blood glucose levels often lag by 30–45 minutes behind peripheral blood glucose levels and so there are inherent discrepancies in the periphery versus the cerebral circulation almost all of the time. Rapid-changing blood glucose levels, of course, also may cause confusion with such symptoms. Many patients also lose their ability

to detect hypoglycaemia because of a condition called hypoglycaemic unawareness syndrome and this makes detection and treatment of such hypoglycaemic episodes that much more difficult and also more necessary to rely on actual blood glucose levels since symptoms are missing.

Symptoms of Hypoglycaemia

The clinical features of hypoglycaemia can be sorted into those associated with low cerebral glucose levels, so-called neuroglycopaenia, and those peripheral effects of hypoglycaemia that are mostly related to the neuroendocrine and autonomic nervous system, especially adrenaline. Neuroglycopaenia includes difficulty concentrating or making decisions, confusion, inability to perform usual tasks (i.e. at work or school, driving a car), changes in mood especially when out of context with the situation at hand, irritability, inconsolable crying, blurred vision, double vision, loss of vision, disturbed vision, difficulty hearing, slurred speech, unsteady gait or dizziness, nightmares or odd dreams, loss of consciousness, coma or seizures and death from respiratory or cardiac arrest. Other symptoms and signs of hypoglycaemia may or may not be present. These symptoms sometimes are present for several years and then are lost if hypoglycaemic unawareness occurs, perhaps as an early manifestation of diabetic neuropathy. These would include tremors, rapid heart rate (tachycardia), pounding heart (palpitations), sweating, pallor, unusual or inconsolable hunger and/or nausea with or without vomiting. Cardiac arrhythmias also can be associated with hypoglycaemia and another syndrome called 'dead-in-bed' syndrome can occur presumably when cardiac arrhythmias occurs during sleep and death occurs from cardiac arrest without any warning.

DCCT-style Grading of Hypoglycaemia

The DCCT was a multicentred special treatment trial that also helped define severity of hypoglycaemia in a standardised fashion in the 1980s. This system has been widely accepted around the world and adopted for routine care as follows.

- **Mild hypoglycaemia:** occurs by definition when a patient recognises hypoglycaemia and is able to self-treat without the assistance of others. By definition, very young infants and many young children can never have such mild episodes since they are unable to self-treat. Blood glucose values are approximately less than or equal to 3–4 mmol/L (60–70 mg/dL). Sometimes, there is discordance with blood glucose levels when they are rapidly dropping and symptoms or signs of hypoglycaemia may occur, of course.
- **Moderate hypoglycaemia:** occurs by definition when the patient is aware of, responds to, and treats the hypoglycaemia but requires someone else's assistance. Blood glucose values are again approximately less than or equal to 3.9 mmol/L (70 mg/dL) but the person is not able to help himself or herself during this episode. Moderate hypoglycaemia is not related to a specific blood glucose level but to the need for someone else for help in treatment.
- **Severe hypoglycaemia** is defined when the patient either loses consciousness or has a convulsion (seizure; fit) associated with the low blood glucose and like moderate hypoglycaemia is not defined by a specific blood glucose level but rather by the occurrence of coma or seizure.

Hypoglycaemia Management

Ideal hypoglycaemic management includes knowledge about the causes of hypoglycaemia so such episodes can be minimised. It is never possible to 100% exclude hypoglycaemia even with insulin pump or multidose insulin analogue treatment coupled with frequent blood glucose monitoring, since counterbalance of insulin, food and activity is never perfect.

Modern intensified T1DM management includes frequent blood glucose monitoring not only to identify periods of hyperglycaemia but also to identify periods of hypoglycaemia. It is also now well known that there are numerous times during the day and especially during the night when hypoglycaemia occurs without signs or symptoms and that hypoglycaemia unawareness syndrome is a common and early co-morbidity of T1DM.

1. RECOGNITION

First, teach the patient to recognise hypoglycaemia. Parents, siblings and other family relatives, friends and teachers all need to know this as well since sometimes they can recognise hypoglycaemia, when the person with diabetes cannot. Learning about hypoglycaemia involves paying attention to timing and amount of food, timing and duration and intensity of activity, timing and types of insulin being provided and coupling this with sufficient blood glucose monitoring to identity patterns and make adjustments accordingly. Under optimal circumstances, blood glucose levels should confirm hypoglycaemia but if blood glucose testing is not available, treatment should be based upon symptoms, reinforcing that not all hypoglycaemia produces symptoms and that cerebral hypoglycaemia may show up differently than peripheral hypoglycaemia.

2. HYPOGLYCAEMIA TREATMENT

The goal of treatment of hypoglycaemia is to get glucose values back to normal and to prevent progression to loss of consciousness or convulsions/seizures. This is achieved by providing fast-acting, simple sugars or glucose. Sugar drinks or soda (Coca-Cola, Pepsi Cola, 7 Up, ginger ales and similar flavours), fruit juices, glucose or fructose-flavoured drinks all can work as can simple table sugar, glucose tablets, honey or maple syrup, sucrose containing sweets (i.e. LifeSavers or other similar hard candies) all have rapid-acting simple sugar that works within 10—15 minutes to be absorbed and to raise the blood glucose levels. Any foodstuff with fat, i.e. chocolate, peanut butter, cheese, is a poor choice for hypoglycaemia treatment — unless nothing else is available — because the fat slows down the absorption of whatever sugars are also present. Usually, between 5 and 15 g of such simple carbohydrate is needed to treat hypoglycaemia, with or without symptoms. The lower the blood glucose, the more carbohydrate that is needed. Dose titration can stipulate, approximately 5 g to raise the glucose levels ~1 mmol (~15 mg/dL) so dose titration of 5—10—15 g of sugar equivalents can be worked out for different blood glucose levels. The lower the glucose value, the more glucose is needed. Usually, it takes 10—15 minutes for symptoms to abate as the blood glucose levels respond to the fast absorbed carbohydrates. The slower the carbohydrates, the more fibre in the carbohydrates, and the more other protein and fats that also slow down the absorption, the slower will be the biochemical raising effect and, concurrently, the slower will be the symptom response. Repeat fast-acting carbohydrate supplementation is occasionally needed but usually one dose will work unless there is some delay in starting treatment or more prolonged exercise has been the cause hours earlier. Common errors include using such high-fat chocolate treats which then do not work so quickly or not waiting sufficiently long to see the symptoms abate and thus mistakenly taking more and more food to 'feel better'. These types of errors eventually raise the blood glucose levels.

If there are significantly sustained exercise effects causing the hypoglycaemic episode, consideration for providing a higher fat and/or higher protein food for more sustained caloric provision should be discussed. High-fat foods such as ice cream and/or peanut butter are particularly well suited for many youngsters to prevent overnight hypoglycaemia, especially when basal insulin such as NPH — but also

some of the other basal insulins like detemir or glargine — peak post-dancing or late afternoon/early evening sustained sports such as football, lacrosse, track etc. Previously, many diabetologists automatically taught that every episode of hypoglycaemia should be treated with fast-acting carbohydrates but also with slower acting carbohydrates. This has turned out not to be needed, as it only raises the blood glucose levels hours after such episodes and does not make one feel better. Added calories, obviously, is also a problem and so this treatment protocol has been changed in recent years. Emphasis should always be on learning why such an episode occurred in the first place and what might have been done differently so that it can be avoided in the future, if possible.

If a child or adolescent is having severe symptoms (is not able to eat, severely nauseated or vomiting or acting belligerently), is unconscious or having a convulsion/seizure, anything provided by mouth is potentially dangerous and could be aspirated. Therefore, oral treatment of moderate to severe hypoglycaemic episodes is more problematic. Treatment requires parental glucagon, either intravenously, intramuscularly or subcutaneously — or intravenous treatment with a slow infusion of glucose:

- intravenous glucose (e.g. 10% glucose drip or 1 mL/kg of 25% dextrose)
- IV, IM or subcutaneous glucagon (0.25 mg for small children; 0.5—1 mg for larger children and adults).

After an injection of glucagon, the blood glucose would be expected to rise within 10—15 minutes. Intravenous glucose would expect to produce an even more rapid rise in blood glucose levels. If one were unconscious or convulsing, there is some lag between peripheral blood glucose levels and cerebral glucose levels so that the full clinical effect may not be so instantaneous.

In circumstances where neither glucagon nor intravenous glucose is available, a 'rapid-acting' carbohydrate, preferably a liquid or gel (e.g. honey, sugar syrup, pancake syrup) can be placed in the mouth alongside the cheek, with the child or adolescent placed in a side-ways lying-down position to minimise the dangers of aspiration especially if there are concomitant severe symptoms, convulsions or hypoglycaemic coma. In adolescents or young adults especially, if there is no appropriate response to documented hypoglycaemia, look-ing for other causes or contributors (alcohol, marijuana or other drugs) should be a consid-eration. Insulin overdoses, either purposeful or unintentional, may explain such prolonged episodes.

Hypoglycaemia Prevention Should be a Priority

Periodic refresher education about causes, signs and symptoms of hypoglycaemia should occur at least twice a year and be documented in the education flow sheet records.

There needs to be specific teaching about missed meals or snacks or late meals/snacks including what to do if food is financially unaf-fordable or otherwise unavailable. Assessment and advice includes the following.

- Obvious changes in schedule, i.e. weekends or summer vacation.
- How to handle sleeping late.
- Attention to peak and trough effects of insulins being used, particularly older basal insulins such as NPH or lente compared to the lower-hypoglycaemic profiles of newer analogues.
- High risk associated with new activities, more sustained or intense activities.
- Special risks and periodic monitoring needs for overnight hypoglycaemia.
- Special risks associated with those who have hypoglycaemic-related seizures.
- Consideration for anti-seizure medications especially if recurrent hypoglycaemic seizures are documented.

- Review of potential dangers with alcohol and marijuana as well as other drugs which interfere either with hypoglycaemia recognition or adrenergic responsiveness to hypoglycaemia.
- Illness-associated hypoglycaemia, most often viral, and other gastroenteritis associated with nausea and vomiting.
- Blood glucose (BG) monitoring is key to establishing patterns and to learning about such hypoglycaemic problems.

A number of factors can predict the occur-rence of hypoglycaemia: age (increased in infancy because communication is, by defini-tion, more difficult and in adolescence associ-ated with compliance issues as well as activity changes), longer duration of diabetes, presum-ably with known or unknown diabetic auto-nomic neuropathy, higher doses of insulin, lower HbA1c values, inconsistent meal plan-ning, timing or amounts of food, activity increases especially if activity occurs irregularly, recent changes in treatment regimen, lack of symptoms (hypoglycaemia unawareness), dur-ing sleep, alcohol use blunting hepatic gluco-neogenesis (not causing the hypoglycaemia per se) with alcohol effects notoriously occur-ring hours after ingestion and lasting for many hours as well (i.e. next morning sleeping late), other drug use (i.e. marijuana) which interferes with proper treatment decisions (i.e. what to eat, whether to test) as well as how to interpret what has occurred, what a blood glucose level indicates, correct insulin dosing or taking insulin far in advance of food as well as too close to food intake, lack of routine monitoring so no patterns can be understood, prior history of hypoglycaemia problems, poor proactive planning because of intellectual compromise in understanding such physiology or because of psychosocial barriers to using such information.

Repeated episodes of hypoglycaemia require a thorough review by the entire family and diabetes management team looking to identify patterns that may respond to change in any or all of the above factors. This is especially true for adolescents who are learning to be self-responsible but not always able to carry this out. Too early transfer of self-care by many parents, even too-early recommendations for such transfer by diabetes treatment teams, contribute to Figure 12.1 MedicAlert® identification bracelet poor overall diabetes outcomes but especially too frequent hypoglycaemia. Children or adolescents troubled with other minor or major psychosocial issues (psychological or sexual trauma, learning problems and attention deficit as well as executive dysfunction, single-parent or impoverished families) as well as families who are enmeshed and where poor adult supervision has been observed, are prone to problems with severe hypoglycaemia as well as hyperglycaemia.

MedicAlert® Identification Bracelet or Necklace

Since people with diabetes can become unconscious or unable to communicate their problem when they develop hypoglycaemia, it is ideal for them to carry a card, a bracelet or a locket , as shown in Figure 12.1, which says, 'I have diabetes.' This would allow emergency personnel or even teachers or coaches to recognise that the child or teenager has diabetes and consider that loss of consciousness may be due to hypoglycaemia, which can be treated by giving glucose or food.

REGULAR T1DM TREATMENT

After initial diagnosis and education, regular follow-up visits should be established with the diabetes management team as well as the entire family, parents and child/teenager. Inviting extended family members, i.e. siblings, grandparents and other relatives commonly involved with home care, would be wise to consider. Relying only on mothers to provide such adult supervision is also problematic since it gives a false message to many children and teenagers that this is not so important since father is not involved. Special invitations to fathers may be necessary to attend clinic and ambulatory follow-up and teaching sessions.

In the DCCT, support visits and review occurred monthly but this is often not possible because of cost and travel to the diabetes centres. Alternatives to such support include telephones, faxes and more recently email and other social network sites as well as mobile telephones that allow questions to be posed and answers provided, problems to be solved and overall improved health for the person with T1DM. Whether the physician, nurse, dietician or other healthcare workers are the focus of such follow-up is less important than that the entire team works closely together with the same philosophy of management and the same treatment goals. This was learned quite eloquently in the DCCT and emphasises the goal-driven proactive response to problem solving that empowers change to be initiated and hopefully be sustained.

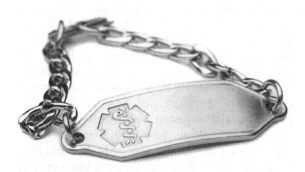

FIGURE 12.1 MedicAlert® identification bracelet. *Reprinted with permission from The Diabetes Control and Complications Trial Research Group. The Effect of Intensive Treatment of Diabetes on the Development and Progression of Long-Term Complications in Insulin-Dependent Diabetes Mellitus. New Engl J Med 1993;329:977-86. Copyright 1993, New Engl J Med.*

Choosing and Using Insulins

As there are different insulins available in different parts of the world, decisions about which insulin to choose are sometimes not based upon what is ideal but more practically what is possible. Older insulins cost less than newer analogues but tend to have more variable peak and valley effects as well as producing more hypoglycaemia and hyperglycaemia as a result. Such older animal-source or human regular and NPH insulins are associated with less flexibility and greater rigidity of food and activity timing than with newer — but more costly — analogues. In previous decades without much monitoring possibility, more rigid food and activity schedules attempted to compensate for such lack of flexibility but glycaemic control was also less optimal so there were more short and long-term complications.

In practice and because of government, insurance and financial constraints as well as inconsistent availability of insulin in many parts of the world, patients and prescribers may have to use a variety of available or donated insulins. While not ideal, this adds more learning difficulties and more problems teaching changing balancing requirements. Hence it is necessary to be familiar with the range of insulins available on the market and adapt the patient's doses to the medications available locally even if they may change far more than is ideal. It is also true that food availability, unfortunately, in many parts of the world is also not guaranteed and so insulin dose adjustments could be designed accordingly based upon blood glucose monitoring results and algorithms created just for such purposes.

Most diabetes specialists and most guidelines acknowledge that the improved control possible with modern diabetes regimens is partly attributed to the improved insulin profile available with newer but costlier analogue insulins, using MDI regimens or pumps. It should be remembered that insulin pump therapy is not the only way to have excellent glucose control.

Targeted blood glucose control as proven by the landmark DCCT studies remain the essential element of T1DM care if resources can be provided for such monitoring and insulin delivery coupled with educational, nutritional and psychosocial support for the child and adolescent.

1. Fast-Acting (Regular) Insulins

Regular insulins previously were derived from cows or pigs. Over time, they were improved upon and purified to be closer to human insulin. Regular insulins usually had to be injected about 30–60 minutes ahead of food but this was rather inconvenient and so almost always was never timed correctly. Peak effects occur about 2–4 hours after injection and duration lasts 6–8 hours. Regular insulins were somewhat more variable in their action than newer analogues, a reason for their replacement by the newer rapid-acting insulin analogues.

2. Rapid-Acting Insulins

Rapid-acting analogue insulins (insulin aspart [Novorapid® or Novolog® by NovoNordisk], insulin lispro [Humalog® by Eli Lilly], insulin glulisine [Apidra® by Sanofi Aventis]) have been synthetically modified to better provide immediate postprandial coverage of glycaemia. They have faster peak effect, shorter duration and shorter tail effect. Onset of action with the rapid-acting analogues is in 15–30 minutes with peak effect at 1–2 hours and duration of effect about 3–4 hours. Usually, such rapid-acting analogue insulins are given as part of an MDI regimen with meals and snacks covered accordingly and with basal insulins such as detemir or glargine. Most commonly these are available by insulin pens but can also be given via syringe. They are, of course, also used effectively with insulin pumps for combination bolus and basal insulinisation. Rapid-acting analogues can be used with NPH or any other basal insulin regimen and can also be mixed in a syringe either in premixed ratios (least flexible style) or with NPH via syringe adjusted accordingly.

For very young children, especially those who are picky eaters, irregular eaters or very slow eaters, such analogues can be given just prior to food or even just after food is completed to better allow balancing of actual food or snack intake with less guessing. Such analogues, when affordable and available, have replaced the older synthetic human regular insulins or the animal-source regular insulins because of more reproducibility and less hypoglycaemia associated with their use.

3. Intermediate-Acting Insulin

Previously, basal insulin effect was provided either by lente or NPH (Neutral Protamine Hagedorn) insulin (Insulatard® or Humulin®). Lente insulin is much less available in recent years and had a slightly longer duration of effect than NPH. NPH insulin had an onset of action about 2–4 hours after administration, variable peak effects from 3–8 hours and variable duration effects of 10–18 hours. When used as a basal insulin, lente and NPH usually needed to be given at least 2 if not 3 times a day in overlapping dosage. Many healthcare teams used them as background (basal) insulin in 3 or 4 times-a-day MDI regimens to try to minimise peak effects, minimise hypoglycaemia and optimise insulin availability coupled with faster regular or rapid-acting analogues around meals. In some circumstances, they were used only twice a day particularly when there was little blood glucose monitoring or education services available. Such dosage systems frequently were insufficient to control hyperglycaemia and have mostly been supplanted by better MDI basal insulins, as described below.

4. Long-Acting Insulins (Duration 18–24 Hours)

Detemir (Levemir® by NovoNordisk) and glargine (Lantus® by Sanofi-Aventis) are the currently available longer acting insulins that have often replaced NPH or lente or ultralente insulins in most modern MDI regimens. Both detemir and glargine produce lower peaks, more reproducible peaks and have more sustained and day-to-day reproducibility than prior intermediate acting or long-acting insulin. Both detemir and glargine insulins begin to have an effect from 2–4 hours after injection, reach modest peaks around 8–12 hours after injection and tend to wane after 18–24 hours. Glargine is a bit longer lasting than detemir but in smaller doses typically used in children; both may need to be given twice a day, most usually at breakfast and again at bedtime. Overnight monitoring helps to determine exact schedule needs since dosing always must be individualised. Most children and adolescents need relatively more basal insulin at bedtime compared to morning doses because of a prominent dawn effect attributed to early morning insulin resistance. Some need just the opposite distribution. Some need only a morning long-acting insulin and none at bedtime. All such decisions should be made based upon actual blood glucose monitoring profiles and not by preformed dogmatic ideas about which is a better or worse pattern. Style and amount of food and activity, of course, influence such decisions enormously.

5. ultra-Long-Lasting Insulins

Ultralente is rarely available these days but previously was used as a once-at-bedtime basal insulin to avoid extra injections and couple with meal-time bolus insulins. It had some success with frequent blood glucose monitoring despite having wide variability in its peak as well as duration effectiveness. More recently ultralente has been off most markets and replaced either by insulin pumps or by glargine or detemir basal insulin preparations.

6. Mixing Insulins in the Same Syringe

It is very common to combine intermediate-acting with either regular insulin or rapid-acting as an attempt at convenience. For instance, regular and NPH at breakfast, regular alone at supper and NPH alone at bedtime; analogue plus NPH at breakfast, analogue plus NPH at suppertime. The regular or rapid-acting insulin is always drawn into the syringe first to mini-mise any contamination of the faster insulin with protamine. The rapid-acting doses can be adapted/adjusted every day or every meal and snack to food intake and physical exercise. Regular or rapid-acting insulin is not recom-mended for mixing with either glargine or dete-mir insulin because of potential changes in action characteristics.

7. Fixed Ratio Combinations

Fixed ratio combinations also are available on the market especially in vial as well as pen formulations. They are much more commonly used with T2DM rather than T1DM but sometimes they are used when they are the only insulins available in different parts of the world. They are much more diffi-cult to provide food flexibility since both types of insulin change in amount when the dosage changes and this occurs in fixed proportion to their formulations. Because there are two types of insulin present from the manufacturer, both types must be adapted if dose changes: the rapid-acting peak and duration effects and the more prolonged protaminated compo-nent peak.

Choosing the Best Insulin for a Patient

There is no perfect insulin preparation but good glycaemic control can be reached with any insulin, even though some protocols and regimens offer more or less flexibility even as the work required to make them successful changes with patient and family interest, quality of life choices, healthcare team options and financial considerations. The choice of insulin should be individualised and based on the patient's needs, the desired characteristics of the insulin as well as the availability and cost

of the insulin and desired treatment goals and target blood glucose levels.

Adherence to treatment is a key success factor of diabetes control as is frequent blood glucose monitoring and self-analysis with an emphasis on proactive adaptation of food, activity and illness for that individual's require-ments. Most intensive insulin treatment regi-mens currently prefer using insulin analogues since they offer faster action profiles, less wait-ing between insulin and food, better postpran-dial glucose coverage and less chance of hypoglycaemia without any compromise in overall glucose control as measured by HbA1c results. In many developing countries such analogues remain out of reach because of finan-cial difficulties or simple unavailability.

Dangers of Insulins Bought on the Informal Market or Black Market or Obtained from Donations

- **Integrity of the cold chain:** insulin needs to have been stored properly at $2-8°C$, without having been frozen or overheated at any time after it leaves the factory and before it reaches the final consumer. Insulin bought from alternative channels may not have been stored properly and may have lower potency.
- **Mislabelling:** different products may have similar names and packaging in different countries.
- **Counterfeit goods** may be diluted or lose potency because of improper handling or storage.

Blood Glucose Testing Strategies

In many parts of the developing world and even in some parts of richer countries, limited blood glucose testing occurs because of unaf-fordability of such testing, lack of strips and/or lack of batteries or even blood glucose meters themselves. The purpose of blood glucose testing is self-learning for the child, adolescent or family in addition to maximising day-to-day flexibility and adjusting food and insulin for optimal glucose control, prevention of acute complications such as DKA and hypoglycaemia and ultimately prevention of long-standing diabetes complications.

What Affects the Blood Glucose Reading?

The blood glucose reading is affected by:

- the dose injected
- how fast insulin was released from the injection site
- presence of lipohypertrophy or lipoatrophy
- the amount of food consumed
- how fast the food was digested, fibre content, fat content, glycaemic index
- how much glucose was used by the muscles/ activity effects
- how fast the glucose is being converted to glycogen
- effects of stress hormones like adrenaline and cortisol
- effects of growth hormone and testosterone or oestrogen
- illness effects
- obesity-related insulin resistance.

Almost all blood glucose meters are sufficiently accurate so that, with proper technique, a very small drop of blood can be applied to the blood glucose test strip and a reproducible and accurate blood glucose reading can result. If the patient's blood glucose data is not useful to the clinician in its present form, the doctor or nurse must encourage a change in the frequency or pattern of testing, the quality of accompanying information about diet, dose and activity or all of the above. If a patient does many blood glucose readings but does not know how to interpret them and does not change either the dose of insulin, the pattern of eating or activity in response to the glucose levels, testing the glucose readings becomes a futile and wasteful exercise. This becomes a focus of education to figure out barriers to home adjustment either for the child, the adolescent or the family members helping in the care of such patients.

Because of the relatively high cost of blood glucose testing strips, it may be necessary to make treatment decisions and change insulin doses on the basis of just a few blood glucose readings. This section will run through the principles of designing a glucose-testing strategy that will maximise returns for the individual patient while conserving scarce resources. Since the blood glucose level may be affected in so many ways but patients especially in the developing countries are usually on a relatively fixed dose of insulin, the patterns of blood glucose levels are generally more important than individual glucose readings.

- If a pattern of BG readings is always high, the dose most likely to be operating at that time is not sufficient.
- If a pattern of BG readings is always low, the dose most likely operating at that time is too high.
- If a BG reading is sometimes very high or very low, either insulin, food or exercise are not consistent and some problem-solving discussions should occur to determine the cause and make corrections accordingly.

Consideration if BG Strips are Available and no Financial Rationing is Needed

The following may be considered:

- frequent pre-meal and post-meal BGs: pre-breakfast and 2 hours post-breakfast (mid-morning), pre-lunch and 2 hours post-lunch (mid-afternoon), pre-dinner and 2 hours post-dinner plus at bedtime and sometimes also nocturnal monitoring as well
- home logbooks for visual analysis
- colour-coded home logbooks for pattern identification
- computer-downloaded analysis of BG results with modal day data, averages by time of day, bar graphs and pie chart analysis and trend analysis

- Education includes not only record-keeping but also goals for analysis, understanding of insulin kinetics, understanding of meal planning, carbohydrate counting and glycaemic index as well as understanding of activity effects as well as sick-day guidelines. All this can be done even with limited facilities.

Consideration if Four BG Strips are Available Each Day

The following may be considered:

- routinely checking pre-meals and at bedtime
- occasional checking post-meals
- problem solving if hypoglycaemia occurs, nocturia or enuresis occurs etc.
- similar home logbook, colour-coded home logbooks and computer-downloaded analysis and education options as with more testing each day but obviously less information available so more guesswork occurs
- some families and some patients even when financially able to monitor more often will obviously elect to not monitor at all, only monitor occasionally and refuse to keep any kind of home records so that their own ability to analyse their own data is limited.

Consideration if Three BG Strips are Available Each Day

The following may be considered:

- routinely checking pre-breakfast and then learning about different meals of the day with pre-meals and post-meal BG checks for several days in a row to identify any patterns
- intermittent checks in the middle of the night to be sure that there are no missed hypoglycaemic patterns
- some testing for hypoglycaemia episodes
- some testing with sick days.

If glucose strips are in short supply, the aim should be to gain at least a working knowledge of the patient's key problems. Some examples follow.

If Only 10 Strips a Month are Available

Do three pre-main meal glucose level tests on 3 consecutive days and a late-night glucose level on one of the nights. As activity often is different on weekend days, it is useful to then check to see if the weekend appears to be the same pattern or a different pattern related either to time of going to sleep, getting up, sports activity etc.

For 5 Strips/Month

Pick one typical day of activity and food and do a series of different days each month utilising pre-breakfast, pre-lunch, mid-afternoon, pre-dinner and post-dinner/bedtime test periods. The aim is to identify any patterns of hypoglycaemia or hyperglycaemia, with the understanding that most youngsters with T1DM will have very different BG readings on each day so that this only provides a cursory evaluation possibility.

Urine Glycosuria Testing with Benedict's Solution or Urine Strips

Although BG testing is felt to be optimal, if there is no financial possibility of BG testing, discussions about the possibility of urine strip testing or use of Benedict's solution should not be eliminated. While urine tests do not provide immediacy of glucose evaluation results, they do provide some ability to look for patterns and trends. If all the urine testing results for several days done with very inexpensive Benedict's solution showed high levels of glycosuria, the insulin dose is either too low or the food being provided too rich in carbohydrates − or some combination − so that changes would be needed on this basis. Similarly, if there were hypoglycaemic episodes and they were associated with urine sugar-free time periods so that a pattern could be recognised, adjustments of the food upwards and/or insulin downwards would be indicated. Totally eliminating urine glycosuria assessments when BG monitoring is unaffordable and not provided by the health-care systems does not make much sense.

Meal Planning, Exchange Concepts, Carbohydrate Counting and Glycaemic Index of Food

Children with T1DM need to eat in a healthy fashion in amounts and proportions appropriate for their age and stage of development. During the pubertal growth spurt, obviously there are needs for increased calories and this too should be not so different from peers. Because the person with T1DM does not make insulin suffi-ciently for their own needs and needs to take insulin by injection, the food must be balanced with the insulin provided and further balanced for activity that occurs, illness etc. Similarly, if the child or adolescent with T1DM is also over-weight or obese, caloric restrictions will also need to be considered and this also is not much different than those without diabetes except that the insulin dose must also be balanced. If financial constraints also make food scarce or erratic, this is an added burden, but it must be discussed openly and honestly and balancing attempts optimised. Different insulin schemes may be provided for different circumstances with the hope for sufficient BG monitoring to allow better estimation of need instead of totally guessing. As the child assumes more self-management as an older child and adolescent, all such teaching should be repeated and individualised so that repetitive education efforts are also part of nutrition planning. More activity and more exercise means more caloric intake or lowered insulin doses are needed to counterbalance the effects of such activity. This too should be taught and ongoing education efforts stress such teaching points.

Nutrition
- An individualised daily nutrition history and review should be done shortly after diagnosis

and used as a basis for initial nutrition advice. Highlights would include type and amount of simple sugars ingested, sources of dietary fibre, vitamins and minerals, amount of saturated fat, amount and quality as well as quantity of protein, financial issues with food availability and consistency, local family and community customs and whether or not there are specific religious feasts or fast-days that need to be considered and balanced.
- A 24-hour dietary recall is useful at diagnosis and repeated at least once a year or if questions/problems arise before then.
- If the child or adolescent is not overweight or obese, caloric restriction is not at all part of the meal plan whereas timing and balancing of insulin and activity always will have to be taught and reviewed.
- Empowerment methodology for questions and interactions is often an ideal way to gather such typical food information, especially about health beliefs. This should be balanced with the new information provided about activity and insulin vis-à-vis BG results and effects. Offering choices rather than 'dictating' change should be strongly considered as more efficacious.
- Understanding of local traditions and customs also would establish a collaborative relationship and increase trust for future questions and problem solving.
- Ideally, a trained paediatric dietician or nutritionist should be part of the multidisciplinary T1DM team, but if this is not possible or available because of government health ministry policy, local hospital availability or other financial constraints, either the physician or the nurse working on the diabetes team will have to assume this role.
- At a minimum, such dietary review should be documented and take place in a formal fashion every year. If specific problems arise, this may be needed more frequently.

- Mothers and grandmothers but also fathers and siblings should be invited to learn about proper nutrition and especially about diabetes-related nutrition needs. This can help open up avenues of discussion, identify cultural and societal food issues and help the child or adolescent with diabetes in a supportive fashion.
- School and peer food-related issues, timing of school meals, quality and quantity of school meals also need to be discussed.
- If there is concomitant hyperlipidaemia, saturated fats may also need to be restricted.
- If there is renal disease as a diabetes complication related to hypertension or oedema, protein restriction or salt restriction may also be reviewed.
- While more common in the developed rather than the developing world, anorexia and bulimia also can co-exist with T1DM so awareness by the medical team is important. A particularly risky situation has been dubbed 'diabulimia' and is deemed to take place when purposeful omission of insulin because of emotional turmoil, especially prior sexual or physical abuse, occurs resulting in extremely high and out-of-control chronic hyperglycaemia. This can be associated with omitted insulin doses, falsified or omitted glucose monitoring and binge eating with risks for severe hypoglycaemia as well as ketoacidosis.

Specific issues with lack of food, lack of consistency of food and the finances of obtaining food are also important topics for discussion in developing countries because poverty is such a big issue. Adjustments of insulin and activity must take this into account and efforts to have open and honest discussions of the possible solutions should also take place instigated by the diabetes team.

Lack of appropriate nutrition and caloric intake may be the main cause of poor growth and development around the world, unrelated at all to T1DM. Rather than focus on the idea of diet as being a restriction, a term such as meal planning is more positive and produces the concept of balance between insulin, activity and food amounts. Food portions, exchange lists and carbohydrate counting are all part of systems designed to teach ways to determine how much food should be supplied at a given time of the day. Food can be separated into carbohydrate, protein and fat components to sort them for ease of teaching and thinking about how they can be offered. Parents and perhaps also grandparents and other family members, particularly older siblings, can be involved with the meal planning since they often are the purchasers and suppliers of food. Parents also have a critical role in supervising consistency from meal to meal and day to day.

- Different insulin regimens have different food requirements. Insulin should be adapted to food intake if possible, rather than food 'forced' against insulin effects if possible. Review of the insulin regime should be done as often as possible to minimise the risk of hypoglycaemia and the need for large snacks as much as possible.
- More rigid dietary requirements are necessary when premixed insulins are the source of insulin used since flexibility is much more restrictive.
- In between insulin regimens such as a twice-a-day regular and NPH regimens must take into account the peak and trough effects of both the regular and NPH insulin types; and frequently this demands three meals and three large snacks. Further flexibility occurs when the second insulin dose is split and this involves three injections per day: regular and NPH pre-breakfast, regular alone pre-dinner, and NPH alone at bedtime to better deliver insulin overnight, compensating for the pre-breakfast dawn phenomenon and help avoid middle-of-the-night insulin-induced hypoglycaemia. All such insulin styles can be

balanced with meal plans appropriately spaced to help avoid the extremes of low and high glucose levels.

- MDI, multidose insulin regimens include pre-meal and pre-snack regular or analogue insulins coupled with longer-lasting analogues such as glargine or detemir (or insulin pumps) provides the most food flexibility and mimics normal pancreatic function but at added cost and complexity.
- Plan for an overall breakdown of 50—60% carbohydrates, 15—20% protein and less than 30% fats.
- Estimated calorie needs are 1000 calories for a 1 year old with an additional 100 calories per year of age until approximately 10—12 years.
- Girls then often need some caloric restriction and attention to BMI to prevent puberty-related obesity. An intake closer to 1000—1600 calories/day may be more appropriate under these circumstances, except if peripubertal and pubertal girls are exceptionally active.
- Peripubertal and pubertal boys often need continued caloric increases as their own testosterone levels increase throughout puberty but paying attention to activity energy requirements and BMI is imperative.
- Special attention to sick-day food and liquid management associated with illnesses, especially the need for increased fluid and salt intake with respiratory illnesses causing hyperglycaemia and ketonuria/ketonaemia as well as the need for higher sugar intake (maybe also temporarily lessening insulin doses) associated with gastrointestinal disturbances. Optimally, such decisions should be based upon BG and ketone monitoring.

Carbohydrates

Complex carbohydrates require less insulin because of how they are digested and absorbed, and therefore have less likelihood of causing extremely high post-meal hyperglycaemia. Increases in dietary fibre not only promote optimal bowel function, but also may help with glycaemic outcome. Legumes, beans, pulses and bran-containing foods fall into this category, in contrast to faster-digested simple carbohydrates such as juices and fruits, milk sugars, and simpler carbohydrate foods such as corn and potatoes. Exchange lists often utilise the 'rule of 15' where one exchange portion provides approximately 15 g of carbohydrates. Thus, one slice of processed bread, one-half cup of dried cereal, one small fruit or one glass of milk all provide approximately 15 g of carbohydrate. This is a simple fact that can be taught whether the patient or family are literate or illiterate. Consistency may be obtained using such exchange concepts.

Dietary Behaviour and Compliance Issues

The interaction of the family with the infant, child or teenager with T1DM closely relates to the control of blood glucose levels. How the young person eats, whether the same or different from the rest of the family and his or her friends, is important in this relationship. Food behaviour is expressed through family, societal, religious, nutritive and emotional components and all must be acknowledged and addressed with appropriate education and discussion. Paying attention to individual needs and wants also is important. Children and adults with a medical illness are not required to fast during Ramadan, for example, if they have diabetes mellitus. However, older children, adolescents and adults may choose to observe the Ramadan fast. People of other faiths may also want to fast for religious reasons at various holiday celebrations, e.g. Yom Kippur. Dietary non-compliance is often a key problem area either through mis-education or direct confrontation and inconsistent messages from family, society or healthcare professionals. Interference with optimal glucose control is often diet-related. How food has been used within a family unit in the past could be an important factor in changing food-related behaviour and choices as part of a diabetes treatment programme.

Poverty-Related Nutrition Issues: Lack of Food, Lack of Consistent Food

In certain parts of the world and in certain countries, improved diabetes care is at least partly hampered by economic constraints. Food is simply not always available, too costly or too inconsistently supplied. This presents a major barrier to improved diabetes care, since deciding how much insulin to supply is essentially impossible without knowing how much food will be supplied at that moment. In most such situations, because of the financial problems, not only is food unreliably available but monitoring is virtually nonexistent. Whether or not insulin is available in these places is also doubtful. The combination of all these factors places the child or adolescent with T1DM at high risk of chronic hyperglycaemia, because a reasonable response to inadequate food is to under-dose insulin, thus avoiding hypoglycaemia from inadequate food supply or snack supply. Efforts to address these issues are complex, societal and governmental-related and remain extremely difficult for the diabetes specialty healthcare team as well as the family.

Activity and T1DM

Exercise is a good thing. Exercise and physical activity is a common part of children's lives and should be encouraged for those with diabetes. In addition to an improved sense of well-being, exercise may help with weight control; it limits the rise in glucose after meals, keeps the heart rate and blood pressure lower and helps keeps blood lipid levels normal. These factors may reduce cardiovascular risk and may be associated with a lower HbA1c.

Effect of Activity on Diabetes

Children and adolescents with T1DM are not able to automatically regulate insulin effects during exercise because their insulin has to be adjusted by either themselves if they control their treatment or by their parents. They commonly have unrecognised glucose dysregulation involving counter-regulatory hormones like glucagon and adrenaline in addition to their direct β-cell insufficiency. These factors frequently result in **hypoglycaemia** during or after activity. Hypoglycaemia is more likely to occur with prolonged or intense activity. Hypoglycaemia may also occur many hours after prolonged activity, particularly if there is a delay in replacing glycogen stores in the liver. However, excessive intake of carbohydrate, decreased insulin doses and the emotional responses to activity and competition may result in **hyperglycaemia**. Excessive sweating and decreased fluid intake may cause dehydration during activity. In the case of poor control and high glucose values, the exaggerated effects of counter-regulatory hormones may cause increased production of **ketones**.

Factors Affecting Glucose Response to Exercise

1. Duration.
2. Initial adrenaline surge.
3. Intensity of activity and effect — soon or later — on glucose levels.
4. Type of activity: anaerobic activity (e.g. sprinting) vs aerobic activity with different immediate and longer term glucose effects.
5. Metabolic control: poor metabolic control often results in high blood glucose values and low circulating insulin levels. Exercise under these circumstances can cause ketonuria and continued hyperglycaemia rather than hypoglycaemia.
6. Type and timing of insulin injections. Peak or waning insulin effect of type of insulin.

7. Absorption of insulin, sites and ambient temperature.
8. Type and timing of food, carbohydrate effects, glycaemic effects of fat and stomach emptying.
9. Degree of stress/competition involved in the activity.

Managing Exercise and Activity

With the large number of variables that can affect glucose values during exercise, it is not surprising that activity can produce very variable values in different children and teenagers. While there are a few guidelines that need to be followed, having an individualised way of dealing with activity would be helpful with key emphasis on understanding insulin, food, stress and activity effects in a theoretical sense and then applying such knowledge to the specific situations coupled with frequent BG monitoring to learn how best to counterbalance exercise effects, optimise insulin administration and prevent both extremes of hyperglycaemia and hypoglycaemia accordingly. For longer activities, BG monitoring can and should be allowed and utilised to learn best responses, and coaches and peers should be aware of the rationale for such monitoring, potential need for extra food or rapid-acting sugar containing balancing and how to assist should hypoglycaemia occur anyway.

Tracking Growth: Height and Weight

Children and adolescents with T1DM should achieve normal growth targets for their ethnic group and the community in which they live. Ideally, children should be measured for growth using population-specific charts. Where these charts are not readily available, the United States Centers for Disease Control and Prevention (CDC) charts or comparable charts available in Canada, Australia, Japan, Israel, France, Germany, Italy (and many other countries) may be used for plotting height and weight for age. Many including the CDC charts are available for free downloading on the Internet. If normal growth and pubertal staging is occurring, this is a powerful indicator of adequacy of diabetes care. Chronic hyperglycaemia often is associated with growth slowdown, growth failure and pubertal delay (Mauriac syndrome) so growth itself can be utilised as a quality of care indicator.

As weight gain occurs, it should be expected that insulin doses will comparably need to be increased using approximately 0.6–0.8 units/kg/day for an average prepubertal and postpubertal insulin dose requirement and increase insulin dosage up to 1.3–1.5 units/kg/day during the pubertal spurt. Slowdown in height velocity and/or unexpected changes in weight should prompt an enquiry into the cause, for instance, Hashimoto's thyroiditis and hypothyroidism, adrenal insufficiency (Addison's disease), coeliac disease. However, the worse the overall glycaemic control, the higher the A1c values, and the more negative the growth evaluation, the more likelihood that the cause for the poor growth would be diabetes itself.

Glycosylated Haemoglobin (HbA1c)

The red blood cells contain the oxygen-carrying protein compound called haemoglobin. Since the red blood cells are always surrounded by blood plasma, which contains glucose, some glucose molecules will stick onto haemoglobin by a process known as 'non-enzymatic glycosylation'. This makes a new substance called glycosylated haemoglobin. We can measure the haemoglobin A1c (HbA1c or HgbA1c). The reaction is non-enzymatic, slow and irreversible so that the HbA1c level in the blood reflects the average blood glucose level during the life of the red blood cell (approximately 120 days). It actually reflects the more recent average blood glucose levels a bit more strongly than the entire lifespan of the red blood cell but nevertheless measuring A1c levels can provide us with a time-average estimate of glucose control that is extremely objective, reliable, reproducible and that also can be used for assessing long-term complication risks such as growth, pubertal timing, eye disease (retinopathy), nerve disease (neuropathy), kidney disease (nephropathy) and hypertension, cardiac complications etc. (see below).

What is the Normal or Ideal HbA1c Level?

If the blood glucose levels are often high, more glucose molecules will stick onto the haemoglobin, and the HbA1c level will be high, while if the blood glucose levels are usually low, fewer glucose molecules are stuck onto haemoglobin and the HbA1c level will be low. Normal HbA1c is about 4–6%. Ideal target A1c levels are not known but efforts to keep the A1c levels below 7–7.5% are considered reasonable targets as long as there is not excessive or severe and repetitive episodes of hypoglycaemia.[4] In very small babies or where optimal food and monitoring are unavailable, modifications of such targets have been proposed, i.e. aiming for values below 8%. Table 12.1 shows the relationship between estimated average glucose (eAG) and A1c.

If the patient has severe anaemia, sickle cell disease, some types of thalassaemia or a shortened red blood cell lifespan due to abnormal red blood cells, the HbA1c may not reflect the true average blood glucose level in the body.

Large-scale studies (such as the DCCT and United Kingdom Prospective Diabetes Study [UKPDS]) have shown that the HbA1c level correlates with the risk of diabetic complications and the risk of hypoglycaemia (see the two DCCT figures below: 12.3 and 12.4). The various expert bodies such as the International Diabetes Federation, the American Diabetes Association and ISPAD have made recommendations about target HbA1c levels. Target A1c levels should be established by the diabetes team and all members of the team should be aware of these

targets as well as when they may need to be modified (i.e. recurrent severe hypoglycaemia or hypoglycaemia unawareness). One of the key success factors when comparing different centres may well be a uniform philosophy of diabetes care especially in evaluating BG monitoring and results as well as A1c results. In the DCCT, A1c was obtained monthly and feedback provided not only to the entire diabetes team but also the patient and his or her family. Most guidelines suggest at least getting an A1c done every 3 months. If this is not financially possible, the diabetes team will need to ascertain what is an initial goal (i.e. annually, semi-annually) based upon what the patient can afford, what the government will allow or what insurance systems and healthcare systems will permit. Quality control efforts should include not just individual assessment of A1c levels and whether or not improvement or deterioration occurs but also clinic-wide average A1c levels, trend analysis and barriers to improvement.

T1DM CHRONIC COMPLICATIONS ASSESSMENT AND PREVENTION: METABOLIC CONTROL MATTERS!

T1DM is a chronic disease which needs to be controlled since there is no currently known cure. Good control of T1DM can only be achieved by a well-designed care plan which is carried out not only by a team of healthcare professionals working in a coordinated fashion with similar goals and dedicated to this effort but with close collaboration of child and adolescent, family and society. T1DM can result in complications such as high blood pressure, high cholesterol values, damage to the nerves causing constant burning pain (neuropathy) or absent deep tendon reflexes, damage to the kidneys (nephropathy with protein leakage and ultimately kidney failure and death) and damage to the eyes (retinopathy and ultimately blindness). Longer term damage to the macrovascular system is associated with early heart attack and stroke as well as amputations. These complications directly correlate with glucose control, although there clearly are genetic and family factors that explain their distribution and issues like cigarette smoking or drug use/abuse that specifically worsen the prevalence of such complications. In developing countries and in association with significantly worse overall glucose control, not only do children and adolescents die earlier from DKA and severe hypoglycaemia but all the long-term complications also seem to be more prevalent as a direct result of lack of education, lack of medical equipment and medications and all the myriad interactions of these factors.

These complications may take many years to develop and may not be obvious until adulthood but the precursors to such problems are already present in children and adolescents with T1DM in many instances. However, if the diabetes developed when the child was very young or if the diabetes control has been very poor, diabetes complications can already appear in the childhood and adolescent years. In richer countries, this fact was known several decades ago, but with improved education and care as well as improved treatment intensification, this problem has declined in an extraordinary fashion. In the developing world, such improvement has not taken place.

The DCCT and other studies show that improved glucose control (as measured by HbA1c) will reduce the incidence and progression of these long-term microvascular as well as macrovascular complications. This is the concept of 'metabolic memory'. The challenge is to find ways to achieve good glucose control all over the world and to provide education, support, appropriate monitoring and appropriate treatment techniques throughout the world. **Metabolic control matters!** If blood glucose control is good, growth in height and weight, and the age of onset of puberty and the menstrual periods will be no different from that of other children and adolescents without T1DM. If blood glucose control is improved, early blindness and cataract formation should be avoided almost completely.

Retinopathy

Past surveys show that people with T1DM have a 5–10% chance of becoming legally defined as blind. After 10 years of having T1DM about 50% of patients will have some diabetic retinopathy. Usually, severe and clinically significant types of diabetic retinopathy that interfere with vision are not present before puberty but the years before puberty still count in setting up the small-vessel damage that causes cataracts and retinal blood vessel haemorrhages and ultimate scarring and blindness. Most guidelines recommend direct ophthalmoscopy at least annually after 5 years' duration of diabetes and/or the onset of puberty. Stereo fundus photography and/or fluorescein angiography are also very sensitive methods for detecting early retinal abnormalities. Newer special cameras can save a lot of healthcare money and are used for satellite and central eye evaluations to detect the earliest signs of micro-aneurisms or haemorrhages. A skilled ophthalmologist should be consulted with any abnormal symptoms (e.g. floaters, persistent blurry vision) or physical signs (e.g. haemorrhage, exudates,

TABLE 12.2 Estimated Average Glucose (eAG) Conversion Chart

A1c %	5	5.5	6	6.5	7	7.5	8	8.5	9	9.5	10	10.5	11	11.5	12
eAG mg/dL	97	111	126	140	154	169	183	197	212	226	240	255	269	283	298

Adapted from ADA. http://www.diabetes.org/living-with-diabetes/treatment-and-care/blood-glucose-control/estimated-average-glucose.html

cataracts, new retinal blood vessel formation). Any rapid improvement in glycaemic control, especially when starting with extremely poor glucose control (A1c greater than 10%), can be associated with very rapid worsening of retinopathy so caution should always occur when making changes in someone who has had long-term chronic poor glucose control so that improvements can happen slowly and steadily, thus decreasing the risks of rapid deterioration of eye function. Diabetic eye damage causes new blood vessels to form, known as proliferative retinopathy. Often they bleed easily and can cause scar tissue, with sudden blindness and the need for emergency operative repair and laser treatment to save vision.

Nephropathy

Damage to the kidneys will result in an increase in the protein leakage and this can be

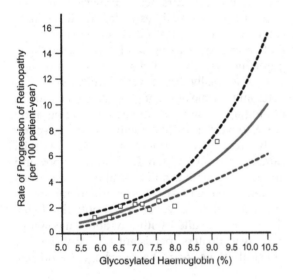

FIGURE 12.2 Rates of progression of retinopathy. *Reprinted with permission from The Diabetes Control and Complications Trial Research Group. The Effect of Intensive Treatment of Diabetes on the Development and Progression of Long-Term Complications in Insulin-Dependent Diabetes Mellitus. New Engl J Med 1993;329:977-86. Copyright 1993, New Engl J Med.*

detected with urinary measurements far before any signs or symptoms occur. Early in the development of nephropathy, the amount of protein in the urine will be slightly increased. This is called microalbuminuria. Treatment can be started at this stage to slow down the progression of the kidney disease, improving glucose control with more intensified treatment and using either diuretics such as hydrochlorothiazide or furosemide as well as newer medications called angiotensin-converting enzyme inhibitors (ACEi) such as enalapril, captopril or lisinopril. Later on, a larger amount of protein will be lost and this is called macroalbuminuria or just albuminuria/proteinuria. This later stage is frequently associated with hypertension, although hypertension can also occur much earlier in the adolescent and young adult years. Family history of hypertension and kidney problems as well as smoking will increase these kidney risks just as high A1c and chronic hyperglycaemia clearly cause such problems. Further progression of kidney damage will result in kidney failure. It is therefore important to detect signs of kidney damage as early as possible and to start treatment to prevent the progression to kidney failure.

Up to 30–40% of patients with T1DM may eventually develop end-stage renal failure and require dialysis or kidney transplantation – or else early death will occur. Poor glucose control, worsened by smoking, untreated hypertension and untreated hyperlipidaemia will increase these renal risks. The DCCT showed an 83% long-standing risk reduction in kidney disease sustained for up to 8 years post-study and some more recent renal follow-up data suggests that improved glycaemic control happening in many parts of the world in the past two to three decades is already producing significantly less end-stage renal dysfunction than in years past. Whether this can also happen in the developing world is unknown but will clearly depend upon bringing more modern technology and treatment options there as well.

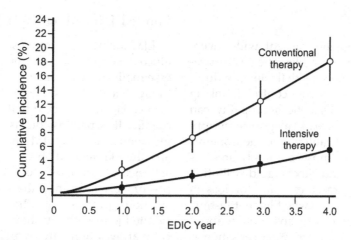

FIGURE 12.3 Rates of progression of renal disease (conventional vs intensive treatment). *Reprinted with permission from The Diabetes Control and Complications Trial/Epidemiology of Diabetes Interventions and Complications Research Group. Retinopathy and Nephropathy in Patients with Type 1 Diabetes Four Years after a Trial of Intensive Therapy. New Engl J Med 2000;342:381−89. Copyright 2000, New Engl J Med.*

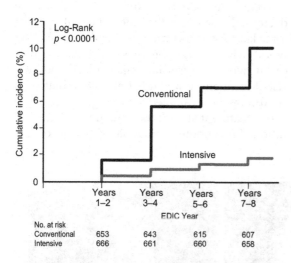

FIGURE 12.4 Cumulative incidence of new cases of proteinuria with time (years). *Reprinted with permission from Writing Team for the Diabetes Control and Complications Trial/ Epidemiology of Diabetes Interventions and Complications Research Group. Sustained Effect of Intensive Treatment of Type 1 Diabetes Mellitus on Development and Progression of Diabetic Nephropathy, The Epidemiology of Diabetes Interventions and Complications (EDIC) Study. JAMA 2003;290:2159−2167.*

Beginning at puberty, or five years after diagnosis of type 1 diabetes mellitus, urinary protein should be screened annually using urinary microalbumin tests or protein dipsticks. Treatment with ACE inhibitors or diuretics can help reduce proteinuria, even in the absence of hypertension. Reducing total protein intake, especially animal-source protein, to less than 20% of calorie contribution has also been shown to reduce microalbuminuria. Blood pressure should be checked at least annually and compared to age and sex-matched normative standards, with aggressive early treatment considered when hypertension is present. Any improvement in hyperglycaemia often will help renal function, slow down further deterioration and often produce improvements in hypertension and renal status. Cessation of smoking likewise will only be a positive consideration. Consultation with a nephrologist may be important especially if there is progressive and uncontrolled hypertension or protein leakage associated with increasing blood urea nitrogen or creatinine levels.

Neuropathy

Occasionally, teenagers present with severe painful neuritis or with problematic gastroparesis. This is usually in those with the longest duration and/or the worst glucose control. Smoking increases these risks. Diabetic neuropathy can be classified into two broad categories: peripheral neuropathy and autonomic neuropathy. Peripheral neuropathy most commonly presents in a typical 'glove and stocking' distribution involving pain, hyperaesthesia and/or loss of sensation to pinprick or plastic filament testing. Deep tendon reflexes can be absent or reduced in the lower extremities. Vibration sensation is decreased or absent, usually symmetrically. This helps distinguish such problems from unilateral spinal or peripheral nerve disorders since most diabetes-related nerve damage occurs in a bilateral fashion. Carpal tunnel syndrome is a sign of median nerve involvement and is also increased in long-standing poorly controlled T1DM but also with some history of repetitive motion damage. Autonomic neuropathy can include gastroparesis, bloating with decreased appetite, significant constipation and/or diarrhoea, heart palpitations, urinary retention and impotence, abnormal sweating and absent or abnormal pupillary responses. Consultation with a neurologist or an adult diabetologist may be very helpful.

Limited Joint Mobility (LJM)

LJM mobility[3,9] is often seen when the blood glucose control is poor for a long time. It is essentially never seen prior to puberty and is thought to be caused by glycosylation of the skin collagen associated with chronic hyperglycaemia. It is painless but is a marker for poor glycaemic control. LJM increases the risk of all the known diabetes complications by 400–600% compared to those without LJM, presumably indicating the same type of glycosylation process of the microvasculature. Limited joint mobility should be assessed clinically at least annually by placing the hands in a 'prayer' position and can be staged as shown (Figure 12.5). Similar to other such issues, written documentation and sequential follow-up is important.

Complications Screening

Follow-up data from the DCCT shows the decreased risks and that these benefits persist for at least 7-8 years post-study. In the developing world where it can be presumed that significantly worse control has taken place and persisted for many years, it is imperative that such conditions be evaluated and sought out, since early treatment still offers some hope of amelioration. Prevention is possible if the resources

FIGURE 12.5 Limited joint mobility. *Photos courtesy of Stuart Brink.*

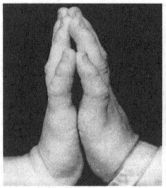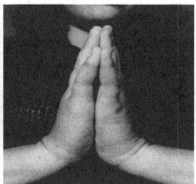

and education can be tied together in a meaningful manner. A good diabetes centre will have a systematic programme of measuring lipids, thyroid function, renal function, urinary protein and microalbumin excretion, blood pressure, weight, height and growth as well as HbA1c. Regular eye examinations with a direct ophthalmoscope and perhaps even fundus photography screening should take place. Establishment of links with an ophthalmologist who is familiar with diabetic retinopathy screening and treatment is an important aspect of diabetes follow-up and treatment. Foot examinations and neurologic examination should also be part of the treatment and evaluation package particularly in those with the longest and worst glycaemic control and, as with ophthalmologists, establishing links for ongoing consultation will be important to consider. Baseline and follow-up HbA1c would be obtained at least annually if not more frequently (optimally at least quarterly) and written medical record documentation would allow quality-control assessments. Tracking of sequential follow-up with the expected improvement from the use of a multi-disciplinary team, use of a common and more modern education empowerment philosophy and treatment schemes that optimise care to the extent possible given the lack of healthcare infrastructure and lack of funding from government sources would add to such improvement despite ongoing poverty in the developing world. Partnerships with pharmaceutical and diabetes-related device companies (meters, syringes and pumps) and funding from many worldwide foundations including Life for a Child and the International Diabetes Federation (IDF) should help this process as well.

CO-MORBID CONDITIONS WITH TYPE 1 DIABETES MELLITUS

The issues of cost of screening and cost of testing remain major barriers to identification and treatment of these T1DM co-morbidities. Some can be diagnosed when healthcare professionals working with T1DM pay more attention to their existence, even though many of the more subtle conditions are without major symptoms until late in their development; others remain asymptomatic under most conditions and many remain undiagnosed even where healthcare is otherwise affordable because of inattention by the healthcare teams. T1DM is associated with other autoimmunopathies (thyroid disease, coeliac disease, vitiligo and adrenal insufficiency). Such disorders are *not* caused by having diabetes or by poor diabetes control but reflect the common genetic predisposition with such autoimmune diseases and the association with autoimmune T1DM. It is not usually possible to identify exactly which children or adolescents are most susceptible to these conditions so that clinical laboratory screening is recommended if available and affordable. Simple measures such as taking a good history, obtaining family histories in a readily reviewable format, charting the growth of the child and noting actual versus expected physical growth, and looking for an abnormal increase or decrease in pigmentation and looking for development of a goitre will help to identify many such cases. Coeliac disease is caused by intolerance to gluten, a protein found in wheat and wheat products and will result in poor growth and sometimes poor glycaemic control. In some but not all studies hypoglycaemia is also increased in untreated coeliac disease. It is more common in Caucasians with T1DM but less information is known about other populations around the world. Many children, adolescents and adults who have coeliac disease are asymptomatic or only have very mild symptoms so that diagnosis is problematic unless laboratory testing is available and index of suspicion high. It is estimated that coeliac disease co-exists with T1DM in about 5–10% of the population so that most guidelines suggest optimal screening should occur annually using transglutaminase or endo-mysial antibody sampling. Adrenal insuffi-ciency (Addison's disease) may occur in 1—2% of youngsters with T1DM confirmed by low cortisol levels, raised ACTH levels and positive anti-adrenal antibodies. It should be suspected if there is an unexpected or unexplained decrease in insulin requirements as well as unexplained hypoglycaemia or severe hypogly-caemia. Hyperpigmentation and unexplained weight loss may be clinically apparent findings. Chronic vitamin D insufficiency and/or defi-ciency are increased with poorly controlled T1DM so that osteopaenia is more likely, partic-ularly in children and adolescents with darker skin pigmentation.

Thyroid Disorders

Thyroid dysfunction includes euthyroid goitres, Hashimoto's thyroiditis and

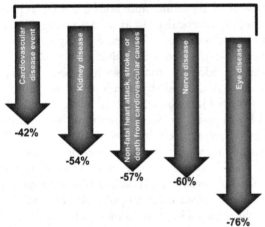

FIGURE 12.6 Intensive blood glucose control reduces the risk of major diseases. *Adapted from The Diabetes Control and Complications Trial/Epidemiology of Diabetes Interventions and Complications (DCCT/EDIC) Study Research Group. Intensive Diabetes Treatment and Cardiovascular Disease in Patients with Type 1 Diabetes. New Engl J Med 2005;353:2643—53.*

compensated as well as symptomatic hypothy-roidism. These problems are all more commonly seen in patients with T1DM. Thyroid conditions overall can affect 20—40% of people with T1DM, if thyroid antibody positivity only is counted, in an otherwise euthyroid child or adolescent, and in about 20% if only those with clinically impor-tant hypothyroidism or hyperthyroidism are included. Hyperthyroidism also occurs more frequently in association with T1DM and may even precipitate DKA. Any child or adolescent with TIDM who suddenly loses weight should be assessed for possible hyperthyroidism.

Most guidelines suggest routine thyroid function screening with free or total T4 as well as TSH, or even TSH alone, depending upon cost and availability of laboratory support. Many also add thyroid antibodies (thyroglobulin antibodies and thyroid peroxi-dase/microsomal antibodies) since the pres-ence of positive antibodies even with normal thyroid function per se would identify that patient as having higher future risks for clin-ical thyroid dysfunction. Both hypothyroidism and hyperthyroidism may be associated with positive thyroid antibodies for many years before clinical thyroid functions change and goitre occurs. However, not all thyroid dysfunction is associated with Hashimoto's thyroiditis. If thyroid functions and thyroid antibodies are negative for the first 2—3 years, less frequent monitoring may also be consid-ered. Treatment of thyroid disease is no different when one has T1DM than in the general population.

Hyperlipidaemia

Elevated total and LDL cholesterol are common but made worse by chronic hypergly-caemia. The higher the usual blood glucose levels, the worse will be the triglyceride levels. Improvement in glucose control is associated with improvement in triglyceride abnormalities and some improvement in total and LDL cholesterol levels as well. Ideally, lipid levels should be drawn at least annually.

Lipohypertrophy (or Hypertrophy)

When insulin is injected in the same sites time after time, localised subcutaneous scarring may occur that produces lumps of fatty-like tissue that is non-tender and not red or otherwise irritated. It can occur in any injection site that is overused. Lipohypertrophy is not age-specific or sex-specific nor is it related to any particular type or brand of insulin, although older less pure insulins in the past seemed to produce more lipohypertrophy than do current highly purified human or synthetic analogue insulins. Cow-derived insulin seemed to also produce more lipohypertrophy in prior decades than pig-derived insulin. Lipohypertrophy must be a cosmetic issue but it may also hamper insulin absorption or cause erratic insulin absorption. Rotation of injection sites usually prevents the problem. It is thought that overuse of the same injection areas decreases local pain of syringe or pen needle injections and that is sometimes felt to be more important by patients than the future possibility of hypertrophy itself. Patients and parents should be taught to avoid injecting into the lipohypertrophied areas to minimise absorption problems and associated increased hyperglycaemia as well as hypoglycaemia. Avoidance of the hypertrophied areas for many months or even years may be needed for resolution to occur so prevention is better than treatment.

Lipoatrophy

In the lipoatrophic region, there is localised loss of subcutaneous fat so that the skin has the appearance of a small or large indentation. Usually, there is no actual ulceration or infection but there may be cosmetic problems and interference with insulin absorption since there is significantly less subcutaneous tissue present.

Sometimes specifically injecting insulin into the rim of the depressed area of lipoatrophy has been successful and this is thought to produce a localised lipohypertrophied area. Corticosteroids have been tried without much success as have various oils and skin lotions. Avoidance of the lipoatrophic area for years sometimes also will allow some resolution.

LEARNING TO COPE WITH DIABETES: THERAPEUTIC EMPOWERMENT-BASED EDUCATION

Education is a key component of T1DM treatment. It has to be reinforced during each visit and ideally should include methods of empowerment to optimise behavioural change that is often required by parents and patients alike. Education is more than information: it is a long-term process providing regular support to the child, teen and his or her extended family. What to talk about with the family and patient, what myths exist and how to dispel them, what local traditions must be addressed concerning T1DM and T2DM (since they are often misunderstood and mixed up), what other childhood and adolescent illnesses may co-exist, how specifically to deal with nutrition, how to store and sustain insulin supplies, all must be considered. If possible, written materials can and should be provided for home-learning and for clinic-teaching purposes. Some facilities will have these available only for clinic and hospital use while others will have the possibility to have these for home use as well. Some donor institutions, especially local pharmaceutical companies, may have printed material in local languages available that will support initial instruction in insulin giving, syringe and pen use, meal planning, blood and urine glucose testing as well as exercise and sport participation. Some will have more of a focus on the psychosocial aspects of diagnosis and ongoing care. Some will focus more on family issues while others will be involved with young children or adolescents. Being aware of what is available either on the Internet or from local sources will be invaluable to diabetes staff as well as to children and teenagers and their families and friends.

Myths and Fallacies

Local customs, regional factors, myths and fallacies relating to diabetes are likely to exist and all must be addressed in an open and educational discussion orchestrated by the healthcare team dealing with T1DM in children and adolescents. Families must be involved, including siblings, parents, grandparents and perhaps entire extended families and villages, schoolteachers etc. These should be addressed as soon as the emergency situation of diagnosis is under control. These should also be periodically updated and questions posed to ensure optimal understanding. It is imperative that healthcare professionals not be rude, condescending or disrespectful of the parents or others who should be encouraged to discuss their concerns and the opinions of those around them and in this way help to sympathetically open up such dialogues to ensure safety and adequate treatment while applying appropriate modern scientific technology.

Myths and fallacies are often centred around the following areas:

- causes of diabetes
- differences between T1DM and T2DM
- blaming one side of the family
- curing diabetes
- alternative treatment options including witchcraft and holistic options
- distrust of 'Western'-style medicine(s)
- toxicity of insulin
- hypoglycaemia fears
- why pills cannot be used instead of insulin
- 'catching' diabetes

- embarrassment and social stigma/discrimination.

Coping with Acute Illnesses: Sick-Day Guidelines and DKA Prevention

Acute illness affects blood glucose control. The consequences of acute illness include having high glucose values (hyperglycaemia) and the appearance of ketones, progression of this condition to DKA, coma and death as well as low blood glucose (hypoglycaemia). Early detection of changes in glucose values and active management will prevent these acute complications of diabetes from escalating and getting out of control and also help prevent recurrent hospitalisation. Children and adolescents with well-controlled diabetes should not experience more frequent or severe illness or infections than children without diabetes. However, children and adolescents with poorly controlled diabetes may experience more infections because of interference with the general immune system function and therefore decreased ability to ward off common illnesses. Many illnesses, especially those associated with fever and the respiratory tract, increase blood glucose values because of the effects of stress hormones and the insulin resistance that occurs concomitantly. This can also induce ketone production, associated nausea and eventually ketoacidosis and metabolic decompensation if sufficient insulin is not provided in addition to the usual insulin doses and if sufficient fluid and electrolytes are not replaced. Lack of monitoring for financial or other reasons increases such risks; more monitoring is often needed during sick days to allow proper identification of the insulin needs. Gastrointestinal symptoms (e.g. diarrhoea, nausea and vomiting) may lead to lower blood glucose values and hypoglycaemia due to decreased food intake, poor absorption and changes in intestinal motility. With such hypoglycaemia, there may also be ketonuria so much confusion may occur during sick days. In fact, changes in blood glucose values may precede an acute infection especially if they are caused by viral illnesses. In the days prior to actual symptoms showing up, the virus is multiplying in the body and starting the insulin-resistant phase before such hypergly-caemia actually is apparent. Alterations in glucose values may also persist after the resolution of an acute illness as the body readjusts to the effects of that particular illness. Most illnesses are viral in nature but attention to those requiring antibiotics (i.e. strep throat, otitis media, bacterial pneumonias) and those associated with malaria or HIV/AIDS is important.

Illness in a Child or Adolescent with T1DM: Sick-Day Guidelines or Rules

- Do not stop insulin delivery. Insulin doses may need to be increased or decreased based on the blood glucose and food intake but should not be stopped.
- If there are no facilities for home glucose monitoring of glucose or ketones, the child or adolescent should be seen at a healthcare facility for evaluation and testing as well as consideration for transportation to a higher level treatment facility.
- Increase BG monitoring of blood glucose at least every 3–4 hours and more frequently if there is no response to extra insulin, fluid and electrolyte treatment or if there are wild fluctuating changes
- Monitor ketones at least 1–2 times or more each day as a guide to how much extra insulin is needed. This too may be done at the local healthcare facility when the family does not have access to ketone monitoring. Blood ketones or urine ketones are both available for home monitoring as well as emergency room and hospital monitoring.
- Evaluate and treat the acute illness and source of the emergency situation. Where

possible use sugar-free medications or tablets. Avoid antibacterial medication unless a specific bacterial infection is diagnosed (urinary tract infection, strep throat, otitis media, bacterial pneumonia, severe skin infection etc.) If no sugar-free medications are available then use the locally available medications. Avoid steroid use since corticosteroids will inevitably raise the BG levels.
- Provide, or ensure that the family is able to provide, appropriate supportive care including:
  - access to easily digested foods when there is a loss of appetite
  - adequate fluid intake (fever and hyperglycaemia can cause increased fluid losses; oral rehydration fluid provides both a source of fluid and energy)
  - treat fever with antipyretics (e.g. paracetamol) and treat or prevent vomiting by using small volumes of fluid more frequently
  - if these supportive measures cannot be ensured as an outpatient, the child or adolescent may need admission to a healthcare facility.
- Adjust insulin doses for illnesses as required during the acute illness. Often this will require 10% more regular or analogue fast-acting insulin given above the usual dosage and given every 2–4 hours around the clock including in the middle of the night. Such decision would be based upon degree of hyperglycaemia documented as much as possible by frequent BG monitoring.
- Twenty percent more regular or analogue fast-acting insulin in similar fashion every 2–4 hours given around the clock including in the middle of the night would be provided if there is hyperglycaemia as well as concomitant ketonuria or ketonaemia based upon not only BG monitoring but also ketone monitoring.

- Admission to the local healthcare facility or transfer to the nearest healthcare facility available would occur under the following circumstances:
  - very young children with diabetes where risk of dehydration and DKA is higher
  - inability to check glucose at home
  - inability to check ketones at home
  - when supportive care cannot be ensured at home for any reason, financial or psychosocial
  - if the acute illness is severe
  - there is persistent ketonuria unresponsive to treatment
  - if there is ongoing non-response including ongoing weight loss, uncontrolled dehydration or other symptoms
  - if there is suspicion of another illness that may require surgical intervention, i.e. appendicitis.
- Respiratory illnesses are more likely to cause hyperglycaemia and ketosis. However, with poor oral intake and tachypnea, dehydration and hypoglycaemia can also occur.
- Gastrointestinal disorders (viral or parasitic) often cause hypoglycaemia.
- Malaria can co-exist in anyone with T1DM.
- Similarly, HIV/AIDS can also co-exist with T1DM and treatment with anti-retroviral drugs can cause the metabolic syndrome and increase insulin resistance.
- Sick-day guidelines should be provided to the patient and family at the time of diagnosis with thorough education about their rationale and appropriate follow-up teaching should occur at least annually. These guidelines should be in written format and the entire medical staff should be well-versed in their application. These guidelines should also ideally accompany the child and family to any other healthcare facility to ensure that they are also followed at that location where expertise in childhood or adolescent T1DM may not be apparent.

Dealing with Diabetes at School

Rights and Responsibilities

The challenging task of caring for a child and teenager with diabetes extends to all areas of that child's life. Education for children with a chronic disease is a crucial part of a child or teen's life throughout the developed and the developing world. Therefore safe attendance at school is an important consideration in the care of a child and adolescent with diabetes. As diabetes is becoming more frequent among children throughout the world, it is increasingly likely that schools are going to be placed in situations where the staff will be responsible for a child with diabetes. For this reason it is desirable that all responsible individuals who are involved in the care of a child with diabetes become familiar with the illness, its complications and are able to deal competently with acute complications. Poor management of emergencies may place the child at considerable additional risk. As an unremitting, chronic illness, diabetes places considerable psychological stress on the child and family, and this stress may influence his or her behaviour at school. Teachers are often filled with anxiety and nervousness when they are faced with a child with diabetes in their class.

The Rights of the Child and the Adolescent

The child and the adolescent have a **right to be admitted** to a school despite having diabetes. However, in societies where diabetes has a stigma and where school authorities are anxious about having to be responsible for the child's diabetes, school attendance can still be denied to those with diabetes. The child has the right to receive **appropriate care** for diabetes while at school. The child and the adolescent have the right to be **fully integrated** into the school environment by ensuring the safety of the child, involvement in all school activities, attainment of developmental goals, development of self-esteem and acceptance by peers.

The Responsibility of the Parent and Care Team

Educate those at school who will be caring for the child and the teenager with diabetes. Teachers and other responsible carers need to be educated on aspects of the child's care, including need for insulin, regular meals and snacks and to be able to test blood glucose. The school personnel need education on appropriate management of acute complications (including hypoglycaemia and hyperglycaemia). Education *must* be done by the parents or care team and not by the child. Support must be given to the school and teachers in their efforts to care for diabetes in school. Details of management regimens, and contact details for parents and emergency care, need to be provided to the school. Make sure that there are enough supplies for the care of the child and teenagers in school including (where needed) insulin, glucose meters and food in case of hypoglycaemia.

Issues to be Discussed with the School Staff

Issues include:

- general information on diabetes and its management
- information on recognition, treatment and prevention of hypoglycaemia
- information about illnesses
- information on hyperglycaemia and ketones
- practical knowledge and practice in testing and insulin injections
- information on the effects of diet and activity on diabetes
- information on the social and psychological impact of diabetes.

PSYCHOSOCIAL ISSUES

Diabetes and Adolescence

Type 1 diabetes mellitus in adolescents may be one of the most common teenage chronic illnesses after asthma and epilepsy. Treatment goals for teenagers with type 1 diabetes are the same as those for younger children, and include lowering glucose levels without causing excessive or severe hypoglycaemia, efforts to set up a balanced meal plan against which insulin can be delivered, and promotion of normal growth and development. General goals of therapy must take into account:

- pubertal status and weight
- insulin requirements and how insulin works for that individual
- nutritional requirements for growth and well-being
- ethnic and family cultural traditions about feeding
- likes and dislikes
- eating patterns and provision of food at home and during the day (i.e. at school)
- activity patterns
- what insulin is available
- psychosocial concerns, including appropriate limit-setting, how other members of the family can be helpful, who assumes the responsibility for diabetes care at school and after school hours etc. Blood glucose monitoring, while expensive, is a key component of such decisions because general rules about diabetes can be tailored for individual circumstances.

In those adolescents who have had diabetes for longer duration and especially if also associated with years of chronic hyperglycaemia, the diabetes-related complications may occur. Systematic and planned monitoring for eye, renal, cardiac, neurologic and other problems must be planned. Appropriate attention to history and physical examination and specific monitoring for retinopathy and cataracts, hypertension, protein leakage and kidney failure, as well as lipid and neurologic problems, must be addressed by healthcare providers working with adolescent diabetes patients. Knowing about the prior degree of glucose control helps to place such patients into risk categories and helps to identify complications as well as to initiative appropriate individualised treatment.

Teenagers need to be retaught the 'rules' of diabetes and to begin accepting more responsibility for self-care while parents and other adult supervisors need to change their roles and accept more of a secondary, rather than primary, caretaker role. At the same time, particularly when self-care is not adequate or when other complications occur, parents and others in the family may need to step back in and directly supervise healthcare if long-term complications are to be minimised or treated.

Taking Responsibility for Self-Care

Parents must change over time from a direct caring role to a supervisory role but must nevertheless remain in the picture for many adolescents to sustain difficult efforts needed for effective self-care. Giving too much responsibility to children too early is a common mistake, but not giving appropriate responsibility as children manoeuvre their way through adolescence and become more independent self-care providers also can cause problems.

Awareness of specific ethnic and cultural patterns with food as well as family health issues must take place. Education and re-education for the adolescent on a routine basis should be considered for the adolescent and attention to peer influence issues such as alcohol, cigarettes, marijuana and other issues must be added to the curriculum. Adolescents begin to have some concepts woven into their awareness of the future but many do not act as if their decisions have long-term consequences. Issues of sexuality and contraception as well as pregnancy prevention and treatment for young women also become important to think about and should be addressed systematically by healthcare providers. Meeting with other

teenagers also can be extremely helpful and a sense of isolation can be overcome, either in a camp setting or at the clinic where informal or formal support can be offered and a sense of isolation can be overcome. Internet web sites can allow some exchange of information and support related to diabetes.

Poor Glycaemic Control

Explanations for chronic and sustained poorly controlled diabetes, with chronic hyperglycaemia and/or excessive or severe hypoglycaemia, are the same in adolescents as in other patients. Any severe non-compliance, lack of education about treatment and goals or concomitant illnesses including psychological problems, depression, learning problems, physical or sexual abuse can also contribute to poor glycaemic control, as can economic or psychological problems in other members of the family. Table 12.3 lists some specific clinical causes of uncontrolled diabetes in adolescents. Those in italics are also associated with DKA. Re-education and/or insulin adjustment must involve the adolescent as well as the parents since 'non-compliance' of one kind or another is common if sufficient insulin otherwise is available and provided. If healthcare systems are problematic and insulin is not always available or affordable, similar problems of chronic poor glycaemic control are more likely.

Re-education and/or insulin adjustment must involve the adolescent as well as the parents, since non-compliance of one kind or another is common if sufficient insulin is otherwise available and provided.

CONCLUSIONS

T1DM is a disease often misdiagnosed or frequently diagnosed very late and, as a consequence of such problems, is associated with

TABLE 12.3 Diabetes Control Issues

- Intercurrent infections — the most frequent cause of DKA

- Lipohypertrophy interfering with insulin absorption

- Failure to increase insulin for growth spurts, or lack of medical follow-up

- Inadequate routine monitoring (poverty)

- Abnormal counter-regulation causing poor or absent hypoglycaemia recognition

- Surgery or severe trauma

- Cortisone-like medications (even if used for legitimate medical reasons)

- Major emotional turmoil (parental divorce, child abuse or neglect, parental alcohol or drug abuse, depression)

- Hypoglycaemia fears (and thus inadequate insulin provision)

- Insulin being bound and released sporadically by the body

- Other serious concomitant illnesses (i.e. sickle cell anaemia, malaria, coeliac disease)

- Alcohol, marijuana and other substance abuse

- Pregnancy

Source: adapted from Brink.[3]

high morbidity and mortality as a result of its relative rarity in paediatric and adolescent medicine around the world. In the developing countries where financial and social upheaval is a major factor in child and adolescent health and where major infections, disease and sanitary problems persist, HIV/AIDS and malaria as well as gastrointestinal bacterial and parasitic illnesses abound, T1DM diagnosis and treatment issues often become secondary ones not

readily apparent. Being aware of new nocturia, polyuria, enuresis, unexpected weight loss and even ants around toilet facilities allows earlier diagnosis to occur. Healthcare professionals involved with triage and screening as well as provision of actual care who think about the possibility of T1DM in the differential diagnosis will make a huge difference in the health and well-being of children and adolescents. Knowledge about insulin and meal planning, psychosocial issues of growth and development, exercise and other associated conditions and risk factors will provide a means to improve diabetes-related healthcare and make appropriate newer treatment modalities available at the same time as optimising current options.

References

1. Brink SJ, Lee WRW, Pillay K, Kleinebreil L. *Diabetes in Children and Adolescents: basic training manual for healthcare professionals in developing countries.* Baegsvard, Denmark: NovoNordisk; 2010.
2. ISPAD. ISPAD. Declaration of Kos. *J Paed Child Health* 1995;**31**:195.
3. Brink SJ, Serban V, editors. *Pediatric and Adolescent Diabetes.* Timisoara, Romania: Brumar; 2004.
4. Hanas R, Donaghue KC, Klingensmith G, Swift PGF, editors. *ISPAD Clinical Practice Consensus Guidelines 2009 Compendium. Pediatr Diabetes* 2009;**10**:1–210.
5. IDF Pediatric Guidelines (2011).
6. Allgrove J, Swift PGF, Greene S, editors. *Evidence Based Paediatric and Adolescent Diabetes.* Oxford, UK: Blackwell Publishing, BMJ Books; 2007.
7. Chiarelli F, Dahl-Jorgensen K, Kiess W, editors. *Diabetes in Childhood and Adolescence.* Basel, Switzerland: S. Karger AG; 2005.
8. Hanas R. *Type 1 Diabetes: A Guide for Children, Adolescents, Young Adults and Their Caregivers.* New York: Marlowe & Co; 2005.
9. Chase HP. *A First Book for Understanding Diabetes.* Denver: Children's Diabetes Foundation; 2007.

APPENDIX: INTERNATIONAL STUDY GROUP OF DIABETES IN CHILDREN AND ADOLESCENTS DECLARATION OF KOS

International Study Group of Diabetes **ISGD** Groupe International d'Etude du Diabète
in Children and Adolescents de l'Enfant et de l'Adolescent

STUART BRINK, MD
SECRETARY-GENERAL, ISGD
c/o NEW ENGLAND DIABETES & ENDOCRINOLOGY CENTER (NEDEC)
25 BOYLSTON STREET, SUITE #211, CHESTNUT HILL, MA 02167-1710 USA
TELEPHONE 1 617 232 6709   FAX 1 617 232 6797

ISPAD DECLARATION OF KOS

On September Fourth, Nineteen Hundred and Ninety Three, on the island of Kos, the members of the International Study Group of Diabetes in Children and Adolescents (ISGD), assembled at our nineteenth annual international scientific meeting and in the process of transforming ISGD into the International Society of Pediatric and Adolescent Diabetes (ISPAD), renew their Hippocratic Oath by proclaiming their commitment to implement the St Vincent Declaration to promote optimal health, social welfare and quality of life for <u>all</u> children and adolescents with diabetes around the world by the year 2000. We take this unique opportunity to reaffirm the commitments by diabetes specialists in the past and, in particular, unanimously pledge to work towards the following:

1. to make insulin available for <u>all</u> children and adolescents with diabetes

2. to reduce the morbidity and mortality rate of acute metabolic complications or missed diagnosis related to diabetes mellitus

3. to make age-appropriate care and education accessible to <u>all</u> children and adolescents with diabetes as well as to their families

4. to increase the availability of appropriate urine and blood self-monitoring equipment for <u>all</u> children and adolescents with diabetes

5. to develop and encourage research on diabetes in children and adolescents around the world

6. to prepare and disseminate written guidelines and standards for practical and realistic insulin treatment, monitoring, nutrition, psychosocial care and education of young patients with diabetes - and their families - emphasizing the crucial role of health care professionals - and not just physicians - in these tasks around the world.

Signed:

Bruno Weber, MD   Stuart Brink, MD
President, ISGD   Secretary-General, ISGD/ISPAD

Witnessed:

Christos Bartsocas, MD   Kirsten Staehr-Johansen, MD
XIXth ISGD Convener   WHO Regional Adviser

Hypoglycaemia

John Gregory

CLINICAL SETTING

Hypoglycaemia may present at any age but is more common in infancy and early childhood. Recognition that a child is presenting with symptoms or signs of hypoglycaemia is clinically important, as certain causes of hypoglycaemia, particularly those associated with deficiencies of alternative metabolic fuels such as ketone bodies (as may occur in hyperinsulinism), may be associated with adverse effects on cerebral functioning including loss of consciousness in the short term and adverse neurodevelopmental consequences in the longer term. Prompt clinical intervention and provision of glucose may therefore prevent these adverse consequences.

Furthermore, recognition that a child is presenting with symptoms of hypoglycaemia allows blood sampling for relevant investigations before administration of glucose. The results of these tests may retrospectively produce diagnostic evidence as to the cause without the need to resort to a planned fast and induction of hypoglycaemia for diagnostic tests at a later date with all the attendant risks therein.

DEFINITION

Hypoglycaemia has been defined in many ways, including the presence of symptoms

Practical Pediatric Endocrinology in a Limited Resource Setting
http://dx.doi.org/10.1016/B978-0-12-407822-2.00013-X

and the occurrence of adverse effects on neurophysiological and neurodevelopmental outcomes.

- There is a general consensus that blood glucose values below 2.6 mmol/L are associated with evidence of both adverse effects on neurophysiological functioning in the short term as well as adverse effects on neurodevelopment in the longer term in certain at-risk patient groups. This value is taken, in many centres, as one that requires both investigation into the cause and urgent therapy, particularly when symptoms are present.
- However, in the absence of symptoms, clinically significant hypoglycaemia has been defined at a lower blood glucose value, less than 2.0 mmol/L.
- Importantly, in hyperinsulinism when there is an absence of alternative fuels for cerebral function, action is required and hypoglycaemia is defined when blood glucose values fall below 3.5 mmol/L.

PHYSIOLOGY

Control of the processes of gluconeogenesis, glycogenolysis, glucose uptake and metabolism via endocrine and neural mechanisms is governed by substrate availability. During feeding, blood glucose concentrations increase. In response to rising intracellular ATP concentrations, closure of the K_{ATP} channel leads to β-cell membrane depolarisation and calcium influx with subsequent release of insulin through insulin granule exocytosis. Insulin is a potent anabolic hormone, facilitating glycogen, protein and fat synthesis.

With fasting, glucose levels fall, leading ultimately to suppression of insulin secretion. Once insulin levels have been suppressed, lipolysis occurs and through the process of mitochondrial β-oxidation and generation of ketone bodies from fatty acids. To avoid hypoglycaemia, a series of counter-regulatory hormones (including cortisol, growth hormone, glucagon and adrenaline) are released which stimulate glycogenolysis and gluconeogenesis.

Substrate availability varies widely at different times of life, with a high glucose requirement in infants of around 8 mg/kg/minute compared with adults at 2–3 mg/kg/minute. The infant is more vulnerable to hypoglycaemia in the first year of life, during which time the ability to generate ketone bodies provides an important alternative fuel source for cerebral metabolism. The ability to tolerate a fast improves with time, with increasing glycogen stores and reducing rate of glucose utilisation over the first 12 months.

SYMPTOMS

Symptoms of hypoglycaemia change with age (see Table 13.1), being generally more non-specific in neonatal life and infancy. As blood glucose levels begin to fall, initial symptoms are caused by the stimulation of the autonomic nervous system, but should glucose concentrations continue to fall, then the consequences of neuroglycopaenia start to predominate, rendering it increasingly difficult for the older child to respond appropriately and to take appropriate measures to reverse the hypoglycaemia.

CAUSES

A key distinction in understanding the aetiology of hypoglycaemia is the recognition that causes of hypoglycaemia can be broadly subdivided into two groups:

- those causes that are associated with excessive glucose consumption
- other causes of hypoglycaemia where there is largely a failure of fuel supply (glucose production) (Table 13.2).

TABLE 13.1   Symptoms of Hypoglycaemia

Neonate	Older infant or child
Autonomic	Autonomic
Pallor	Anxiety
Sweating	Palpitations
Tachypnoea	Tremor
Neuroglycopaenic	Neuroglycopaenic
Jitteriness	Hunger and abdominal
Apnoea	pain
Hypotonia	Nausea and vomiting
Feeding problems	Paraesthesiae
Irritability	Headache
Abnormal cry	Weakness and dizziness
Convulsions	Blurred vision
Coma	Irritability
	Mental confusion and
	unusual behaviour
	Fainting
	Convulsions
	Coma

TABLE 13.2   Causes of Hypoglycaemia

Increased glucose consumption	Other causes
• maternal diabetes • maternal drugs (dextrose, chlorpropamide, benzothiazides, β-sympathomimetics) • congenital hyperinsulinism • Beckwith–Wiedemann syndrome • insulinoma • Rhesus haemolytic disease • perinatal asphyxia • malaria	• ↓ glucose production • small for gestational age • accelerated starvation • inborn errors of metabolism • fatty acid oxidation disorders • gluconeogenic disorders • glycogen storage disease • galactosaemia • maple syrup urine disease • propionic acidaemia • others • hypothermia • sepsis • adrenal insufficiency • growth hormone deficiency, hypothyroidism • glucagon deficiency • polycythaemia • limited glycogen supply • prematurity • perinatal stress • starvation • glycogen storage disease • drugs (alcohol, aspirin, ß-blocker) • liver dysfunction • congenital heart disease

Most causes of hypoglycaemia due to increased glucose consumption are due to hyperinsulinism and commonly present in neonatal life.

- Neonatal hyperinsulinism as occurs in poorly controlled maternal diabetes. It is often associated with macrosomia. It may be severe in nature but is usually relatively short lasting, resolving within days of delivery.
- By contrast, congenital hyperinsulinism is rarer but longer lasting in its effects and has been shown in many cases to be due to mutations of genes whose products are involved in the regulation of insulin release from the pancreatic ß-cells. Insulin release is initiated following closure of the inward rectifying potassium channel (KIR 6.2), which is closely associated with the sulphonylurea receptor (SUR) and results in membrane depolarisation, calcium influx and subsequent insulin release (see Figure 13.1).

Mutations of the ABCC8 and KCNJ11 genes, encoding the sulphonylurea receptor and the potassium channel respectively, produce so-called 'channelopathies' and are relatively common causes of congenital hyperinsulinism.

- Rarer genetic causes of congenital hyperinsulinism include mutations of several genes (see Figure 13.1): the GCK gene encodes the enzyme glucokinase, GLUD1

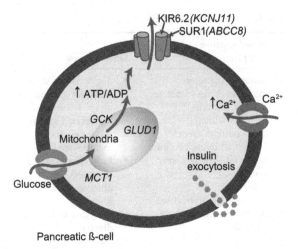

FIGURE 13.1 Glucose-stimulated insulin secretion in the pancreatic ß-cell (regulatory genes shown in italics).

encodes glutamate dehydrogenase, HADH encodes hydroxyacyl-coenzyme A dehydrogenase, HNF4A encodes hepatocyte nuclear factor 4 alpha and SLC16A1 which encodes the monocarboxylate transporter 1. Glucokinase is the rate-limiting enzyme for glucose metabolism in the β-cell and plays a key role in regulating insulin release. Glutamate dehydrogenase is an intramitochondrial enzyme which regulates protein (leucine)-mediated insulin release. Mutations of GLUD1 present with hyperinsulinism and plasma ammonia levels three to eight times normal, although mechanisms causing the rise in ammonia are not clearly understood.

The incidence of hyperinsulinism varies widely around the world, with particularly high rates in communities in the Middle East where consanguineous marriages are relatively common.

DIAGNOSTIC APPROACH

As indicated above, an important initial diagnostic step is to try to establish from a careful

history and clinical observation whether there is evidence that hypoglycaemia occurs in the presence of excess glucose requirements or only when there is a disruption in fuel supply as arises with fasting or as often happens with intercurrent illness.

HISTORY

When hypoglycaemia occurs in neonatal life, history is of paramount importance.

- Careful details should be obtained regarding the pregnancy including its duration (prematurity is a risk factor for hypoglycaemia) and the mode of delivery (breech presentation is said to be more common in cases of hypopituitarism).
- Presence of any maternal history that might have suggested gestational diabetes should be obtained.
- Details of birth weight should be sought as intrauterine growth retardation predisposes to hypoglycaemia.
- Particularly important is to establish how feeding is taking place to clarify whether there is insufficient nutrition or excess glucose requirements.
- The presence of prolonged jaundice might suggest hypopituitarism.
- Given that several causes of hypoglycaemia are familial in origin, a careful family history is also important. This includes consanguinity and previous unexplained neonatal deaths.
- Presentation with unexpected clinical deterioration and delayed onset of hypoglycaemia hours to weeks after birth should increase suspicion for an inherited metabolic condition.

In an older child, precise details of the circumstances leading up to the episode of hypoglycaemia should be sought, including what was last eaten and when in relation to the symptoms, and there should be specific enquiry for symptoms that might suggest any of the causes listed in Table 13.2 above. For example, hypoglycaemia after introduction of lactose should suggest galactosaemia or after introduction of solids or fructose may indicate organic acidurias or fructose intolerance. Late hypoglycaemia many hours after a meal may indicate failure of gluconeogenesis. It is particularly important not to overlook potentially life-threatening adrenal insufficiency and the presence of symptoms only with intercurrent illness, early morning lethargy, headaches or a past medical history of other autoimmune disease should raise concerns.

EXAMINATION

As in all good clinical examinations, the child should be initially inspected from the end of the bed, looking for dysmorphic features suggesting syndromic causes of hypoglycaemia. Overall growth and nutritional state must be more formally documented by height and weight measurements, plotted on relevant centile charts.

- The presence of macrosomia and hepatomegaly may indicate hyperinsulinism. Associated features of macroglossia, hemihypertrophy, umbilical abnormalities and ear creases would suggest Beckwith—Wiedemann syndrome, a cause of hyperinsulinism.
- Abnormalities of the midline of the craniofacial skeleton, neonatal jaundice, visual impairment or optic atrophy and poorly formed genitalia including micropenis are findings which may be associated with hypopituitarism.
- The presence of increased skin pigmentation, hypotension or genital ambiguity may suggest primary adrenal insufficiency to be the underlying cause.

- Hepatomegaly is a feature of inborn errors of metabolism including glycogen storage disease.

INVESTIGATIONS

The most important investigation is to obtain a blood sample at the time of hypoglycaemia prior to correction of the hypoglycaemia. Obtaining a blood sample at this time does not delay subsequent resuscitation significantly. More importantly, it prevents the need for a potentially dangerous planned fast at a later date, which would otherwise be required to induce hypoglycaemia for investigative blood sampling.

A urine sample can be obtained at any time later after resuscitation and correction of hypoglycaemia has occurred. This should be the next urine passed after the hypoglycaemic event.

A potentially large number of investigations can be undertaken where relevant laboratory assays are available and there is no limitation of resources (see Table 13.3).

However, in a resource-limited setting, careful consideration of what is essential to perform is necessary.

- In the presence of a history of excess glucose requirements being needed to avoid hypoglycaemia, hyperinsulinism is the likely explanation.
- Documentation of either excess insulin levels or suppressed non-esterified fatty acids and ketone bodies will provide confirmatory evidence.
- If these assays are not available locally, establish the absence of evidence of ketonuria, which can be measured using bedside 'stick' testing. This provides supportive evidence of the presence of hyperinsulinism at the time of hypoglycaemia.

TABLE 13.3   Potential Investigations of Hypoglycaemia

Blood	• intermediary metabolites (glucose, lactate, pyruvate, alanine, free fatty acids, glycerol and ß-hydroxybutyrate) • electrolytes, liver function, acid-base status • ammonia • amino-acids • total and free carnitine and acylcarnitine profile • insulin, C-peptide • growth hormone, cortisol, thyroid function • galactosaemia screen
Urine	• ketones by dipstick, reducing substances • dicarboxylic acids, glycine conjugates, carnitine derivatives • toxicology screen
Others	• ophthalmic exam • cranial ultrasound or MRI

• However, where glucose requirements to avoid hypoglycaemia exceed 10 mg/kg/minute, no other explanation other than hyperinsulinism is likely. Given the limited availability of insulin assays, it would not be unreasonable to make a diagnosis of hyperinsulinism on clinical grounds and consider undertaking a trial of medication to suppress insulin secretion accordingly.

If hypoglycaemia is occurring in the presence of an interrupted fuel supply during fasting, other causes are more likely to be responsible.

• It is important not to overlook a diagnosis of adrenal insufficiency and so measurement of cortisol should be prioritised, particularly where symptoms occur in the presence of intercurrent illness.
• Growth hormone deficiency is unlikely to cause hypoglycaemia beyond infancy or to be present in a normally grown child and, therefore, formal measurement of serum growth hormone concentrations during hypoglycaemia is often unnecessary.

• The presence of an inborn error of metabolism can often be diagnosed only by the presence of unusual patterns of intermediary metabolites and, in a resource-limited environment, discussion should take place with both biochemical colleagues and colleagues with an interest in metabolic disease as to which individual metabolites should be prioritised for assay. In the absence of locally available assays, the possibility of tandem mass spectrometric analysis of dried blood spots collected onto filter paper and sent to another centre now exists for a number of causes of inborn errors of metabolism which cause hypoglycaemia. Samples such as these can, in addition, often be used for extraction of DNA for further relevant investigations.

RATIONALE FOR MANAGEMENT

Urgent treatment to reverse hypoglycaemia is important in the short term, primarily to prevent more significant acute effects such as convulsions or to terminate these symptoms, should they already be occurring. The use of anticonvulsants to terminate hypoglycaemic convulsions will not prevent the development of adverse neurodevelopmental consequences in the future. This serious problem has been shown to affect between 14 and 42% of cases with an underlying cause of hyperinsulinaemia.

Treatment should be initiated as soon as diagnostic blood samples have been collected.

1. Acute

The acute management of hypoglycaemia requires normalisation of blood glucose values through administration of glucose.

If the patient is still conscious, he or she should be offered drinks or granulated sugar containing 10—20 g glucose followed by food containing more complex carbohydrates to prevent recurrence of hypoglycaemia in the longer term. Approximately 10 g glucose is available in 2 teaspoons of sugar, 3 sugar lumps or 100 mL of non-diet versions of Coca-Cola. A semi-conscious patient who is still capable of protecting their airway may be safely treated by the administration of an oral glucose gel, which does not need to be swallowed to be effective but may simply be smeared around the buccal mucosa, across which direct absorption of glucose can rapidly occur.

If an oral approach to therapy is deemed inappropriate, the patient should be treated with an intravenous bolus of 0.2–0.4 g glucose/kg body weight in the form of 10% dextrose (2–4 mL/kg) administered slowly over 4–6 minutes. Thereafter, an ongoing intravenous infusion of dextrose providing 10 mg/kg/minute should be established until the patient is fully recovered. There is no need to induce blood glucose concentrations much in excess of 4 mmol/L.

The failure of a patient to recover consciousness for some time after blood glucose values have been normalised raises the possibility of an underlying inborn error of metabolism, an acute intracranial event or adrenal insufficiency. In these circumstances, empirical administration of an intravenous bolus of 50–100 mg hydrocortisone is recommended. Children with hyperinsulinism may require large amounts (up to 25 mg/kg/minute) of glucose to reverse and prevent further episodes of hypoglycaemia, but the use of concentrated forms of 50% dextrose is contraindicated as it is associated with an increase in mortality.

In the event that intravenous access proves impossible, the administration of subcutaneous or intramuscular glucagon (20 µg/kg in infancy, 500 µg from 1 month to the age body weight exceeds 25 kg, above which 1 mg should be used). Larger doses than these may be needed if the child has hyperinsulinism. Once the child has recovered consciousness, oral carbohydrate should be provided, although this may prove practically challenging as vomiting following glucagon is not uncommon.

2. Long Term

The clinical approaches to the management of hypoglycaemia in the short term are similar, regardless of the underlying cause. In the longer term, avoidance of further episodes of hypoglycaemia can be facilitated by a number of measures.

- Provision of regular, frequent snacks and meals and the avoidance of any prolonged periods of fasting are important.
- Administration of complex carbohydrate in the form of uncooked cornstarch at bedtime (1–2 g/kg) may help avoid nocturnal hypoglycaemia.
- Once a diagnosis of the underlying cause has been made, specific additional therapies may need consideration to prevent recurrent episodes of hypoglycaemia.

Hyperinsulinism

Hypoglycaemia which is a consequence of maternal gestational diabetes is likely to resolve within a few days, whereas that due to mutations of genes involved in the regulation of insulin release is likely to be more persistent.

- **Diazoxide:** A trial of specific anti-insulin therapy is also indicated using diazoxide 5–25 mg/kg/day subdivided 8 to 12-hourly along with chlorothiazide 20 mg/kg/day subdivided 12-hourly. Occurrence of hyperglycaemia while receiving conventional doses of medication is a good sign that the underlying hyperinsulinism has resolved and that therapy may be cautiously weaned off. Unfortunately, diazoxide is associated with side effects including hypertrichosis, fluid retention and tachyphylaxis. Lack of development of lanugo-type body hair should raise concerns about adherence to therapy.

- **Somatostatin:** Should there be a failure to respond to diazoxide, a somatostatin analogue (Sandostatin®) at a dose of 6–40 μg/kg/day subdivided into 4-hourly subcutaneous injections should be added.
- **Glucagon:** If Sandostatin is not available, an alternative additional therapy is intravenous infusion glucagon given at a dose of 1–18 μg/kg/hour (maximum 50 μg/kg/hour) in neonates or 1–10 μg/kg/hour adjusted as necessary in children aged 1 month to 2 years.

Failure to respond to medication can occur and is an indication for pancreatic surgery in a specialist centre. Modern imaging techniques (e.g. [18F] fluoro-L-DOPA PET scanning) are slowly becoming available that allow differentiation between focal and diffuse forms of hyperinsulinism, which guides the extent of surgery. Diffuse forms of the disease are caused by mutations of the ABCC8, KCNJ11, GCK, GLUD1, HNF4A, HADH and SLC16A1 genes whereas focal forms are associated with a paternal mutation in ABCC8 and KCNJ11 genes or paternal uniparental disomy of chromosome 11p5.1 to 11p15.5. In the absence of [18F] fluoro-L-DOPA PET scanning facilities, mutational screening of candidate genes may provide useful information about the likelihood of focal or diffuse forms of the disease and the reader is recommended to make contact with a centre which has expertise in screening for these mutations (e.g. www.projects.exeter.ac.uk/diabetesgenes/geneticslab/clinicalgenetic/hyperinsulinism.htm). This information is important to obtain as it helps direct the required surgical procedure most likely to be successful. Surgical excision of a focus of hyperinsulinism is likely to be curative with minimal adverse consequences, whereas the near-total pancreatectomy required in diffuse forms is associated with high risks of pancreatic exocrine deficiency and insulin-dependent diabetes mellitus in the longer term and is therefore best avoided if at all possible.

Hypopituitarism or Adrenal Insufficiency

If hypopituitarism or adrenal insufficiency is diagnosed, hypoglycaemia can be prevented by the administration of hydrocortisone 10–15 mg/m^2 body surface area/day subdivided into 2 or 3 doses. At times of significant intercurrent illness, as may be associated with pyrexia for example, the dose of hydrocortisone may need to be increased two- or threefold and even given parenterally if there is vomiting. (*See Chapter 1, Growth, and Chapter 4, Adrenal Disorders, for further information.*)

Growth hormone deficiency is an unlikely cause of hypoglycaemia outside of infancy. However, should treatment with hydrocortisone in the very young child with hypopituitarism fail to prevent further episodes of hypoglycaemia, replacement with growth hormone at doses of 23–39 μg/kg/day given as a subcutaneous injection may be necessary in infancy before evidence of growth failure has arisen.

Inborn Errors of Metabolism

The principles of treatment to prevent hypoglycaemia involve prevention of a catabolic state by avoidance of prolonged fasting and provision of regular, frequent high carbohydrate-containing meals. Cornstarch at bedtime (see above) may also prove helpful to avoid nocturnal symptoms.

3. Follow-Up Plan and Expected Outcomes

Children with hypopituitarism, adrenal insufficiency or inborn errors of metabolism require lifelong follow-up to monitor their growth and therapy and to make appropriate adjustments to medication dosages as they increase in size. By contrast, congenital hyperinsulinism often resolves on long-term medication, which may ultimately be stopped.

Infants and children who have experienced recurrent or severe episodes of hypoglycaemia, particularly where hyperinsulinism was the underlying cause, are at increased risk of adverse neurodevelopmental consequences and should undergo longer term monitoring of their development with appropriate support for their needs being provided where necessary.

Finally, the hereditary associations of hyperinsulinism and many inborn errors of metabolism mean that the parents may be at risk of future affected children and they should be offered genetic counselling regarding these risks.

COUNSELLING AND EDUCATION

Useful information about the investigation and management of hypoglycaemia and links to relevant high-quality web sites including those of other professional societies and patient support groups can be found on the web site of The British Society for Paediatric Endocrinology and Diabetes (http://bsped.org.uk/professional/resources/endocrine.htm).

References

Champion MP. An approach to the diagnosis of inherited metabolic disease. *Arch Dis Child Educ Pract Ed* 2010;**10**: 40–46.

Kapoor RR, Flanagan SE, James C et al. Hyperinsulinaemic hypoglycaemia. *Arch Dis Child* 2009;**94**:450–57.

Paediatric Formulary Committee. Treatment of hypoglycaemia. In: *British National Formulary for Children 2010–2011*, London: BMJ Group, 2010:439–42.

Palladino AA, Bennett MJ, Stanley CA. Hyperinsulinism in infancy and childhood: when an insulin level is not always enough. *Clin Chem* 2008;**54**:256–63.

Raine JE, Donaldson MDC, Gregory JW, van Vliet G. *Practical Endocrinology and Diabetes in Children*, Chichester: Wiley Blackwell, 2011.

van Veen MR, van Hasselt PM, de Sain-van der Velden MG et al. Metabolic profiles in children during fasting. *Pediatrics* 2011;**127**:e1021–27.

Wilcken B. Fatty acid oxidation disorders: outcome and long-term prognosis. *J Inherit Metab Dis* 2010;**33**: 501–06.

CHAPTER

14

Clinical Scenarios

Margaret Zacharin, Michele O'Connell, Martin Ritzen,
Annemieke M. Boot, Vijayalakshmi Bhatia, Anna Simon,
Leena Patel

This chapter aims to provide the reader with a broad range of typical clinical scenarios that may be met in everyday practice of paediatric endocrinology. They are written by a number of different endocrinologists and thus reflect a variety of methods of evaluation, judgement and practice management strategies. No attempt has been made to unify the format of these brief vignettes, so that they can give a real impression of varied working methods and approaches required in clinical practice. For brevity, question marks have been used throughout the scenarios,

to indicate that consideration should be given to the proposed point.

The scenarios are designed to be used either for assistance in judging a specific clinical problem or can be used as an exercise in developing clinical skills.

Some scenarios also add brief additional information as to technologies that are available in some countries for specific diagnosis of difficult cases. The reader is referred to the general text for a more extensive discussion of management details.

Practical Pediatric Endocrinology in a Limited Resource Setting
http://dx.doi.org/10.1016/B978-0-12-407822-2.00014-1

BONE HEALTH

> A 14-year-old girl with 1-year history of Crohn's disease. On steroids for 3 months. She presents for assessment of BMD Z-score −2.5 at lumbar spine.

Assess and Manage

Assessment

Clinical assessment for height and pubertal status are required before any comment can be considered as to bone mass.

- BMD assessment for body size and bone age, *not* for chronological age.
  Using volumetric (BMAD) calculation:
- assess vitamin and calcium status and intake
- consider other causes of possible low BMD; even though she has inflammatory bowel disease she might have a primary bone disorder, immobility etc. as well.

Treatment

- Ensure normal calcium and vitamin D intake.
- Wait 1 year before repeat BMD, unless she has very high steroid needs over many months, in which case early reassessment may be useful, to assess for rapid ongoing loss of bone.
- Anticipate spontaneous puberty if health good and no steroids *or* there may be a possible need to induce puberty at more than 14.5 years if progress does not take place. Given that 50% bone mass is accrued during puberty, this is very important.
- Bisphosphonate *not* indicated.

> A 14-year-old girl with 5-year history of Crohn's disease. Multiple relapses including recently. Corticosteroid use for 3.5 of 5 years. BMD Z-score −3.5 at LS.

Assess and Treat

Assessment

Assess clinical status:

- assess for nutrition, calcium, vitamin D
- onset of puberty, ? any progress or arrest
- look at growth chart for evidence of growth arrest and/or weight loss, as indicators of poor bone health
- ? are other agents adding to bone problems, e.g. methotrexate
- BMAD – adjust for height, age, pubertal status
- do thoraco-lumbar spine X-ray for evidence of crush fracture.

Treatment

- Use vitamin D, calcium and induce puberty, but *only* at a time of 'good' health, i.e. low steroid needs and low ESR – to obtain best outcome in terms of growth potential.
- If puberty does not commence spontaneously, start HRT at very low dose oestrogen, as per normal protocols. Take through puberty completely unless sudden miraculous, in which case pubertal change vastly exceeds the expected appearance via exogenous oestrogen administration.
- If she is already showing some pubertal signs (probably from a past time of better health), can start HRT at a slightly higher dose.

Consider bisphosphonate if:

- vertebra crush fracture present
- BMD fails to increase or reduces, in the face of pubertal advance.

> A 12-year-old boy with a quadriparetic cerebral palsy. Puberty started at age 8 but has progressed slowly. Tanner stage 3 genital development currently. He has had one femoral fracture recently, when at school. No previous fractures. BMD Z-score LS −2.8. Referred for bisphosphonate treatment.

Assess and Advise

Assessment

- Assess for place and circumstance of fracture injury, e.g. trampoline etc. at school, i.e. is this fracture due to innate bone fragility or secondary to trauma? May not get an answer from carers/school.
- Clinical height, weight, pubertal status.
- BMAD (volumetric adjusted). A standard areal BMD (aBMD) is very misleading. If the child is short the BMAD will probably be considerably higher — in this case it is likely to be higher than expected for a child with cerebral palsy; this is due to bone accrual during his early onset puberty. However, hip BMD will remain very low, due to immobility and non-weight bearing.
- Check vitamin D, calcium intake. If gastrostomy fed these will be normal. If orally fed, virtually certain to be low.
- ? anticonvulsant as additional risk factor for low BMD.

Treatment

Probably no need to do anything except D/Ca, as puberty will add a further 25% of bone mass and strength, thus reducing future fracture risk.

Talk to family about the following:

- In a child with CP there are multiple lifetime risks for fracture — poor muscle bulk, inability to protect self during a fall, immobilisation osteopaenia.
- Puberty — there may be unrelated concerns that are not immediately obvious and are unlikely to be spontaneously mentioned, e.g. sexualised behaviour in pubertal child.

> **A 16-year-old female with quadriparetic cerebral palsy on Epilim® and Lamictal®. Pre-menarchal, breast stage 2–3, pubic hair stage 2. No history of fractures. BMD Z-score LS −4.5. Referred for ? bisphosphonate.**

Assess and Advise

Assessment

- Assess in terms of height and pubertal status.
- ? gastrostomy fed.
- ? Vitamin D and calcium status — should be normal if PEG fed. Probably low if not.
- History of zero fractures is important, i.e. BMD is low but is related to age, size, degree of immobilisation and does not necessarily represent very high risk.
- Anticipate a future decrease in risk once puberty is completed.

Treatment

- Vitamin D and calcium if needed.
- Await normal pubertal progress.
- Treat if pubertal arrest. This is more likely if remains underweight.
- Bisphosphonate not indicated.

Literature is sparse: one randomised trial, very small numbers.

Non-randomised trials demonstrate increased BMD with bisphosphonate **without** decreasing fracture risk i.e. fracture risk is more related to poor mobility, low muscle bulk, falls from precarious positions or by accidental trauma by carers.

Anticonvulsant effects on bone interfere with vitamin D metabolism and some have a direct osteoblast-inhibiting effect.

> **An 8-year-old girl with Rett syndrome, four low-impact lower limb fractures over 18 months.**
> **Referred for ? bisphosphonate.**

Assessment

- Clinical assessment of height and pubertal status.
- Precocious puberty is very unlikely with this condition as most are extremely thin.

- Usually very thin and poor muscle bulk, further predisposing to fracture.

Acute, severe immobilisation with low-impact fractures x 4 suggests that anticonvulsants are significantly worsening a situation where tiny fragile bones and low muscle bulk are already high risk.

Treatment

- Calcium and vitamin D status — as required.
- Bisphosphonate may be indicated as it will increase BMD until puberty takes over bone accrual.
- Cease bisphosphonate when pubertal, with a BMD Z-score approximately 0 for volumetric BMD (BMAD) *not* aBMD.

A boy of 15 years referred because of fractures. At age 12 years he had a fracture of his thumb when somebody hit him. One year later he fractured his left forearm when hitting a ball and at age 14 he fractured his right lower leg when he fell off his motorcycle. He had some muscle pain. He did not drink milk but ate six double slices of bread with cheese daily. He had no medication. His mother was Dutch and his father Egyptian. Family history was unremarkable.

He had a normal height and weight, brown skin, white sclerae, normal mobility, Tanner stage G5P5, testes 25 mL. The rest of the examination was unremarkable.

Assessment

Most likely to be vitamin D deficiency in healthy postpubertal male.

- Check time outdoors, lifestyle.
- Ask about muscle pain — associated with vitamin D deficiency.
- Exclude hyperparathyroidism, systemic disease including coeliac disease as risk factors for fracture.

- Mode of fracture important — all with injury, no evidence for minimal trauma or ligamentous laxity contributing.
- Check BMD for possible low level: if mild could be simple vitamin D deficiency. If surprisingly severe, reconsider pathologic cause — including $1,25(OH)_2D$ defect, i.e. mild vitamin D resistance.

CALCIUM DISORDERS

Male baby aged 35 days, with failure to thrive.

Total calcium 3.0 mmol/L (NR 2.1–2.6), PTH 5–7 pmol/L (NR 2–6.8), urinary calcium persistently in normal range.

Diagnosis and Management

Main Issue

Is this hyperparathyroidism or familial hypocalciuric hypercalcaemia?

Differential Diagnosis

Infantile:

- familial hypercalcaemic hypocalciuria (FHH)
- hyperparathyroidism: primary/secondary (e.g. renal failure)
- hypervitaminosis D.

Neonatal:

- FHH
- secondary hyperparathyroidism due to maternal hypocalcaemia
- subcutaneous fat necrosis
- Bartter syndrome
- Williams syndrome
- breast milk-induced rickets of prematurity (induced by relative phosphate deficiency from breast milk)
- infantile hypophosphatasia (severe form).

Diagnoses such as immobilisation, malignancy, MEN 1 and 2A, hyperthyroidism and secondary to drugs (milk alkali syndrome, thiazides etc.) are more relevant to an older age group.

Clinically

Weakness, anorexia, polydipsia, polyuria, although some infants may well be asymptomatic with this calcium level.

Investigations

- With raised calcium, PTH should be suppressed; therefore this is a state of relative hyperparathyroidism.
- PTH levels are not very high — unlikely to be primary parathyroid overactivity.
- Rather, it fits with an inactivating Ca receptor mutation on the PTH gland resulting in resetting of the set-point of Ca level and PTH secretion.
- Hypercalcaemia and hypocalciuria result from increased proximal tubular reabsorption of calcium.
- The urinary calcium in the 'normal range' is inappropriately low considering the underlying hypercalcaemia. This is consistent with FHH.
- Magnesium concentrations may be 'high normal', phosphate level mildly low.

Treatment

Nil/observe, no reduced skeletal mass or increased incidence of fractures.

Prognosis

Extremely good.

Family Studies

(FHH = AD)-double dose (homozygosity) for the mutation causes severe neonatal hyperparathyroidism. Gene map locus 3q13.3-q21, Ca^{2+}-sensing receptor gene CASR or PACR1. The Ca^{2+}-sensing receptor belongs to the superfamily of 7-membrane-spanning G protein-coupled receptors.

Note: Activating mutations in the same gene cause autosomal dominant hypocalcaemia.

Neonatal hypocalcemia due to maternal vitamin D deficiency: a 12-day-old infant, born full term, birth weight 3.0 kg, breast-fed, presented with seizures. The mother had not taken prenatal supplements. Her skin colour was dark. Systemic examination provided no clues towards the aetiology. Blood counts, blood sugar, serum creatinine, Na/K and CSF analysis were normal. Low total serum Ca 1.72 mmol/L (6.9 mg/dL) and iCa 0.8 mmol/L (3.2 mg/dL), elevated serum phosphate 3.04 mmol/L (9.5 mg/dL) and alkaline phosphatase of 800 IU/L (normal: less than 450 IU/L) were consistent with the diagnosis of vitamin D and calcium deficiency.

Investigations

25(OH)D and PTH were costly investigations for this family from an underprivileged background. Since vitamin D and calcium deficiencies are so common in infants born to dark-complexioned mothers not supplemented antenatally, no further investigations were undertaken.

Treatment

After stabilisation with infusion of 10% calcium gluconate, oral cholecalciferol 30,000 IU once every month under observation for 4 doses to the baby and 120,000 IU orally once to the mother, followed by 60,000 units once in 2 months thereafter, were prescribed.

Learning Points

- The vitamin D status of an infant, for the first 2 months approximately, depends on the amount of 25(OH)D transferred from the mother prenatally.

- Human milk contains less than or equal to 25 IU of vitamin D per litre unless the mother receives adequate vitamin D supplementation antenatally and postnatally (approximately 4000 IU/day) from supplements or from sunshine.
- Neonatal hypocalcemia due to vitamin D deficiency may be accompanied by high serum phosphate.
- For neonates oral vitamin D doses of the order of 300,000 to 600,000 units, which are often prescribed by paediatricians, may cause serious hypercalcemia, and are not needed to achieve sufficient 25(OH)D concentration.

> **A term neonate with birth weight 2.8 kg, born to a mother with pre-existing type 1 diabetes mellitus, developed respiratory distress and jitteriness at 30th hour of life. Glycaemic control of the mother during pregnancy was fair. There was no history of birth asphyxia. The neonate was jittery on examination with tachypnoea and mild respiratory distress. Blood glucose was normal and chest radiograph was suggestive of signs of transient tachypnoea of the newborn.**

Since this was an infant of a diabetic mother, samples for serum calcium and magnesium were collected and infusion of calcium gluconate was started.

Serum Ca (1.6 mmol/L) and iCa (0.78 mmol/L) were low, as was Mg (0.49 mmol/L). Inj. MgSO$_4$ 50% (0.2 mL/kg IM 12-hourly) was given, with frequent monitoring of serum Ca, Mg and iCa. Normalisation of the above parameters was obtained 24 hours after initiation of treatment. No further doses of Mg were required and the calcium infusion was tapered and switched over to oral calcium for a week.

Learning Points

Transient early-onset hypocalcemia is a well-known feature in infants born to diabetic mothers. This complication should be anticipated and managed appropriately. Magnesium deficiency leading to decreased secretion of PTH and resistance to its action has been proposed as one of the aetiologies.

> **A term neonate weighing 3 kg was admitted to the NICU with history of birth asphyxia with early features of hypoxic ischaemic encephalopathy (HIE). At 30 hours of life subtle seizures in the form of twitching of eyelids and cyclical movements of the limbs were noted.**

After documenting a normal blood glucose, anticonvulsants were administered, with partial control of the seizure activity. Calcium infusion produced cessation of convulsions. Low serum Ca (1.8 mmol/L) and iCa (0.78 mmol/L) were documented on the pre-treatment sample. Septic screen, Na/K, and CSF analysis were unremarkable.

The seizures were attributed to HIE with concomitant hypocalcemia. IV calcium was given for 24 hours. Anticonvulsants were gradually tapered and were omitted on documenting a normal neurological examination at discharge. Normal serum calcium was documented at discharge and on follow-up in the developmental clinic.

Learning Points

Transient hypocalcemia occurs in neonates with birth asphyxia due to an exaggerated physiological fall in serum calcium and endogenous phosphate load due to breakdown of glycogen and proteins leading to impaired functional capacity of the parathyroid glands temporarily.

> A 6-year-old boy presented with chronic diarrhoea, poor growth, proximal muscle weakness, reduced muscle bulk along with perioral tingling and numbness. Examination revealed short stature, wasting, pallor, positive Gower sign, positive Trousseau sign and Trendelenburg gait, and Bitot spots.

A clinical diagnosis of malabsorption was considered. Microcytic hypochromic anaemia, low serum albumin, low serum Ca 1.85 mmol/L (7.4 mg/dL), iCa (0.8 mmol/L) and P 0.7 mmol/L (2.2 mg/dL), elevated alkaline phosphatase, 25(OH)D 6.7 nmol/L (less than 3 ng/mL) were documented, and radiographs were consistent with active rickets.

Failure of serum Ca to normalise even after 48 hours of IV calcium suggested an associated magnesium deficiency. Serum Mg was low (0.53 mmol/L) and serum Ca reverted to normal after two doses of 0.2 mL/kg of 50% $MgSO_4$ IM.

Intramuscular cholecalciferol 100,000 IU IM produced symptomatic improvement in his muscle weakness.

The patient was referred to paediatric gastro-enterology department for further evaluation of the cause of malabsorption where a diagnosis of coeliac disease was made and the patient was subsequently put on a gluten-free diet. In long-term follow-up, he needed only ordinary preventive doses of vitamin D, and a nutritious diet containing calcium and iron in adequate amounts.

Learning Points

- Magnesium deficiency usually presents as hypocalcemia refractory to treatment and requires an index of suspicion for diagnosis.
- Intermittent parenteral calciferol is mandated for vitamin D deficiency associated with malabsorption.

- IM vitamin D produces a gradual rise of serum 25(OH)D in contrast to oral vitamin D administration, so larger doses may be used.

> A 4-year-old boy from a lower socio-economic group family was brought with complaints of poor growth, recurrent respiratory infections and bony defor-mities. His birth history was uneventful and he was breast-fed till 1 year of age. His motor milestones and tooth eruption were delayed and his activities were confined to the indoors. Bony deformities in the form of bending of legs were noticed since he started walking. He was always irritable. His overall nutritional intake including calcium was low. He weighed 10 kg.

Examination revealed short stature, frontal bossing, widening of wrist, rachitic rosary, Harrison's sulcus, bilateral genu varum, dental caries and proximal muscle weakness, sugges-tive of rickets.

Investigations showed normal serum alka-line phosphatase (140 IU/L), low calcium 1.97 mmol/L (7.9 mg/dL) and low phosphorus 0.74 mmol/L (2.3 mg/dL) levels. Serum 25(OH)D was not tested, due to financial constraints.

Radiography confirmed active rickets.

Treatment

Nutritional rickets being the most common cause of rickets, the child was treated with vitamin D 60,000 units once-monthly for 3 doses and oral calcium (50 mg/kg/day of elemental calcium), in addition to protein, energy and other micronutrients including zinc. Proper die-tary advice was given. Clinical, biochemical and radiological improvement was documented on follow-up, alkaline phosphatase at 1 month showing an initial rise to 700 U/L with fall to normal by 2 months. Subsequently, the child was put on a preventive regimen of 60,000 U of vitamin D every 3 months for the next 1 year, pending improvement in sun exposure with general well-being, outdoor activity and thus sun exposure.

Learning Points

- Rickets in this case is due to both calcium and vitamin D deficiency due to nutritional inadequacy complemented with poor sun exposure.
- Although a normal or low normal serum calcium with low phosphorus and markedly elevated alkaline phosphatase typifies the biochemical picture of vitamin D deficiency rickets, at times phosphorus levels can be elevated due to a state of transient pseudohypoparathyroidism.
- Also in severely malnourished children with rickets, alkaline phosphate may be inappropriately normal due to associated micronutrient deficiency especially zinc.
- During treatment there can be an initial elevation of the alkaline phosphatase before the actual fall starts due to rapid healing of the rachitic bony lesions.

A 10-year-old boy born to third degree consanguineous parents was brought with complaints of poor growth, generalised weakness and polyuria. He had bilateral lower limb deformity since early childhood. There was one episode of passing stones in urine. Birth history was normal. There was no bony pain, proximal muscle weakness, muscle cramps, tetany, seizures or malabsorption symptoms. One of his elder siblings died at 4 years of age. Two of his elder siblings have similar bony deformities. There was no deafness in the family. He had been on calcium and vitamin D supplementation for more than 5 years. He had also received a trial of phosphorus supplementation for 6 months.

Examination findings included waddling gait, bilateral genu valgum, wrist widening and dental enamel hypoplasia.

Investigation reports showed elevated alkaline phosphatase (1490 IU/L), normal calcium 2.28 mmol/L (9.1 mg/dL) and low phosphorus 0.9 mmol/L (2.8 mg/dL) indicating secondary hyperparathyroidism. In addition he had hypokalemia (serum potassium 2.8 mmol/L). His renal function was normal (serum creatinine 61.9 μmol/L [0.7 mg/dL]). Blood gas analysis showed compensated metabolic acidosis with normal anion gap.

An abdominal ultrasound revealed bilateral medullary nephrocalcinosis.

Subsequently an acid loading test with ammonium chloride failed to acidify urinary pH below 5.5, confirming distal RTA.

Both siblings also were evaluated and found to have distal RTA.

Wilson's disease was ruled out by normal serum caeruloplasmin levels and slit lamp examination. All three children were started on bicarbonate therapy (2–3 mmol/kg/day) and potassium supplementation (1–2 mmol/kg/day). Clinical and biochemical improvement was seen in all. There was no progression of nephrocalcinosis on subsequent sonography.

Learning Points

- Both proximal and distal renal tubular acidosis can result in rickets. In proximal RTA, the primary defect is failure of kidneys to conserve bicarbonate.
- In distal RTA, moderate doses of alkali (2–3 mmol/kg) and potassium supplementation are required.
- Higher doses of alkali (up to 10 mmol/kg) may be required to reverse the acidosis in proximal RTA.

- In addition renal phosphate loss as part of Fanconi syndrome will necessitate phosphate supplementation in addition to alkali.
- Both forms of RTA can result secondary to various (inherited) metabolic diseases; screening for these diseases, as well as family screening, must be considered.

A 2-year-old boy born of non-consanguineous union was brought with the complaint of progressive bowing of legs since 1 year of age. He had a normal birth, developmental and nutritional history. There were no symptoms suggestive of hypocalcaemia/proximal myopathy. His teeth erupted normally. His mother also had similar bony deformity and was significantly short. She had complaints of low backache. The child had already received multiple doses of vitamin D and was on regular calcium supplements with no improvement in symptoms.

Examination revealed short stature, frontal bossing and bilateral genu varum, and no rachitic features on the chest or upper limbs. Serum calcium was 2.3 mmol/L (9.2 mg/dL), alkaline phosphatase was mildly elevated (650 IU/L, normal less than 450 U/L) and fasting serum phosphorus was low (0.48 mmol/L [1.5 mg/dL]). X-ray of long bone showed mild rachitic features at knee and ankle, and dense trabeculae. Venous blood gas study was done to look for metabolic acidosis as a part of Fanconi syndrome; this was normal. Glycosuria and aminoaciduria were also documented to be absent. Urinary phosphate wasting was confirmed by estimating the percentage tubular resorption of phosphorus (TRP) and tubular threshold maximum for phosphate (TmPO4/GFR). Facilities were not available to evaluate serum PTH, to document that this biochemical picture was not the result of hyperparathyroidism secondary to calcipaenic rickets (such as distal RTA or malabsorption).

Since the clinical picture strongly pointed to hypophosphataemic rickets (sparing of upper part of the body, absence of hypocalcaemia, presence of dense trabeculae), a presumptive diagnosis of hypophosphataemic rickets was made and treatment started. The child was started on oral phosphate supplementation and active vitamin D_3 (calcitriol). Doses were titrated so as to normalise the phosphorus levels without inducing hyperparathyroidism and hypercalcaemia or hypercalciuria. Bony deformities improved over many years, and no surgery was needed.

Learning Points

- X-linked hypophosphataemic rickets is the most common cause of inherited hypophosphataemic rickets in children. Secondary hyperparathyroidism due to vitamin D deficiency can also lead to phosphaturia. In XLH, phosphaturia occurs in presence of a low or normal PTH level.
- Phosphorus supplementation should be started with a very low dose initially (~ 125 mg/day) given as 4—5 divided doses and gradually increased over weeks to reach the optimum dose (20—40 mg/kg/day) to avoid gastrointestinal side effects. However, overtreatment with phosphorus stimulates PTH release and can result in secondary hyperparathyroidism.
- 1,25(OH)D levels are low normal in XLH due to phosphatonin-mediated inhibition of 1α-hydroxylase enzyme and hence requires active vitamin D supplementation.
- If hypercalciuria develops with calcitriol supplementation, thiazide diuretics may be added. Alfacalcidol (1α-hydroxy cholecalciferol) is a preferred alternative due to once-daily dosing (25—50 ng/kg/day).

GYNAECOLOGY

A 14-year-old girl with secondary amenorrhoea, acne and hirsutism.

Diagnostic Approach

Assessment

Clinical assessment should include all causes of secondary amenorrhoea even though PCOS is most likely.

Hence the following:

- Stature in family related to midparental height, growth rate and time of growth spurt, i.e. a girl with CAH may have grown very rapidly at 7–9 years then stopped.
- History of pubertal course including breast, pubic hair onset, i.e. was this menarche or a withdrawal bleed in the early stages of puberty
- Pubic hair very early (at under 6–7) might suggest PCOS or CAH.
- Time span of condition: ? slow evolution, ? very rapid over 1– months: may indicate tumour – adrenal or ovarian.
- Time of onset of acne – premenarchal more often indicates an underlying pathologic cause.
- Family history of PCOS.
- Family history of ? of CAH or suggestion of CAH, e.g. are other siblings very tall etc.
- Evidence for metabolic syndrome, IHD, high cholesterol, diabetes on either side of family.
- Evidence for premature ovarian failure in family – including haemochromatosis, carrier fragile X; boys with fragile X , indicating that there may be carrier fragile X girls
- History that may suggest eating disorder.

Examination

- Position on growth chart currently – if premature epiphyseal fusion and short for

family despite past rapid growth – likely CAH.
- Evidence of virilisation *must* be sought – consider CAH/ tumour.
- Is there genuinely a lot of acne/hair? Some girls have a severely distorted body image and very little real medical evidence for the complaint.
- Turner syndrome features?
- Location of hirsutism – androgenic or not.
- Type of acne – comedomal/cystic etc., ? hidradenitis suppurativa
- ? body weight for height.
- Other features to suggest long vs short duration of virilisation, e.g. poor quality breast development in CAH in presence of high androgen levels.
- ? galactorrhoea (plus any clinical association with acromegaly – rare but not unheard of). Prolactinoma is clearly associated with PCOS.

Investigations that May Help with a Diagnosis

- 17-OHP, androstenedione, testosterone, FSH/LH, DHEAS.
- Prolactin.
- Either baseline 24-hour steroid profile or synacthen test – the latter may be preferred in this case.
- Pelvic ultrasound – transabdominal only.
- Karyotype if Turner syndrome, gonadal dysgenesis is considered.
- Other as indicated, e.g. MRI etc.
- OGTT – if indicated, can check insulin at each time point to ascertain extent of hyperinsulinaemic response.

Management

1. Ascertain the girl's wishes! (Provided this is PCOS – clearly, it is necessary to treat an underlying condition if it is found.)
2. Weight management if needed: diet and exercise +/− metformin – this may be

enough to resolve amenorrhoea and significantly reduce acne and aromatisation of oestrogen to androgen in peripheral fat.

3. Start spironolactone 150–200 mg/day – start slowly to minimise risk of headache (could treat acne with antibiotic first but usually not needed).

4. Use OCP – non-norgestrel-containing as that is very androgenic – best to start with a pill using norethisterone as the progestogen. Try not to use cyproterone containing OCP as this can cause weight gain and depression.

5. Best to start androgen blockade then ovarian suppression consecutively so you will know if any side effects – counsel patient to call if she has any adverse effects as they are very easy to manage by a change of medication.

6. Counsel regarding need for at least 2 years of combined treatment prior to dose reduction or OCP alone; likelihood of relapse.

7. Counsel regarding fertility as some internet sites and well-meaning friends suggest infertility is the rule (nonsense!); also re lifestyle to avoid excess weight, chance of future lipid, diabetes etc. problems.

8. Occasionally, may need dermatologist for an opinion regarding use of Roaccutane® and/or laser hair removal.

A 14-year-old girl with spastic quadri-plegia, cerebral palsy and menorrhagia.

Assessment of this girl includes the following:

- General features of nutritional status.
- Whether she is gastrostomy fed or orally fed which will reflect vitamin D status as a specific risk factor of bone health.
- Calcium intake.
- ? presence of epilepsy and use of anticonvulsant; both are detrimental to bone mass accrual and maintenance.

- Time of onset of puberty. Some children with cerebral palsy have a very early puberty which relates to the brain damage or malformation, with disinhibition of the hypothalamic pituitary axis. While difficult for families, bone mass accrual certainly improves and fracture risk concomitantly decreases with pubertal progress – an advantage under these circumstances.
- Time of onset of menarche, menstrual irregularity and whether menorrhagia is of recent onset or a chronic problem if the adolescent is very thin and only halfway through puberty.

The appearance of apparent 'menorrhagia' may actually indicate lack of oestrogen, with pubertal arrest (depending on parental concept of this event!) but this is much less likely than true heavy menstrual loss. Usually, if vaginal bleeding occurs due to pubertal arrest it is minimal or light, although it might be recurrent, by comparison with a heavy true menstrual bleed.

Treatment

Menorrhagia is relatively common in a normal adolescent, with heavy frequent bleeds at less than 21-day intervals with menstruation lasting 7–10 days or more.

In the short term, use of high-dose proges-togen will usually stop the period and may return the cycle to normal. In the longer term, consideration for intervention should be discussed with the family.

The management of menorrhagia in a severely intellectually and physically disabled adolescent can be difficult. Use of the oral contraceptive pill on a continuous basis without withdrawal bleeds is possible but is dependent on regular medication and may be interfered with by anticonvulsant use, with increased hepatic metabolic excretion of oestrogen.

A progestogen-bearing IUD is a useful alternative, providing 5 years' amenorrhoea and contraception as a side benefit. Use of implantable progestogen or depot progestogen is contraindicated as causes bone loss unless transdermal or oral oestrogen is added in addition to the progestogen.

SALT AND WATER

> **A 10-year-old girl with head injury and polyuria.**

Evaluation and Management.

Central DI most likely — time of onset: ? immediate vs delayed is important to ascertain.

Differential Diagnosis

1. Possibility of postoperative offload of extra fluid after 12—24 hours (if child has had surgery).
2. Particularly if the patient is obese, onset is over days rather than hours and if on dexamethasone, the possibility of diabetes mellitus should be considered.
3. Possible cerebral salt wasting if later onset.

Initial confirmation of diagnosis — u/serum Na and osmol — recognition that delay in assay alters osmolality.

Urgent assessment for other pituitary hormone deficits if DI confirmed — awareness that low T_4 or cortisol causes poor free water clearance and DI may worsen when treated for these deficits.

Note: value of good clinical exam to see if she is in puberty, in which case would expect to see FSH/LH +/− oestradiol measureable — if they are extremely low in the face of pubertal changes, they act as another indicator of hypopituitarism.

Awareness that dexamethasone is *not* measured in a cortisol assay *but* that dexamethasone rapidly and powerfully suppresses adrenal axis so a cortisol test may be useless; so how to diagnose ACTH deficiency? Assume it to be likely in presence of other panhypopituitarism.

Use of basal GH/IGF1 — testing is valuable during early stress, but a low value is common with chronic stress.

Management of DI

Options include intranasal or oral desmopressin (DDAVP) or intravenous vasopressin.

Intravenous therapy may be needed if blocked nose (e.g. nasal intubation if very unwell), or nasal injury etc.

? How often to administer: initially, fluid balance varies every few hours so a dose should only be given once there is onset of further polydipsia and polyuria, over half to one hour.

Note: Pitfalls of DDAVP in the ward! Staff are often busy — onset of polyuria can be missed or not attended for 2—3 hours, by which time the Na is already high and the patient may become dehydrated. Parents are helpful to detect and alert staff who *must* respond immediately. In the initial phase, regular serum sodium measurements will ensure patient is not over or undertreated.

Timing of Resolution of DI Following Head Injury?

Usually, 4—6 weeks max if it is a temporary phenomenon; otherwise damage may be permanent. Note: to monitor for triple response at 3—10 days after injury, with SIADH, then relapse of DI at around 14 days.

Main differential diagnosis is cerebral salt wasting, which also results in polyuria but it more commonly occurs days to weeks after the head injury. *Hyponatremia and high urinary sodium concentrations* are characteristic.

Treatment of Cerebral Salt Wasting

The principal goal is replacement of lost fluid and sodium (as compared with SIADH where hyponatraemia secondary to relative fluid overload responds to fluid restriction).

Sodium can be replaced with oral salt supplements; however, intravenous therapy often required if child very unwell/unwilling to drink in initial phase. Three per cent saline may be required but this requires very close electrolyte monitoring due to the risks of sudden fluctuations in [Na] which may precipitate central pontine demyelination.

> A 10-year-old boy with acute onset central DI and normal MRI.

Work-Up and Follow-Up Plan

Issues

- Ensure diagnosis of central DI has been confirmed — consider water deprivation test (including assessment of response to vasopressin) if not previously done.
- Consider causes: Langerhans histiocytosis, germinoma, other midline lesion. Spontaneous onset of DI at age 10 is pathological!
- Main differentials include psychogenic /habitual polydipsia and nephrogenic DI.

History and Examination

- ? anything to suggest any other anterior pituitary hormone deficiency (may be present even without identifiable lesion on MRI), e.g. growth failure or precocious puberty. Note: the latter may give the impression of apparently normal linear growth.
- ? family history of DI (less likely to present at age 10 but some families have accepted a very large fluid intake as normal!).
- ? history of trauma/head injury/diabetes mellitus/visual problems

- Any clinical features of LCH? Less likely at age 10 but rash and osteolytic lesions can occur at any age.
- Clinical growth and pubertal parameters to suggest a long-standing or recent cause or possible cause, e.g. midline lesion, tumour, NF1 etc.

Causes of Central DI at Age 10

Structural changes:

- Neoplasms, e.g. germinoma, may not be identifiable on initial MRI — if resources allow, consider serial imaging/close follow-up to exclude development of abnormality (e.g. stalk thickening).
- Infiltrative/autoimmune/infectious disorders — especially LCH.
- Accidental/surgical trauma to vasopressin neurons.
- Congenital/anatomical hypothalamic/ pituitary abnormalities — especially midline abnormality.
- Increased metabolism of vasopressin.
- Idiopathic: quoted rates vary in series between 10 and 50% although ~ 40% have antibodies to vasopressin and so process may be autoimmune in nature.

Disorders of vasopressin gene structure:

1. Familial autosomal-dominant central DI — generally presents in first half of first decade with gradual decline in vasopressin; would therefore expect symptoms to have been established for a few years in this case
2. Several mutations in vasopressin structural gene have been identified — mutations are in pro-hormone gene resulting in defective pre-hormone and vasopressin deficiency — more than 35 mutations — most within neurophysin domain.
3. Autosomal recessive and X-linked recessive forms are also described but rare. DIDMOAD (Wolfram syndrome) — gene localised to 4p16, mutation in transmembrane protein;

usually present in early childhood but can be missed if not considered.

Treatment

DDAVP — synthetic analogue of arginine vasopressin.

Oral or intranasal: usually twice daily dosing (varies depending on response), await diuresis pre-dose; increase in dose prolongs duration of action rather than increasing effect.

Oral: requirements vary from 100 to 600 µg/day.

Intra-nasal: 5–40 µg/day.

Other possible work-up as required — baseline investigations in addition to MRI:

- Anterior pituitary hormone testing: 08.00 am cortisol, TSH and fT_4, IGF1; if any concern re growth or baseline hormonal levels, proceed to dynamic testing (e.g. glucagon stimulation test).
- Tumour markers: hCG and aFP (serum and consider CSF levels also). Serum levels of βhCG and αFP are also repeated with further testing in CSF. If MRI appearances change, proceed also to CSF cytology +/- biopsy if possible, with targeted therapy thereafter.
- Skeletal survey (assessing for LCH).

Follow-Up

- Any lesion treated on its merits: if unclear and thick pituitary stalk present, may be LCH or germinoma. MRI mandatory every 3–6 months if available and resources allow. Surveillance MRI scans 4–6 monthly for 2 years, then 6–12 monthly for 2 years, followed by annual imaging if appearances remain unchanged.

Normal baseline MRI in this case should not be interpreted as reassuring, as it has been well established in previous case series that appearances may change over time. Anterior pituitary size may also change over time: increase in size is strongly associated with a diagnosis of germinoma.

- Monitor pituitary function. Rapid evolution of loss of pituitary hormones over months suggests tumour.

HYPOTHALAMIC PITUITARY DISORDERS AND GROWTH

A 12-year-old boy was seen by a paediatrician for short stature. He had a history of abdominal symptoms and anaemia since the age of 7 years. He was seen by a number of doctors and finally the diagnosis of Crohn's disease was made when he had gastro-duodenoscopy and colonoscopy at age 11 years. From then, bowel symptoms were kept under control by the use of an elemental diet. However, growth did not improve and growth failure remained significant.

Q1. Is Growth Failure Likely to be Due to Crohn's Disease?

Answer Chronic inflammatory conditions, such as Crohn's disease, can be a cause for growth failure and short stature. Children often present with poor linear growth at the time of puberty. The underlying chronic illness not only slows growth, but also delays puberty. Growth failure due to chronic illness may become more noticeable in an adolescent at a time when peers are going through a rapid pubertal growth spurt.

Q2. Is the Growth Chart Showing a Flattening of Growth Trajectory Typical of Children with Crohn's Disease at the Time of Puberty?

Answer The flattening of the growth chart suggests growth stasis and a decreased height velocity. In this case, height velocity had been very significantly reduced, well before the time of puberty. The child's symptoms improved on dietetic management, but there was no accompanying improvement in height gain. This suggests that the growth failure was disproportionate to the severity of the chronic illness.

Q3. What Were the Examination Findings? Did they Suggest a Cause for Endocrine Dysfunction?

Answer It is important to assess for any underlying endocrine condition in all cases of growth failure with or without short stature. This is definitely the case for children with constitutional delay of growth and puberty (CDGP), where the diagnosis is by exclusion of any underlying illness. Although CDGP is a common cause of late puberty, just very occasionally, children with a brain tumour, such as a craniopharyngioma, may present with short stature and late puberty.

In this case, physical examination of visual fields, fundi, tendon reflexes, respiratory and cardiovascular systems was within normal limits. Therefore, examination did not suggest any additional cause for endocrine dysfunction. However, it was felt that growth failure could not be explained by the presence of Crohn's disease alone.

Q4. Would it be Useful to Investigate for Growth Failure in a Child with an Underlying Chronic Illness?

Answer Not all children with chronic illness require investigation for growth failure. It is expected that adequate treatment of the underlying chronic illness would lead to improvement in height velocity. However, in this case, growth failure is not commensurate with the severity of the underlying chronic illness. Therefore, further investigation into the cause for short stature is required.

Q5. What Investigations were Performed and What were the Results?

Answer Baseline pituitary function tests (IGF-I, prolactin, thyroid function test, electrolytes) were performed. Serum IGF-I levels were extremely low, while the other tests were normal. On the basis that this boy had significant growth failure and IGF-I was very low, dynamic anterior pituitary stimulation was performed. Growth hormone levels were almost undetectable on an arginine stimulation testing.

Q6. What Investigations would you Consider Next?

Answer Investigations consistent with growth hormone deficiency provide an explanation for the growth failure and short stature in this case. However further assessment is required to investigate the cause of growth hormone deficiency. Therefore an MR scan of the pituitary and hypothalamus was performed. This showed the presence of a variegated sellar mass. There was some compression to the optic chiasm. Although clinical confrontation perimetry was normal, formal visual field examination demonstrated the presence of unilateral upper quadrantanopia. An excision biopsy of the lesion was carried out and histology confirmed the presence of a craniopharyngioma.

Q7. What are the Lessons from this Case?

Answer There are a numbers of lessons to be learnt from this case. First, it is important to plot as many height and weight measurements as possible. Second, the growth chart should be carefully interpreted along with knowledge about pubertal status. Third, it is wise to consider dual pathology even if growth failure could be explained by an obvious cause. Fourth, it is important to consider the possibility of a brain tumour, such as a craniopharyngioma in all children with significant growth failure.

Twin monozygotic girls were referred to the outpatient clinic because of short stature at the age of 5 years and 8 months. They were born after gestation of 37 + 2 weeks, each with a birth weight of 2590 g.

They had always been small with no other health problems.

Father was also small with a height of 168.7 cm (−2.13 SD). He had short legs.

Mother's height was 170.1 cm (−0.10 SD).

Height of both girls was −2.1 SD. They had short legs and the ratio of sitting height and height was +4.1 SD. The rest of the examination was unremarkable. No dysmorphic features.

Assess

For disproportional short stature, consider:

- Turner syndrome
- hypochondroplasia
- SHOX gene deletion.

Check usual causes of short stature including thyroid function but consider bony causes as major likelihood.

Skeletal survey for bone dysplasia.

Note:? typical features of SHOX gene deletion − abnormal distal radial epiphysis likely.

Karyotype with 60 cells may be needed to exclude low level mosaicism − unlikely given they are monozygotic twins.

Diagnosis

SHOX deletion as autosomal dominant is the more likely diagnosis or hypochondroplasia − the latter will be detected on skeletal survey in the children, not the father as he has fused epiphyses.

SHOX abnormalities are GH responsive (where growth hormone is available).

A 2-year-old boy with short stature (height SDS −2.9) and low IGF1.

Interpretation and Approach

Possible growth hormone deficiency but differential diagnosis is important.

History to include prenatal, birth history − birth weight, length.

Postnatal hypoglycaemia may suggest GH deficiency.

Postnatal growth pattern will inform the diagnosis.

- Consider bony dysplasia if always very short from birth.
- IUGR with no catch-up.
- Feeding, chronic illness etc., consider all systems (including renal, cardiac, cystic fibrosis, coeliac early/unusual bowel disease).
- Salient exam features including proportions, head size, hands for signs of brachydactyly or other features to suggest bone dysplasia, as well as midline defect clues.
- ? Preservation of normal head growth − seen in IUGR and GH deficiency.
- Look for central adiposity suggestive of GH deficiency.
- Possibility of cortisol excess, endogenous or administered. If endogenous cortisol excess, likely to be adrenal Ca and associated with virilisation.
- Consider Noonan syndrome with typical features − hard to see at this age; can be obvious in infancy and at mid-childhood.

A low IGF1 reflects poor growth but does not provide a diagnosis. GH testing may be considered after exclusion of systemic disorders.

A 4-year-old girl with multiple pituitary hormone deficiency (GH, ACTH and TSH) and pituitary mass lesion.

Possibilities and Approach

Basic history must include birth, duration of problem of slow growth.

? Presence of DI − if recent onset, much more likely to be space occupying lesion, not congenital.

Septo-optic dysplasia can have DI as part of spectrum but uncommonly seen.

PROP mutation possible but ACTH deficiency usually occurs at late stage, in adulthood.

Differential Diagnosis for an Intracranial, Space-Occupying Lesion

Tumour:

- Be aware of relative likelihood of various pituitary tumours in childhood vs craniopharyngioma (the latter is far more common in this age group and the commonest infra-tentorial tumour of childhood): intrasellar craniopharyngioma is not uncommon.
- If not craniopharyngioma, the next most likely are glioma or germinoma.
- Hamartoma does not present like this.
- Macro adenoma in childhood is vanishingly unlikely; similarly Cushing's and acromegaly are rare in children except in the context of McCune–Albright syndrome.
- Teratoma and pituitary carcinoma are both reported rarely but more likely extending to hypothalamic, not solely a position within the pituitary fossa.

Diagnosis Confirmation

- Use of CT for calcification vs MRI (presumably already done as lesion has been identified). However, if MR is unavailable, use CT not SXR because radiation dose is similar but information better with CT.
- Question of surgical approach — trans-sphenoidal is near impossible in a 4 year old.
- Optic arteries are on dorsal surface of optic nerves so there is an increased risk in surgery from above, with attendant problems with vision preservation.
- Approach to craniopharyngioma: surgical removal/debulking.
- Note: to 'do no harm'. Total removal is associated with a far higher risk for collateral damage. Cranial irradiation may be required in future to reduce recurrence.

Peri-Operative Management

- Adequate steroid cover, management of possible diabetes insipidus postoperatively.
- Family advice needed for future, including advice for family and school re increased steroid cover for stress.
- When to give GH — if available and the lesion is a craniopharyngioma? Some children, particularly those who are obese, continue to grow normally despite GH deficiency
- Understanding of oncologic management if lesion is a germinoma — CXRT vs CSXRT vs chemotherapy — usually is CXRT and chemo because chemo alone is very toxic — awareness of side effects of hypothalamic XRT, including severe adverse effects on memory etc. in a 4 year old.
- Obesity risk: craniopharyngioma risk is far higher than other tumour — management options include later consideration for use of stimulants to aid memory and weight where hypothalamic damage is present.

> A 6-year-old boy with short stature (height SDS −3.2) with normal facies, normal body proportions and screening investigations.

Aetiology and Approach

Issues

Short stature (height less than 1st centile); growth velocity (GV) unknown but likely to have had a prolonged period of poor growth velocity, given height SDS.

Any heights available from the family or school are helpful to establish duration of ? growth failure — including height and growth relative to other prepubertal siblings.

Growth failure is the most important indicator of a medical illness vs constitutional delay vs congenital growth hormone deficiency.

Differential Diagnoses

- Familial short stature
- Constitutional delay of growth and puberty
- Short stature following IUGR/SGA
- Growth hormone deficiency or abnormality of GH-IGF1 axis
- Chronic/systemic disease
- Malnutrition — malabsorption or inadequate nutrition
- Psychosocial deprivation
- Other endocrine causes are unlikely, given normal screening tests (assuming thyroid function normal), normal facies and body proportions (Cushing's disease is extremely uncommon at this age but the typical features of moon face and central adiposity may be absent in a child, with generalised weight gain as the only complaint.)

History

History to include the following.

- Birth history — ? ex IUGR/SGA; check for illnesses in the neonatal period.
- Previous measurements if available to estimate GV as above.
- Family and social history: midparental height and target range; timing of puberty; other, e.g. skeletal dysplasia (less likely given normal proportions), other illness/ deprivation/poor social circumstances.
- Feeding: dietary assessment.
- Neurological symptoms, e.g. headache/ visual disturbance.

Examination

- Assess general examination for indicators of systemic disease.

- Dysmorphism suggestive of chromosomal abnormalities or syndrome (e.g. Noonan syndrome/Russell—Silver syndrome).
- Weight — ? also less than 1st centile (this may indicate primary problem).
- GH deficiency is possible despite 'normal facies', as midface hypoplasia may not be marked and will be absent if GHD is acquired.
- Café-au-lait or other pigmentation changes to suggest NF1 etc.
- Specific features to indicate a midline lesion — single central incisor, dimpled nose, hypertelorism.
- Neurological assessment including fundi and cranial nerves.
- Pubertal assessment — assume prepubertal, given his age and short stature.

Investigations and Monitoring

- Screening tests normal as above — to include ESR and coeliac screen.
- Bone age is the most useful baseline test: likely to be delayed — assess height for bone age. If height/BA is within the expected midparental target range, likely good height outcome.

Assess growth velocity, over at least 6—12-month period. If GV for BA is low (less than −1SDS or 25th centile), this warrants further investigations.

- Consider IGF1 and IGFBP3 if available but they are only general indicators (note IGF1 will be low if malnutrition an issue).
- If ongoing low growth velocity with no identifiable cause, proceed to dynamic testing of GH axis — this can be physiological e.g. exercise stimulation, or pharmacological e.g. insulin tolerance test (requires very close monitoring for hypoglycaemia during test), or glucagon/arginine/clonidine stimulation test.

- Need to ensure full panel has been performed as initial screen for systemic/other cause in child with height below 1st centile: U&E, LFTs, FBE, ESR, coeliac screen, TFTs (and karyotype or micro array, if features suggest need in a male).
- If GH deficiency is diagnosed, MRI head is mandatory.

Treatment and Further Management

These depend on findings.

- If all investigations are normal and bone age is delayed — ongoing monitoring of GV (6—12-monthly to ensure GV remains normal).
- Ensure normal healthy dietary intake.
- If GH deficient — GH replacement therapy, if available, will likely result in significant change in GV and improvement of ht SDS.

ADRENAL/DSD

Two cases that illustrate a logical reasoning in the diagnosis of two different adrenal disorders.

> A 6-year old African girl presents with pubic hair, starting about 1 year ago.

Family History

No known consanguinity, but both parents come from the same region, from villages about 40 km apart. The parents do not recall the age of appearance of their own pubertal signs. Both parents are of average height for their family backgrounds, at −1 and −2 SDS, respectively. Neither parent has excessive hair growth, and both claim to be healthy. A 3-year-old brother is healthy, but tall for age.

Previous Health

At birth she was close to mean length and weight, according to the well-baby growth chart that the mother provides. From 1.5 years of age, height and weight has gradually increased to the present +2 SDS. She has never been hospitalised. She is vaccinated against polio, measles, diphtheria, tetanus, pertussis and rubella.

Present Health Status

She is considered to be very healthy. Her favourite sport is football. She eats well — prefers salty dishes. No gastrointestinal complaints. Normal temperature tolerance. Sleeps 8 hours per night.

Present Medication

None.

Physical Examination

Normal psychomotor development for age. Height +2 SDS. BMI is at the mean for age. Fat distribution, skin pigmentation and blood pressure are all normal. Skin on the nose is oily, about 10 blackheads are seen on the nose. No acne. Breast Tanner stage 1. Pubic hair Tanner 2—3. Clitoris measures 8 mm in length, 4 mm in width. There is no labial fusion. Mucous membranes in vulva are thin, red. No discharge. Bone age is advanced to 8 years.

Impression, Without Lab Tests

A 6-year-old girl with moderate signs of ongoing increased androgen secretion for age (pubic hair, oily skin, blackheads, clitoral size at upper normal range and tall stature). She is tall for parental heights, but at the same SDS as the younger brother. Tall stature, advanced bone age and normal fat distribution speak against excess glucocorticoids as in Cushing's disease, normal blood pressure and her taste for salt speak against excess mineralocorticoids as in 11-hydroxylase deficiency. The younger tall brother should also be examined. If both have the same disorder, and both parents are healthy, an autosomal-recessive disorder should be suspected; the most common being congenital adrenal hyperplasia (CAH) of a mild form.

Next Step

If possible, prove or disprove this hypothesis by lab tests.

Differential Diagnoses

Differential diagnoses include the following.

- 21-hydroxylase deficiency. Confirm or rule out 21-hydroxylase deficiency by morning P-17-hydroxyprogesterone (17-OHP; expected to be high), and P-cortisol (expected to be normal or borderline low).
- 11β-hydroxylase deficiency. In that case, she would be expected to have normal or elevated blood pressure. If lab is available, ask for 11-deoxycortisol; expected to be high. (Note: In some immunoassays, this steroid cross-reacts with 17-OHP). Sodium might be borderline high, but probably not in a mild case like this.
- Adrenal tumour. In most cases, an adrenal carcinoma produces DHEAS as the main steroid, and DHEAS is expected to be very high. However, some tumours produce both excess androgens and cortisol, and may have a picture resembling Cushing syndrome; adiposity of the trunk and neck, suppressed growth rate and signs of androgen excess as above. In the present case, the slow progression, the absence of Cushingoid features and, most important, the presence of a similar problem in the younger brother all speak against adrenal tumour.
- Idiopathic premature pubarche. The absence of a family history for increased hair growth, the increased growth rate, the advanced bone age and the evident signs of androgen over-secretion speak against this benign diagnosis.

CONCLUSIONS

Even without steroid assays, the diagnosis of a relatively mild form of CAH, probably 21-hydroxylase deficiency, is very probable. The most important differential diagnosis to be ruled out is adrenal tumour — which is unlikely in this case (see above). Since the treatment of both non-salt losing 21-OHD and 11-OHD are the same (glucocorticoid substitution), it is not important to differentiate the two from each other.

A 13-month-old boy who presents with pubic hair.

Family History

Third child of healthy Caucasian parents. No consanguinity. The elder two brothers are considered healthy, of average height and weight. No family history of precocious puberty — none of the parents remembers the age at start of puberty.

Previous Health

Both pregnancy and the neonatal period were uneventful. The growth chart shows that the development of length and weight continues to be at +1 SDS.

Present Complaint

From about 9 months of age, the parents have observed increasing pubic hair, and over the past 1–2 months acne has developed over the face and shoulders. He has also developed oily facial skin and obvious growth of the penis over the past 2 months.

Present Medication

None.

Physical Examination

A very active, muscular 13-month-old boy. Walks well, good motor development for age.

Normal body proportions, normal fat distribution, but parents have noticed that his face has become more rounded. This is verified by photos. Blood pressure 110/70, pulse rate 100/min. Abdomen: no palpable masses or organomegaly. Skin: extensive acne over nose and shoulders. Oily facial skin. Normal pigmentation. Genitalia: pubic hair Tanner stage 2–3. Penis measures (stretched) 7 cm in length, 2 cm in diameter. Scrotal skin is thin, reddened. Testes are in the bottom of the scrotum, both 1 mL. Bone age is accelerated to 3 years.

Impression, Without Lab Tests

A 13-month-old boy who had normal development until 9 months of age. Since then, he presents many signs of rapid masculinisation, due to an ongoing over-production of androgens. The only possible sources of androgenic hormones are the adrenals and the testes (provided that external administration of androgens is not the case). The small testes speak against a testicular source. Two causes of adrenal over-secretion of androgens must be considered: congenital adrenal hyperplasia (CAH) and adrenal tumour. In the present case, the rapid progression and intensity of the masculinisation speaks for adrenal carcinoma.

Next Step

Imaging of the adrenals is necessary, by ultrasound or (preferably) by MRI, if available. Measurement of DHEAS is the most important steroid assay; it should be markedly elevated in the case of adrenal carcinoma. 17-OHP is not diagnostic for 21-OHD in this case; it may be elevated also in adrenal cancer. Elevated serum testosterone is proven by the symptoms, and therefore testosterone levels in blood need not be measured if the resources are very limited. Before surgery, selective venous blood sampling from both adrenal veins may be necessary if the imaging does not show an adrenal tumour on one side.

> A 10-year-old boy with unusual movements, loss of memory and sleep disturbance is found to have hyperpigmentation of the skin and buccal mucosa.

The likely cause is primary adrenal insufficiency – Addison's disease.

Commonest cause worldwide is TB, followed by HIV.

Auto-immune disease is probably the next most common but in the context of a male with apparent memory/brain disturbance, adrenoleukodystrophy (ALD) must be considered.

A careful family history is essential as ALD is an X-linked disorder.

Note: girls, as carriers, can have adrenomyelopathy. Late presentation in family members is possible, even to age of 60 years.

How to Diagnose

Need for synacthen testing is unlikely if ACTH assay is available for confirmation. Cortisol may not be strikingly low as child is still walking around!

Causation requires specific testing, e.g. VLCFA, adrenal ab, HIV, TB testing etc.

Hyponatraemia is very unlikely to be seen in the chronic state like this, so its absence does not help.

Awareness of use of MRI in management of ALD, even if such treatment is unavailable in local circumstances.

- Once established changes in white matter have occurred (as is likely with this child), bone marrow transplant will not help.
- Earlier presentation, e.g. at less than 8 years, may occur, with tiredness and a bit of memory loss only – the latter may be due to feeling very unwell, rather than to progression of leukodystrophy.

- Progression to overt rapid neurologic deterioration is less likely over age 8.

If MRI does not show damage this should be repeated with 3–6-monthly MRIs (if resources allow) and consideration for BMTx at *first* sign of any changes – central USA agency for MR review is available. Treatment should only be in specialised centre.

Lorenzo's oil use is controversial; not universally available.

The child should be treated with corticosteroid and mineralocorticoid replacement, and the family advised regarding steroid cover for stress.

Written information should be given to the family, the school staff and a copy should be carried by the child.

> **A 14-year-old male presents with hypotension and hypoglycaemia.**

This suggests the possibility of adrenal insufficiency.

Careful search for hyperpigmentation to indicate an adrenal cause should be made.

While hypopituitarism with ACTH deficiency could present in this way, it would be very unlikely to be associated with hypotension and hypoglycaemia in this age group, although a similar presentation would be common in a very small child or infant.

Assuming adrenal insufficiency, the commonest disorders causing Addison's disease worldwide are TB, followed by HIV, with autoimmune adrenal insufficiency more common in Western populations. Adrenoleukodystrophy presenting as adrenal insufficiency should be considered (see previous scenario).

> **An infant is born at 36 weeks with Prader III ambiguous genitalia.**

Approach to Diagnosis, Family History/Counselling

Consideration

Consideration is for:
Virilised female

- CAH 21-hydroxylase, 11-hydroxylase deficiency (aromatase deficiency, placental oxidoreductase deficiency).

Undervirilised male

- Mixed gonadal dysgenesis, ovotesticular DSD, testicular DSD (e.g. SRY+)
- Androgen biosynthesis defect: 5α-reductase
- Defect in androgen action PAIS, CAH – 3β-dehydrogenase, 17α-hydroxylase, STAR etc.
- Other (severe hypospadias cloacal exstrophy, etc.).

Diagnostic Tests

- Tests include: 17-OHP, karyotype or microarray, FSH, LH, T, DHT, Δ4-androstenedione, urine steroid profile. Many of these are available via international laboratories, filter paper testing.
- Use of genitogram, genitoscopy, ultrasound (+/- MRI if complex) to establish internal genitalia.

Treatment Priorities

- Diagnosis of CAH with adrenal insufficiency is the first essential, due to certainty of adrenal crisis if undiagnosed.
- If CAH confirmed, consensus opinion is for sex of rearing to be female as the girl will have potential for normal fertility.
- Family will need counselling around surgery, timing and extent of and importance of appropriate steroid replacement therapy to suppress adrenal androgen production.
- Close monitoring of growth and bone age is important over childhood, to optimise final height.

> A 20-year-old male with CAH admits that he has not adhered to his treatment regimen for a long time. He is obese, feels intermittently tired and is hyperpigmented.

Assessment

History should include past treatment, side effects, family issues that may have led to compliance problems, family history of CAH and other problems (social, emotional, psychological).

Examination to include evidence for pigmentation to suggest long-standing compliance problems, BP lying and standing, testicular exam — for size, nodules to suggest adrenal rest tissue.

Investigations

Investigations to consider:

- 17-OHP, steroid profile, DHEAS
- FBC, Fe studies etc. for any other reason for tiredness
- FSH/LH, T for hypogonadotrophic hypogonadism (HH) which occurs with long-standing poor control
- Testicular ultrasound for adrenal rests
- Semen analysis for azoospermia secondary to HH or adrenal rests
- Adrenal CT or MRI for hyperplasia or adenomata can be done but often not very helpful.

Treatment

Use of prednisolone or probably dexamethasone may be needed for control (once daily dosing will help with compliance).

Prognosis

Guarded for fertility if he has large adrenal rests, as these are very difficult to resolve, requiring use of dexamethasone for adequate suppression. Nonetheless, prognosis is good for CAH control.

> A phenotypically female infant is found to have inguinal testes and an XY karyotype. The father rejects advice that the child should be raised female on the grounds that the chromosomes and testes indicate a male child and gives a boy's name. The boy returns at age 17 with a male gender identity, a wispy beard and ambiguous genitalia. He is found to have hypertension.

Differential Diagnosis? Investigation? Management?

An Undervirilised Male

Consider possible PAIS but presence of hypertension makes 17α-hydroxylase deficiency more likely. Electrolytes demonstrate high sodium and low potassium, elevated mineralocorticoid metabolites in 24-hour urine GC profile.

BOX 14.1

A SALUTARY TALE

A 7-year-old boy with salt-wasting CAH has a persistently raised 17-OHP level, sexual development and advanced bone age, despite progressive increases in his dose of hydrocortisone.

He had heard so many discussions about the side effects of steroids that he started to believe he was being poisoned and spat every dose into a potted plant, with the result that his CAH got completely out of control. This emphasises the importance of parental supervision of medications; always focus on compliance if sudden deterioration despite adequate dose of steroid replacement.

Treatment

Treatment options are very difficult. He has a male gender identity so use of corticosteroid will reduce androgens and induce need for future corticosteroid cover for stress. Androgen supplementation will then be needed once cortisol treatment is instituted. No other treatment of hypertension is likely to be easily effective. Even steroid use may not control hypertension as it has been long-standing. Fertility potential is unclear.

A 5-year-old boy presents with severe headaches. He is found to have paroxysmal arterial hypertension 180/110.

Any child presenting with headaches may have an intracranial lesion which needs to be excluded. However, in the presence of paroxysmal hypertension, a diagnosis of phaeochromocytoma is likely.

Assessment

Assessment includes:

- Careful family history for any associated cause of phaeochromocytoma as almost 50% of childhood phaeochromocytomas are now known to be associated with a genetic abnormality such as Von Hippel–Lindau syndrome, MEN 2A or MEN 2B or succinate dehydrogenase gene mutations, SDHB and SDHD.
- Bearing in mind the possibility of congenital adrenal hyperplasia with associated hypertension, possible 11-hydroxylase deficiency would be an alternative diagnosis, although the hypertension would not be paroxysmal. In this case the child would be extremely tall with virilisation and severely advanced bone age.

- A history of consanguinity, other affected children or altered growth pattern is essential to consider.

Examination

Examination should be very careful if a diagnosis of phaeochromocytoma is considered, particularly with regard to abdominal palpation which might precipitate a hypertensive crisis. Careful search for papilloedema, angiomatous streaks on the retina to suggest VHL, or ganglioneuromas of eyelids or tongue and lips to suggest MEN 2B should be sought, along with the possibility of a Marfanoid habitus. Virilisation and abnormal tall stature as above, along with hyperpigmentation which would be present if 11-hydroxylase deficiency considered.

Investigation

Twenty-four-hour catecholamines provide evidence of excretion rate of catecholamines, plasma. Metanephrines and catecholamines provide evidence of production rate and are significantly more accurate if able to be obtained.

Preferred imaging utilises MIBG scan to localise a site of a possible iodine avid lesion, followed by focused MRI for structural evaluation.

Management

Preoperative management with alpha and beta blockade requires specialised management and should take place over 2–3 weeks to ensure the patient is completely alpha and beta blocked before consideration for surgery. Surgical removal should only be in a specialised unit.

Follow-Up

Follow-up for possible recurrent phaeochromocytoma in the present of SDH mutations, where lesions can occur anywhere in the aortic, from base of skull to pelvis, requires annual surveillance with ultrasound in early years or with MRI over the age of 10. Annual metanephrines and catecholamines.

A short 10-year-old boy, with obesity.

Obesity or weight gain is usually associated with rapid linear growth in a child. It is important to place the child's height and weight in comparison with midparental expectation when undertaking any assessment of weight gain. A child is usually significantly taller than the expected mid parental height, in the context of weight gain or obesity.

The only two conditions of acute onset that cause slow growth in the context of weight gain are hypothyroidism or cortisol excess.

Much longer standing problems such as Prader–Willi syndrome are highly unlikely to present in this way.

The association of oily skin, acne and pubarche in this child should suggest androgen excess. With weight gain and slowing growth the combination indicates cortisol and androgen abnormalities together, which would indicate either an adrenal lesion of new onset, such as adrenal tumour or, less likely, late onset congenital adrenal hyperplasia due to 21-hydroxylase deficiency or 11-hydroxylase deficiency, with increased appetite causing the weight gain. However, with CAH one would expect rapid linear growth as opposed to cortisol excess, where growth inhibition occurs.

History

History should include:

- tiredness, muscle weakness, symptoms of hyperglycaemia, possible headache.

Examination

Examination looks for:

- signs of proximal myopathy, central adiposity, purple colour to striae, ? abdominal mass.

- In particular, small testes in the presence of virilisation indicate a non-testicular, non-central cause for androgen excess, most likely localised to the adrenal, although possible to be tumour elsewhere.

Investigations

Investigations include:

- 24-hour urinary-free cortisol as screening test
- lack of diurnal variation of cortisol at 8 am and preferably midnight. If this is impractical and not available then 4.30 pm cortisol
- androgen screen including DHEAS as tumour marker
- 24-hour urinary steroid profile will identify abnormal androgens suggestive of tumour (can be done on filter paper and can be sent to appropriate laboratory)
- ACTH should be suppressed if adrenal lesion
- Formal Liddle's test with low dose followed by high-dose dexamethasone suppression. (If there is an adrenal lesion, there is a failure of high-dose suppression of cortisol production.)
- If suspicion of malignancy is present CT/MRI of great vessels and chest is necessary pre-operatively, to define chance of metastatic lesions, particularly in lungs and vena cava.

Imaging

Abdominal ultrasound and/or CT/MRI, to identify a likely unilateral lesion.

Treatment

- Surgical excision, bearing in mind that contralateral adrenal suppression will have occurred over time span of symptoms if more than 6 months' duration. Therefore, pay serious attention to slow response and normalisation of steroid production from the remaining adrenal. This may take many months.

- Corticosteroid cover should commence intra-operatively, before removal of lesion and should be continued at stress doses for 3—5 days, decreasing to maintenance corticosteroid at 10 mg/m^2/day in divided dose.
- Reduction of dose should take place slowly over 2—6 months. Note: suicidal and depression can be a complication of too rapid supporting steroid withdrawal.
- Mineralocorticoid replacement is usually not required where tumour has been present on contralateral side as it is only the adrenal cortex that is suppressed by the lesion.
- Expectation of resolution over several months.

Pathology

Malignancy in adrenal tumours is defined more by size greater than 5 cm together with histological findings of increased number of mitotic figures, range 1—10, 10 being most severe, rather than specific vascular invasion/distant metastases, which are less likely, although possible.

> A 3-year-old boy presents with increased penis size (SPL 7.4 cm) and pre-pubertal testicular volume.

Possibilities and Approach to Diagnosis

Issue

Virilisation in a pre-pubertal boy. Normal prepubertal testicular size indicates this is not a centrally driven process.

Differential Diagnosis

- Previously unrecognised CAH: statistically, this is the most likely diagnosis. Simple virilising 21-hydroxylase deficiency is the most common form. 11β-hydroxylase deficiency, or much more rarely

3β-hydroxysteroid dehydrogenase deficiency, may also present in this manner.

Other less common but possible causes:

- Virilising adrenal tumour
- hCG secreting tumour, e.g. hepatoblastoma, hepatoma, teratoma or chorioepithelioma (unlikely gonadal in this case, as you are not told of asymmetry; this can be situated as mediastinal/pineal/retroperitoneum). Testes can be either less than or greater than 4 mL at various stages in this condition.
- Exogenous androgen exposure
- McCune—Albright syndrome.

Rarer conditions:

- Familial Leydig and germ cell maturation (testotoxicosis or male-limited gonadotropin-independent puberty (GIP).

History

History should include:

- history of tempo of genital changes
- ? pubic hair/sexual hair elsewhere
- ? acne, comedones, oily skin, body odour, voice change, muscular development
- ? bony abnormality/pain/unusual fracture to suggest fibrous dysplasia of McCune—Albright syndrome
- birth/neonatal history: ? micropenis/undescended testes that was overtreated with testosterone or hCG; ? transient salt wasting that may indicate 11β-hydroxylase deficiency
- ? parents using topical testosterone gels for any reason
- ? other possible exogenous androgens, e.g. 'herbal' medications
- family history — ? CAH/testotoxicosis/other
- parental age at puberty — ? history of early puberty/pseudo-puberty.

Examination

- Auxology and height relative to MPH; plot previous measurements if available, to estimate growth velocity; this should be able to pinpoint the time of onset of change.

- Skin exam — pigmentation suggesting ↑ ACTH (e.g. non salt-wasting CAH) or café-au-lait lesions (MAS).
- Blood pressure (hypertension may suggest 11β-hydroxylase deficiency/adrenal tumour).
- Repeat testicular exam is very important.
- Ensure the child is pre-pubertal as described — if testes are actually greater than 4 mL, this suggests true/central precocious puberty (proceed to neurologic exam if so).
- If greater than 2.5 mL and less than 4 mL, he could still possibly have testotoxicosis hCG-secreting tumour or MAS.
- Look for other signs of virilisation (pubic/axillary hair/acne/deep voice).
- ? Cushingoid appearance (most adrenal carcinomas produce excessive glucocorticoids and androgens).
- Skin exam — pigmentation/café-au-lait.

Approach to Diagnosis

Initial investigations, subject to availability:

- androgen profile: 17-OHP, DHEAS, androstenedione, testosterone
- urinary steroid profile (24 hours)
- bone age.

Consider:

- plasma renin activity — may be elevated even if serum Na is normal
- ultrasound adrenal glands.

If 21-hydroxylase deficiency is not evident on above investigations, proceed with:

- synacthen test (250 µg at age greater than 2 years) — stimulated 17-OHP and cortisol levels
- deoxycorticosterone and 11-deoxycortisol levels if available
- hCG
- additional imaging if history suggests possible tumour (more likely to be abdominal

as this is not central precocious puberty — pinealoma is exception as it can produce hCG, causing pseudo puberty, only in boys)
- TFTs +/− prolactin (to exclude chronic hypothyroidism, although age 3 would be young for this).

Treatment

Treatment will be targeted at underlying cause.

1. For 21-hydroxylase deficiency:
   - Commence steroid replacement therapy with hydrocortisone (usually 10–15 mg/m^2/day)
   - Although not frankly salt-losing, low-dose fludrocortisone (e.g. 50–100 µg/day) can help to normalise circulatory volume; its use in virilising form may allow for use of a lower dose of glucocorticoid. Chronic salt loss is also associated with poor linear growth.
   - Long-term follow-up of steroid replacement and growth is required.
   - 3–4-monthly growth velocity, clinical assessment, BP.
   - Annual bone age.
   - PRA and 17-OHP can be checked with intermittent clinical reviews; although 17-OHP has known diurnal variation and also increases in response to stress and so has limitations as a test to monitor adequacy of therapy.
2. If virilising tumour is present, surgical excision is required. The majority are adrenal carcinomas which are not chemosensitive. Prognosis is guarded.

DISORDERS OF PUBERTY

An 18-month-old boy is referred with a paediatrician's letter commenting on enlarged testes and muscular hypertrophy,

> provisional diagnosis precocious puberty. His mother kept a record of his growth and development until he was 12 months old but then stopped measuring him when the next baby arrived. Measurement shows that he is exactly the same length as he was at 12 months. Dentition is also delayed. He has become quiet and doesn't want to play. He is also very constipated.
>
> 1 Differential diagnosis?
> 2 Investigations?
> 3 Why are his testes enlarged?
> 4 Why does he have muscular hypertrophy?

Severe primary hypothyroidism due to unusually early-onset, autoimmune thyroiditis. His level of anti-TPO was 1/1,640,000.

He had bilateral hydrocoeles with normal testes. Muscular hypertrophy was due to myxoedema. Treatment with T_4 produced spectacular growth.

> An 8-year-old boy with tall stature, precocious puberty (SPL 7 cm, testicular volume 10 mL) with nodular testes.

Diagnostic Considerations and Management (This Tests Organisation Skills)

Assessment

History to include stature within the family, aiming to identify duration and extent of T action.

Examination — café-au-lait marks/eye signs, any signs of intracranial lesion — cranial nerve exam etc. Lisch nodules are diagnostic of NF1, as hamartomata in the iris can only be seen with a slit lamp examination.

Currently, he has central precocious puberty because testicular volume is 10 mL bilaterally.

Where did it start, i.e. was it testicular/peripheral initially then secondary central stimulation?

What is the nodularity? Could be testicular tumour if unilateral, McCune–Albright syndrome if bilateral.

Consider the following.

Tumours:

- testicular germinoma, Leydig cell tumour — usually unilateral
- possible MAS with or without Leydig tumour — in this case it could be local GNAS mutation with gonadotropin-independent precocity and testicular microlithiasis or Leydig or Sertoli cell tumour or all three
- Carney complex.

Non-tumour:

CAH with adrenal rests — much less likely at age 8 than in older male with poor CAH compliance.

Issues to consider include the following:

- Understanding of significance of microlithiasis in MAS/CAH (not a sign of tumour in these conditions, is bilateral and does not need surgery, although in MAS there may be separate indications for biopsy, as multiple lesions can occur in one patient).
- Know how to interpret testicular ultrasound — the lesions of MAS are around the rete testis and bilaterally symmetrical.
- Use of peripheral hCG vs CSF hCG measurement — if central intracranial germinoma is considered, neither is very helpful, but CSF levels x20 normal (greater than 200 u/L) are diagnostic.

Treatment

Treatment to include the following.

- Surgery for Leydig tumours (usually benign so local excision probably OK).
- Peripheral and central blockade of puberty may be needed.

- Use of aromatase inhibitors are more effective for control of peripheral precocious puberty in a male, as they prevent androgen to oestrogen conversion and thus slow bone age advance. Tamoxifen (SERM) can be used as an adjunct, to further block peripheral action of oestrogen on epiphyseal fusion.
- If secondary central stimulation has occurred, GNRH analogue may also be needed for adequate control.

> A 16-year-old boy with delayed puberty.
> *Approach, with emphasis on management for different disorders.*
> **Similar superficially to the scenario above but changed emphasis.**

Assessment

- Constitutional — ascertain family history.
- Isolated hypogonadotropic hypogonadism +/− anosmia — consider LHRH stimulation testing +/− MRI brain and pituitary (not always necessary, especially if family history of Kallmann syndrome). Its main use is to exclude tumour as a cause for the problem, not to confirm olfactory bulb absence!
- Hypothalamic/pituitary lesion — tumour including prolactinoma, craniopharyngioma — consider MRI if clinical suspicion.
- Primary testicular cause, e.g. XXY — associated features, small testicular size — confirm with karyotype.
- Chronic disease including Crohn's, coeliac, renal, cardiac etc.
- Rare disorders — adrenal, LH receptor etc.

Management

- Constitutional delay — induction of puberty reasonable, given his age (e.g. intramuscular testosterone injections 50–100 mg 3–4-weekly x 3 doses and monitor response over 6 months).

- Options for treatment of central HH include use of hCG as LH mimic to allow endogenous testosterone production. Current evidence suggests beneficial intratesticular effects in terms of spermatogenesis and ultimate fertility. However, treatment is much more expensive than conventional testosterone replacement (e.g. oral testosterone starting at low dose and increasing over ~ 2 years to full adult replacement; can also then use depot preparations).
- GH if needed (usually not unless central lesion, in which case will need to be delayed until at least 12 months after completion of treatment for underlying lesion).
- ? place for testicular biopsy in XXY for sperm salvage (unproven to date but may be useful in future), future ICSI — this can be discussed in individual cases.

> A 14-year-old girl presented to the paediatrician with concerns about lack of breast development and not starting periods. Parents reported that she had been the shortest in her class since she started school and they put it down to the fact that there are a number of family members who are relatively short. However, now they feel she is not growing at all and appears even shorter because other girls are maturing and getting taller. She has been falling behind with her school work, seems rather withdrawn and no longer wants to spend time with her friends.

Q1. What Differential Diagnosis will you Consider and what Specific Questions will you Explore in the History?

Answer

The presenting history may be explained by familial short stature and constitutional delay in growth and puberty (CDGP), but pathological causes must first be considered.

Turner syndrome must be considered in any girl with short stature.

Other diagnoses in any adolescent with delayed puberty and short stature are autoimmune hypothyroidism, pituitary hormone deficiencies (e.g. due to craniopharyngioma) and chronic systemic illness (e.g. coeliac disease or inflammatory bowel disease).

The problems with school work and being withdrawn may be due to lack of concentration and lethargy from acquired hypothyroidism. Autoimmune hypothyroidism is more common in Turner syndrome and therefore both problems may be present in this case. Thus, a thorough history should be taken to find clues to these pathological causes.

Q2. What Aspects of Physical Examination are Important?

Answer

In the physical examination, the following need careful assessment: pattern of weight and height plotted on a growth chart, height in comparison to parents' heights, nutritional status, status of breast development and pubic hair, general and cardiovascular system examination for features of Turner syndrome, and neck examination for goitre and specific features of hypothyroidism.

Q3. If History and Examination Exclude Chronic Systemic Illness, What are the Most Important Investigations you will Consider?

Answer

- thyroid function tests (TSH and free thyroxine) and anti TPO antibodies for autoimmune hypothyroidism
- karyotype for Turner syndrome
- FBC for anaemia (which may be due to a systemic condition not yet being overt, such as coeliac disease or inflammatory bowel disease)

- coeliac screen (usually a tissue transglutaminase test).

Q4. How was this Case Assessed?

Answer

Examination revealed that the girl was exceptionally short for her parents, prepubertal and relatively overweight. The history and examination suggested hypothyroidism with the following features: a tendency to fall asleep in the daytime for 2 years, no goitre but skin was dry and rough, pulse was 60/minute and knee reflexes showed slow relaxation. There were no specific features of Turner syndrome but finger nails were hyperconvex.

Investigation results showed a karyotype of 45,XO in all cells examined, TSH 115 mU/L and free thyroxine 6 pmol/L. Thus the patient did indeed have Turner syndrome and hypothyroidism. In view of the former, further assessments were undertaken.

Ultrasound abdomen and pelvis showed a small uterus, streak ovaries and no renal tract abnormalities. Cardiac assessment revealed no cardiac abnormalities. Owing to hypothyroidism, thyroid autoantibodies were checked and found to be positive.

Q5. How was this Patient Managed?

Answer

The results and diagnosis were explained to the patient and parents. The immediate priority was management of hypothyroidism with thyroxine replacement and this was started as levothyroxine tablet once daily. Thyroid function was repeated after 4 weeks and then checked at 3 to 6-monthly intervals.

The next priority is managing oestrogen deficiency. Lack of oestrogen beyond age 13 years can have detrimental long-term effects on bone mineralisation and cognitive function. Therefore low-dose oestrogen (a tenth of adult replacement) was started. The dose was gradually increased at 6 to 12-monthly intervals depending on progress with breast development and gain in height. Full adult replacement was given when near final height was attained. At that stage oestrogen was given in combination with progesterone in cycles and this brought about regular periods.

This patient was also given growth hormone treatment to optimise her height.

Q6. What is the Long-Term Management of this Patient?

Answer

This young person will need continued follow-up and at least annual check-ups as an adult. She is likely to need lifelong thyroxine and oestrogen replacement. She will need to be counselled about infertility and options thereof.

> A 15-year-old girl of normal height and appearance presents with primary amenorrhoea and lack of breast development.

Issues

No signs of puberty — ? why. This warrants investigation at age 15 as it is about 4 years later than average. However, if there is a strong family history of severe pubertal delay, it may still be within normal limits.

Approach

- History.
- Pregnancy/neonatal period — any concerns such as dysmorphism, lymphoedema, appearance of genitalia, history of hernia repair.
- Prior illness/therapy (tumours/chemo/radiation/any chronic illness that might be associated with pubertal delay). Symptoms to suggest chronic illness — anorexia, IBD, thyroid etc.
- Growth pattern throughout childhood — is this consistent with family/sibling pattern?
- Family history of delayed or absent puberty/problems conceiving in parents/relatives.

- Sense of smell in patient or family members as Kallman syndrome can have differential expression in family members.

Examination

Assess body proportions, weight for height, breast tissue, genitalia, features of Turner syndrome, neurologic exam for intracranial lesion.

Possible Diagnoses

Hypergonadotrophic states: gonadal insufficiency/failure

- Turner syndrome is by far the most common abnormality although short stature is common feature. However, if there is a tall family, the girl may be of a normal height but very short for her family.

All other causes of primary gonadal failure are much less common (in order of likelihood):

- mixed gonadal dysgenesis
- CAIS or PAIS
- rare adrenal disorders, e.g. 17α-hydroxylase deficiency
- 5α-reductase deficiency.

  Ovarian insufficiency is seen in ~ 1% of females but most do not present in this manner, i.e. usually get some breast development then failure to progress normally/primary amenorrhoea.

  In those who present at puberty — up to 50% will have abnormal karyotype.

  Gonadal dysgenesis

- Mixed gonadal dysgenesis.

  Suspicion if abnormal genitalia, virilisation or lateralising features.

  Genitalia can be normal female or ambiguous (reflects in utero T exposure)

  Gonads often asymmetrical — 'streak' ovaries/dysgenetic testes.

- 46XY gonadal dysgenesis/complete sex reversal.

Delayed puberty in a phenotypic female is a typical presentation. Female genital differentiation is the constitutive result of the complete lack of testicular function. Pubic hair is scanty also. Ambiguous genitalia found only in partial/incomplete forms.

SRY mutations − found in up to 20% of XY gonadal dysgenesis.

Other gene mutations are rarer, e.g. SF1, DAX1, WT1.

- 46XX gonadal dysgenesis

  Pure ovarian agenesis with a 46XX karyotype; rare.

  Characteristics: normal or tall height, no dysmorphic features, normal female external genitalia, hypoplastic/no ovarian development. Can have some small amount of breast tissue but amenorrhoea is universal. Molecular basis remains unexplained.

- Several genes have been identified as causative for premature ovarian failure

  FMR1 gene (Xq27.1) permutations, i.e. fragile X carrier status − 60−200 repeats associated with primary ovarian failure

  AIRE gene (APS) 22q22.3

  X deletions: critical region Xp11.2-p22.1 (numerous candidate genes for POF reported in this area).

Acquired gonadal failure

- Autoimmune − often found in association with other AI conditions, especially Addison's/Type 1 polyglandular syndrome. Common cause of ovarian insufficiency but usually have pubertal arrest/later onset of gonadal failure as opposed to complete pubertal absence. Ovarian autoantibodies are notoriously unreliable.
- Chemotherapy, e.g. nitrogen mustard compounds, alkylating agents, cyclophosphamide − related to dose and age at time of chemotherapy − often recovers later even if help with puberty is needed.
- Post radiotherapy − particularly total body irradiation for bone marrow transplant.

Gonadotrophin receptor mutations

- LH receptor mutation (loss of function mutation) − rare; XY with LH receptor mutation − Leydig cell aplasia/hypoplasia.
- Severe mutations present with female external genitalia, absent Mullerian structures and lack of breast development (or any male or female pubertal development). Vas deferens and epididymis are present. Low testosterone despite high LH/FSH (no response to hCG). Gonads may be inguinal or intra-abdominal − biopsy shows *absence of Leydig cells* but Sertoli cells, spermatogonia and primary spermatocytes. (Less severe mutations can present with male hypogonadism, i.e. assigned male from Day 1.)

Congenital adrenal hyperplasia: 17-hydroxylase-17,20-lyase deficiency

- Characterised by elevated progesterone, pregnenolone, 17-OHP and 17-OH pregnenolone and deficient oestrogen synthesis.
- Female patients are phenotypically normal and present with pubertal delay.
- BP will be high; K^+ may be low.

  *Hypo*gonadotropic states:

  ? is this a delay in normal progression or permanent defect.

- 'Intact axis' but other chronic issue (usually secondary and reversible), i.e. 'functional hypogonadotropic hypogonadism'; e.g. chronic illness such as cystic fibrosis, renal disease, inflammatory bowel disease, excess physical activity such as ballet dancers, anorexia nervosa/ chronic under-nutrition.
- Permanent gonadotropin deficiency:
  - Kallmann syndrome (anosmia)
  - Hypogonadotrophic hypogonadotropism (less common in females than in males)
  - Acquired deficiencies, e.g. post radiation/ trauma/LCH/infiltration.
- Prolactinoma

- Can present with complete pubertal delay (more commonly with arrest).
- Ask about galactorrhoea.

Initial Assessment

This should include the following.

- Height charting with midparental heights to define whether it is physiologic or pathologic delay.
- Bone age for growth potential.
- LH/FSH will provide rapid evidence of primary vs secondary ovarian dysfunction.
- Microarray or karyotype – the latter is better but may not be available. If FSH is raised and microarray is used, add FISH for Y as it will detect even low level Y.
- Ultrasound for gonads and presence of uterus.
- MRI head if indicated, to exclude tumour.
- Biopsy of gonads if needed and removal if Y present.

Treatment

- Ensure gender identity as female.
- Ensure safety, i.e. gonad removal if Y present.
- Undertake feminisation over 2–3 years, adding progestogen at end of this time, if uterus present.
- Support and counselling if needed for patient and family.

A 2-year-old girl presented to the paediatrician with rapid enlargement of breasts and a few pubic hairs. Her mother reported that her behaviour was rather difficult and like that of a 'teenager'. There was no history of accidental ingestion of oestrogen-containing medicines (such as the oral contraceptive pill).

Q1. What were the Concerns at this Stage?

Answer

The presenting complaints and child's parents' concerns in a girl under age 8 years raises the possibility of precocious puberty rather than isolated premature thelarche or isolated premature adrenarche. The history of dramatic breast development along with appearance of pubic hair is suggestive of significant pubertal progress. Isolated premature thelarche is relatively common at this age, but the breast size tends to be asymmetrical and can fluctuate. There would be no breast development in isolated premature adrenarche.

Q2. How did the Paediatrician Address the Problem?

Answer

The paediatrician examined the child and noted definite breast development at Tanner stage 3 on both sides. There were a few short pubic hairs (stage 2), without any evidence of clitoromegaly. The child's height was on the 50th centile, which was appropriate for the midparental height. Examination of the skin did not show evidence of café-au-lait birth marks or other forms of hyperpigmentation. Investigations were organised to check for bone maturation and hormonal evidence for precocious puberty. These included hand X-ray for bone age, basal gonadotrophins (LH and FSH) and oestradiol. A plan was made to contact the family as soon as the results were available and to review changes in growth and pubertal development in 2 months.

Q3. What was the Outcome? What did the Investigations Show?

Answer

Two weeks after the initial consultation, the child presented to the hospital with a large vaginal bleed. Her mother had noted her to be 'miserable' in her behaviour. She was restless at night and sleep was disturbed.

Of the investigations performed at the previous visit, some results were available. The basal gonadotrophins were undetectable, but the serum oestradiol was 2400 pmol/L (normal less than 40 pmol/L in a child).

Q4. How do you Interpret the High Serum Oestradiol Level?

Answer

Interpreting gonadotrophin levels with the oestradiol level together provides information about presence of precocious puberty and also whether it is central or peripheral. At this age, oestradiol is usually not detectable. A level of 2400 pmol/L is extremely high. This in combination with unmeasureable gonadotrophin levels suggests precocious puberty which is gonadotrophin independent. In gonadotrophin-dependent precocious puberty (central precocious puberty), oestradiol can be high but not to this extent. Almost invariably, this oestradiol was produced from an autonomous source in the ovary. In this case, there are two main differential diagnoses. The first is McCune–Albright syndrome and the second is an oestradiol-secreting tumour of the ovary, such as a granulosa cell tumour. The former is less likely as there are no obvious café-au-lait patches.

Q5. What Further Investigations were Performed?

Answer

A pelvic ultrasound scan showed the presence of a large unilateral tumour, presumably arising from the ovary. An MR scan confirmed the presence of an encapsulated ovarian tumour with variegated echo appearances. The tumour was removed surgically and histology was that of a granulosa cell tumour.

Q6. How did the Patient do on Follow-Up Assessment?

Answer

The patient's breast development receded and there were no further vaginal bleeds. Her parents felt that she was 'back to her usual self'.

Q What is the Prognosis for this Condition?

Answer

The child will need follow-up scanning of the contralateral ovary (from which a biopsy was taken and found to be normal). Overall the prognosis is good, but careful watch will be required on a long-term basis.

> **A 2-year-old girl with isolated breast enlargement.**

Evaluation and Management

Perspective

- Likely isolated infantile thelarche – normal variant related to gonadotrophin surge in infancy; needs follow-up to ensure resolution as opposed to progression (up to 10% in some series develop central precocious puberty). As with previous scenario.
- True precocious puberty less common but possible – need to exclude.

Evaluation

History includes the following.

- History usually indicates breast development from early months of life (consistent with the normal infant LH and FSH surge).
- Assess parental impression as to progression or possible regression over intervening period; ? has a growth spurt been documented.
- ? any vaginal discharge or bleeding or features of pubarche (in this age group combined oestrogen and androgen effect suggests adrenal tumour).
- ? associated features, e.g. irritability/other suggesting raised ICP.

- ? bony abnormality/previous fracture/pain suggesting fibrous dysplasia of McCune–Albright syndrome.

  Examination includes the following.

- Breast stage and development (can be useful to measure diameter of breast tissue to allow comparison over time) – ? firm (suggests active oestrogen) or soft tissue.
- Height – ? previous measurements to assess growth velocity.
- Skin – ? café-au-lait spots (NF1 associated with true precocious puberty, usually with chiasmal glioma).
- ? features to suggest hypothyroidism.
- Neurologic exam – ? intracranial abnormality.
- Genital assessment.

Monitoring/Investigations

If no associated/concerning features to suggest true precocious puberty, monitoring/investigations include the following.

- Monitoring of breast tissue, growth velocity and general exam 3–6-monthly is usually all that is warranted. Bone age may be reassuring.
- If history or exam suggests ongoing active oestrogenisation, investigations may include basal LH, FSH to indicate central vs. peripheral cause. High LH more likely to indicate central pathology. If available, this might be followed by GNRH test for confirmation.
- A very high level of oestradiol may indicate ovarian lesion.
- TFTs – hypothyroidism may present with thelarche, usually in later childhood.
- Pelvic ultrasound for ? tumour, ? bilateral follicular activity to indicate central stimulation.

If LH and FSH are low but ongoing oestrogenisation is evident – peripheral precocious puberty.

If other features of McCune Albright syndrome are present, check for up regulation/overactivity of other hormones that involve Gs-α signalling (e.g. hyperthyroidism) – uncommon in this age group.

Treatment of precocious puberty in MAS is difficult – aromatase inhibitors and anti-oestrogen therapy are used but response is poor. Ongoing peripheral precocious puberty can stimulate secondary central activation of puberty, in which case GnRH agonists may be used in addition.

> **A 7-year-old girl with thelarche and tall stature.**

Approach

Approach aims to differentiate between true, established and progressive early puberty that may need intervention and premature onset of thelarche, where puberty will progress at normal tempo and treatment is unlikely to be needed.

Both scenarios arise from premature awakening of the gonadotrophin-gonadal axis.

The decision as to whether treatment is warranted or not depends predominantly on the child and family's ability to manage the emotional upheaval of early puberty and/or menarche.

Treatment of pubertal onset at age 7–8 years is unlikely to have a major effect on final height outcome.

Approach

Thorough history and examination, assessing both puberty and general well-being.

Key questions for assessment:

- Is this true puberty?
- Is it occurring outside normal timeframe? (Yes in this case as less than 8 years.)
- Is rate or tempo of progression abnormal?

- What is the underlying mechanism? Is there a sinister underlying cause?
- Is puberty likely to progress and if so, what impact will that have on physical and psychosocial development?

History

- Timing of onset of breast development:
  - rate of change/progression; may be unilateral in first instance-this is quite normal.
- History of growth parameters over childhood:
  - girls 'programmed' for earlier puberty are often tall throughout childhood years with advanced bone age
  - ? overweight (also advances BA)
  - ? recent growth velocity acceleration.
- Family history of timing of parents' puberty, including maternal menarche; MPH and target range.
- History of CNS infection/head trauma/ perinatal insult, CNS disturbance/raised ICP? Note: IUGR may be associated with early onset of puberty.
  - Café-au-lait marks — NF1
  - History of fracture + café-au-lait marks: ? McCune–Albright.
- ? associated signs of adrenarche (may precede thelarche).
- ? vaginal discharge or bleeding:
  - Early puberty often switches on and off. If endometrium present, withdrawal bleed likely — associated with history of breast decreasing in size or becoming soft and inactive simultaneously. This is *not* menarche.
  - If puberty is advanced and a true menstrual bleed has occurred, it is likely to be heavier, longer. This will be associated with limited growth potential, advanced bone age. It indicates a long-standing, pathologic process.

Examination

- Growth: plot height and weight — if retrospective measurements are available, establish growth trajectory.
- Breast exam: important to *palpate* breast tissue as chest wall adiposity can mimic breast development; true breast tissue of puberty is firm to palpate. Tanner stage.
- Note: breast only may indicate hypothyroidism or ovarian cyst/tumour, i.e. oestrogen only.
- Look for other evidence of oestrogen exposure (vulva/vaginal mucosa).
- Pubic hair/other virilisation — implies androgen production (peripheral).
- Skin exam — ? café-au-lait (McCune–Albright syndrome/NF1)/other stigmata of NF1.

Investigations/Ongoing Monitoring

- If very early breast development (B2), it is reasonable to observe in first instance without additional investigations. However, by definition onset of puberty at under 8 years is not normal. Failure to investigate will miss some pathology.
- Monitor 3–6-monthly — GV and ongoing breast development.
- If breast development is B3 or more, this suggests puberty has either been established for up to 1 year or tempo of progression has been abnormally quick — more likely to warrant additional investigations +/− treatment.
- Do basal (random) LH, FSH, oestradiol, TFTs, PRL.
- +/− LHRH stim test (not necessary if basal levels in pubertal range).
- Ultrasound of pelvis.
- Tumour markers (e.g. hCG and AFP).
- +/− MRI brain as indicated; central pathology that requires specific therapy (e.g. intracranial tumour such as astrocytoma/ glioma/germ cell tumour) is less common in

girls less than 5 years but consider if any suggestion of rapid pubertal progression or CNS disturbance.

Treatment

- Majority of girls will not need treatment for the pubertal progression as tempo of puberty and menarche will be normal with good FH outcome.
- Many girls will have major emotional/social upheaval with such early puberty and may require treatment solely for this reason.
- If final height outcome is poor (less than 3rd centile), or menarche is imminent − treatment with GnRH agonist, e.g. goserelin/Diphereline® 12-weekly can be given.
- +/− specific therapy if alternative underlying cause found.

THYROID DISORDERS

> A 39/40 weeks, 2.8 kg, well baby with cord blood of TSH 95 mU/L and repeat blood tests on day 5 as follows:
>
> - fT_4 = 0.6 ng/dL (0.9−2.2)
> - T_4 = 3 ug% (6.5−16.3)
> - TSH = 150 µIU/mL (1.7−9.1)

What is Your Interpretation?

TFTs show severe primary hypothyroidism: likely agenesis/ectopia/dyshormonogenesis.

Thyroid scan showed athyreosis. The baby was treated with L-thyroxine 12µg/kg/day with normalisation of fT_4 by 4 weeks. Serial TFTs over the next 12 months were normal and there was minimal increase in L-thyroxine requirement.

The patient was lost to follow-up after this and returned after 8 months for review. Though off thyroxine, growth and development was normal.

What is the Likely Diagnosis?

Probable transient hypothyroidism secondary to TSH blocking antibodies.

- Normal thyroid gland can be missed on thyroid scintiscan in the presence of blocking antibodies.
- TSH Binding Inhibitory Immunoglobulin (TSH receptor blockade) is present in maternal thyroid disorders. Transplacental transfer results in failure of iodide trapping by the thyroid gland even if TSH is high. Its presence causes transient neonatal hypothyroidism, without goitre. Apparent 'athyreosis' on nuclear scan.
- Very high risk of recurrence in subsequent pregnancies—parents & doctors to be aware of this condition.

Differential diagnosis of athyreosis on nuclear scan.

- True athyreosis (undetectable Tg).
- Transplacental transfer of TSH- R blocking antibodies; normal gland on USG.
- Na/I symporter mutations (iodide trapping defect); goitre evident clinically or by USG.

> A 6-day-old healthy neonate, 31/40 week with birth weight of 1400 g, exclusively breast-fed, was found to be jaundiced. The results of the thyroid tests done were as follows:
>
> - TSH 5 uIU/mL
> - T_4 3.5 µg/dL
> - fT_4 0.8 ng/dL

What is Your Interpretation?

Immature HPT axis in the preterm.

Decreased TRH production and secretion, immature response of thyroid to TSH, inefficient organification of iodine, low thyroid binding globulin, high Type 3 deiodinase activity, decreased conversion of T_4 into T_3.

Points to Remember

- Compared to term infants, premature infants have lower T_4 and fT_4 with normal to low TSH.
- Lower T_4 correlates with gestational age and birth weight.
- Takes 3–8 weeks for T_4 and T_3 levels to reach same as term infants.
- Usually mild or transient thyroid dysfunction.
- Delayed TSH elevation (up to 3 weeks).
- No long-term or short-term benefits of treating preterms with LT_4.
- Consensus currently recommends not starting treatment unless associated with elevated TSH (Cochrane Database Syst Rev 2007).
- Rescreening is recommended for all infants weighing less than 1500 g after 3 weeks, especially in sick preterms (JPEDS 2010).
- Factors which can affect thyroid functions in the pre-term baby are: immature HPT axis, immature thyroid ability to synthesise hormones, effects of neonatal disease (non-thyroidal illness), dietary iodine deficiency (e.g. TPN), iodine excess (antiseptics, radio-opaque agents), dopamine/dobutamine infusion.

A neonate born at 37 weeks and weighing 2500 g, developed sepsis and marked jaundice. Thyroid functions done on day 4 because of the jaundice demonstrated:

- TSH = 5.4 μIU/mL (1.7–9.1)
- T_4 = 3.2 μg% (6.5–16.3)
- fT_4 = 0.6 ng/dL (0.9–2.2)

How will you Interpret these Values?

Low T_4 and fT_4 with normal TSH.

Differential Diagnoses Considered on these Results

- Sick euthyroid syndrome.
- Secondary hypothyroidism.
- Primary CH with delayed TSH elevation.
- TSH inhibition can also occur with dopamine infusion or high-dose glucocorticoids.

Sick Euthyroid Syndrome

This is cytokine-mediated inhibition of thyroid function and metabolism. There is reduced TRH release, TSH response, T_4 production and release, conversion T_4 to T_3 and production of TBG. Very low fT4 values have been reported to be associated with a poor prognosis.

A term, 3500 g, neonate, operated for duodenal atresia on day 2, recovered well by day 5 and was started on enteral feeding. Jaundice was noted on day 7. Thyroid function then reported as:

- fT_4 = 0. 4 ng% (0.9–2.2)
- T_4 = 1.5 μg% (6.5–16.3)
- TSH = 45.0 μIU/mL (1.7–9.1)

What is this Primary Hypothyroidism Due To?

Transient hypothyroidism, most likely due to excessive iodine exposure with betadine paint during surgery, leading to the Wolff–Chaikoff effect (transient). During excess iodine exposure, when iodine concentration reaches the threshold in serum and thyroid, there is transient inhibition of synthesis and secretion of thyroxine. This is an autoregulatory mechanism to prevent excess trapping of iodide during overload and is more pronounced in immature newborns. It was first described in the 1980s in babies exposed to iodine in antiseptic baths, during procedures, vaginal betadine Rx of breastfeeding mothers etc.

Elevated TSH, Low fT₄, Elevated Urinary Iodine

Common in newborn babies, especially preterms and those in areas with some dietary iodine excess. Preterm babies are particularly susceptible to iodine-induced hypothyroidism because of the immaturity of the autoregulation of the thyroid gland. It may be considered a safe practice to avoid iodine-containing agents in obstetrics and nursery.

An 80-day-old male infant was referred for 'inadequately controlled' congenital hypothyroidism. He was a term baby, born by normal vaginal delivery with birth weight of 3200 g. CH was diagnosed in a local hospital and he was commenced on day 20 with LT4 37.5 µg daily. There was no remarkable family history of thyroid disorder or history of maternal medications. On examination he was a healthy baby with weight of 5 kg and length of 58 cm. The thyroid was not enlarged.

Serial thyroid function tests were done and the results were as follows:

Ultrasonography revealed a normal gland located in the normal position.

TABLE 14.1 Results of Serial Thyroid Function Tests

Age (days)	TSHn µIU/ml 1.7–9.1	T4 µg% 6.5–16.3	fT4 ng/dl 0.9–2.2
20	7	3.5	1.7
50	0. 5	4.5	2.6
64	<0.1	4.0	3.8
78	<0.1	4.8	3.8

TABLE 14.2 Serial Thyroid Profile After Discontinuing LT4

Age (days)	TSH µIU/ml (0.8–6)	T4 µg% (7.5–15.5)	fT4 ng% (0.8–2.0)
80	<0.1	2.4	3.8
94	1.4	3.5	1.9
130	2.0	3.2	1.7

How do you Interpret the Results of Investigations? What is the Diagnosis in this Infant?

Although T4 is low, the fT4 is elevated, with suppression of TSH.

Congenital thyroid binding globulin (TBG) deficiency

- TBG concentration: 5.36 mg/L (Ref 15.5–43.2), partial or complete deficiency.
- Prevalence 1/5000–10,000 newborns (Western data), males affected.
- TBG – the principal transport protein for thyroid hormones in serum. Synthesised in liver.
- Gene locus on long arm of X chromosome.
- No metabolic effect, hence does not need treatment.

Awareness important to prevent unnecessary investigations and treatment for 'hypothyroidism'.

For this infant, LT₄ discontinued on day 80 and serial thyroid profile after discontinuing LT₄ was as follows:

Parents were counselled and reassured.

What are the side effects of thyroxine overtreatment?

- Short term: tachycardia, excessive nervousness, disturbed sleep pattern. Short-term effects are reversed by dosage adjustment and carries little or no long-term risk.

- Long term (3—6 months): osteoporosis, premature cranial synostosis and bone age advancement.

A 5-day-old neonate was found to have elevated TSH on neonatal screening, less than 100 mIU/L.

Repeat thyroid tests were as follows:

- TSH 145 µIU/L (1.7—9.1)
- T$_4$ 4.8 µg% (6.5—16.3)
- fT$_4$ 0.4 ng/dL (0.9—2.2)

There were no dysmorphic features and thyroid scan and ultrasound showed the thyroid gland in normal location, normal-sized gland with increased uptake.

Diagnosed as congenital hypothyroidism, probably dyshormonogenesis. Treatment was commenced with L-thyroxine 10 µg/kg with normalisation of fT$_4$ and T$_4$ by 4 weeks.

At 3 months central hypotonia and delayed motor development was noted. By 2 years of age, there was increasing jerky movements and difficulty in coordination. Diagnosed then as choreoathetoid cerebral palsy.

What is the Possible Aetiology? Inadequate/Delayed Thyroxine Replacement in the Neonatal Period? Are there any other Possibilities?

Likely TTF-1 defect.

Gene involved in thyroid development and function.

Usually, thyroid gland in normal location, size varying from normal to hypoplastic to absent gland.

Autosomal dominant inheritance with variable penetrance.

A 9-month-old infant was admitted for evaluation of protuberant abdomen and constipation. Ultrasound of the abdomen showed multiple haemangiomas in the liver.

Thyroid function tests were as follows:

- TSH 95 µIU/L
- T$_4$ 4.5 µg%
- fT$_4$ 0.6 ng%

Scintiscan showed a normally situated thyroid gland with increased I^{131} uptake.

What is the Diagnosis? How Would you Manage this Patient?

Acquired Hypothyroidism Due to Consumptive Hypothyroidism

Haemangioendotheliomas express Type 3 deiodinase which can result in rapid degradation of T$_4$ and T$_3$. It can require large doses of L-thyroxine (even up to 30 ug/kg/day) to normalise fT$_4$ and is best treated with a combination of LT$_4$ and T$_3$ to achieve euthyroid state. The haemangioendotheliomas may be treated with steroids or alpha-interferon. Regular monitoring of TFTs is crucial for management of these patients. The hypothyroidism resolves with regression of the haemangiomas.

A 10-day-old baby whose mother has Grave's disease is irritable and not thriving.

Clinical Assessment, Investigations and Management

This baby must be presumed to have neonatal thyrotoxicosis until proven otherwise.

Differential Diagnoses

Differential diagnoses include general paediatric conditions that may arise in neonates.

- Sepsis/meningitis/other infection.
- Poor established feeding pattern.
- Other systemic illness (e.g. cardiac defect) causing poor feeding with subsequent irritability and failure to thrive.
- Mechanical problems/other GI tract abnormality.
- Neonatal abstinence syndrome/withdrawal (in setting of maternal substance abuse).
- CAH should be considered in a baby who has not regained birth weight.
- Non-accidental injury.

Neonatal Thyrotoxicosis

- Most commonly secondary to transfer of thyroid stimulating immunoglobulins (TSIs) — (also known as thyrotropin receptor stimulating antibodies) from mother with Graves' disease.
- TSIs may continue to be produced even years after thyroidectomy/radioiodine ablation. It is especially important to identify these women in pregnancy as a predictor of possible neonatal problems.
- When TSI related, thyrotoxicosis is transient, limited by clearance of maternal Ab.

Clinical Features in Neonate

- Can be apparent at birth or delayed for a few days — usually present by day 10.
- Delay occurs either 2^0 maternal anti-thyroid drugs or co-existing TSH receptor *blocking* Ab.
- Levels of TSI from mother in third trimester and from infant correlate well with development of neonatal hyperthyroidism (~ 100% if greater than x5 normal).
- Goitre present in most.
- CNS: irritability, jittery, restless.

- CVS: tachycardia, arrhythmias, cardiac failure (a common presentation by the time the diagnosis is considered!), pulmonary hypertension.
- Hypermetabolism: voracious appetite, weight loss, sweating, diarrhoea.

The following are less likely at 10 days, but possible:

- Bony effects: Advanced bone age (T_4 has an effect on osteoblastic /osteoclastic bone remodelling), craniosynostosis, microcephaly
- Others: hepatosplenomegaly, thrombocytopenia.

Clinical Course in the Neonate

- Initially dependent on control in newborn period — cardiac failure/persistent pulmonary hypertension of the newborn (PPHN)/thrombocytopenia can be life-threatening (12—20% mortality in some series).
- Usually remits by 20 weeks; virtually all euthyroid by ~ 48 weeks.
- Rarely: endogenous TSI production occurs.

Suggested screening investigations (possibly not done in this infant) include the following.

- Some centres check cord blood levels of fT_4, TSH and TSI — not universal practice.
- All infants of mothers with history of Graves' disease should have a clinical examination and bloods taken for fT_4, TSH (and TSI if not done on cord blood) on ~ day 3 (day 2—7) and again between day 10 and day 14.
- If results of thyroid function are all normal, no further treatment/follow-up required.
- If hypothyroid, repeat in further 2—3 days and reassess need for investigation/treatment.
- If hyperthyroid, proceed to treatment as below; check FBE, LFTs also and consider bone age and skull X-ray.

Management of Neonatal Thyrotoxicosis

Medical Therapy of Confirmed Thyrotoxicosis

1. Thionamides — carbimazole/methimazole

   These agents are actively transported into the thyroid gland where they inhibit both the organification of iodine to tyrosine residues in thyroglobulin and the coupling of iodotyrosines, i.e. block *synthesis* of thyroid hormone.

   Propylthiouracil (PTU) is no longer usually recommended for use as first-line agent in children, given concern about serious hepatotoxic effects. It can be used in this particular setting as a short-duration medication, to help reduce T_4 to T_3 conversion during the acute illness.

2. Additional therapies for early symptomatic relief

   When aiming for early symptomatic control, difficulty arises with ongoing release of thyroid hormone that is already formed (can continue for up to 3 weeks — usually less in neonates).

   - Propranolol — controls effects of excessive adrenergic stimulation; dose 0.25—0.75 mg/kg 8-hourly; S/E: bradycardia, hypotension (hypoglycaemia to lesser effect).
   - Iodine solution, e.g. Lugol's iodine solution (5% KI — 8 mg iodine per drop) —give 1 to 3 drops/day.

Work to suppress thyroid hormone synthesis but main reason to use is because it promptly blocks release of thyroid hormone.

Usually only used for first 2—3 weeks, until less clinically symptomatic.

Breast feeding (this is only relevant if the mother is thyrotoxic and needing current treatment)

Both PTU and methimazole (from carbimazole) are detectable in breast milk but appear not to affect neonatal thyroid function if mother's dose is less than 15 mg/day carbimazole or less than 150 mg/day PTU.

PTU — highly protein bound — is excreted into the milk in much lower concentrations (0.025—0.077%) than methimazole (1 : 1 serum to milk ratio).

Follow-Up

If baby treated for thyrotoxicosis, review with clinical exam and TFTs weekly until stable, then 2-weekly, aiming to wean doses when possible. Aim for fT_4 in upper third of normal range — suppression of TSH may take weeks to revert.

Most literature suggests that the majority of cases resolve by 3 months, as maternal antibody titres wane, but can persist out to 12—18 months in occasional cases. If persistent beyond 6 months, recheck baby's antibody levels which should be decreasing. If not, query possible activating TSH receptor mutation (autosomal-dominant condition, although this is unlikely in setting of antibody positive disease originally).

A girl of 15 is irritable and is found to have a 'hot' nodule on scan.

A 'hot' nodule is an isolated lesion with increased uptake to either iodine or technetium, with partial or complete suppression of the remaining of the thyroid gland.

Firstly, this is a relatively rare condition in adolescents or children. It is common in those over the age of 18—20 years and is always a toxic adenoma, benign in nature with minimal risk of malignancy within the lesion. Typical findings on CT scan are of complete suppression of the remainder of the thyroid gland.

In a younger child or adolescent it is important to exclude abnormality of the whole gland, such as an absent contralateral lobe giving the appearance of a hot nodule, when in fact the entire thyroid gland is abnormal. This can occur in the context of dyshormonogenesis in a dysplastic gland or possibly with Graves' disease in a dysplastic gland.

- Thyroid function is likely to be elevated in this, with negative antibodies.
- Biopsy is unnecessary.
- Optimal treatment utilises and ablative dose of I^{131} around 17 mC (750 MBq) which is taken up solely into the hot area, leaving the remainder of the cold unaffected thyroid gland protected.
- After destruction of the hot toxic lesion, the remainder of the gland should recover in 2–6 weeks with normal residual function permanently.
- If I^{131} is not available, surgery for the nodule itself is curative.

A 12-year-old girl has noticed uniform swelling in the front of the neck for 12 months.

Approach

Goitre is common in areas of iodine deficiency, where it may be small, large, multinodular and/or familial.

- If iodine replete, it is most likely that a thyroid swelling will be associated with an auto-immune process, either Hashimoto's disease or, more commonly in children and adolescents, Graves' disease.
- Single nodules are relatively rare in this age group and should be treated with suspicion – thyroid cancer is more common here than adenoma or cyst/colloid nodule.

Initial approach involves careful history.

- Duration, rate of goitre growth.
- ? associated pain or systemic symptoms.
- Was there a short-lived phase of toxicity, poor sleep, weight loss that resolved after around 6–12 weeks?

- Are there severe symptoms suggestive of Graves' disease?

Family History

Goitre, iodine deficiency, cancer, family cancer syndromes, e.g. MEN 2A or B, medullary or papillary Ca.

Examination

- Associated features of hyper or hypothyroidism, including eye signs (proptosis, chemosis, peri-orbital oedema).
- Cervical lymphadenopathy, ? tender gland (thyroiditis).
- Nature of the goitre: firm – Hashimoto's, soft + bruit – Graves'.
- General signs of MEN 2B: tongue, eyelid ganglioneuromata.

Tests

- TFTs – at least TSH if you think she is euthyroid, preferably fT_4 and fT_3.
- Antibodies if available will help: TPO for Hashimoto's – a low titre is very common and unhelpful for future function, Thyrotropin receptor antibody for Graves'.
- Ultrasound for structure – this will define diffuse or focal change.
- The appearance of a lymph node with metastatic disease is characteristic, with chaotic vascular appearance, identifiable by a radiologist.
- Scintiscan for function:
  - if subacute thyroiditis a Tc scan will show zero uptake with toxic biochemistry
  - patchy scan often Hashimoto's but toxic or early phase often diffuse high uptake
  - generally 'hot' scan – more likely Graves'
  - 10–20% uptake on scan and euthyroid tests suggest either dyshormonogenesis or iodine deficiency – impossible to differentiate on scan

- 'cold' area — if solid more likely to be cancer (risk around 17% in this age group).

Action

- FNA if a single nodule but only if adequate histology available.
- Removal if uncertain single nodule, due to high risk.
- If cancer, specific treatment (*refer to section on thyroid cancer in Chapter3 Thyroid Disorders*).

Treatment if Euthyroid

- Iodine supplement if iodine deficiency area.
- Thyroxine will shrink a dyshormonogenetic goitre but not a multinodular gland (less than 2% change in 1 year on average).
- Surgery only indicated for increasing size — partial thyroidectomy, often regrows, ugly result common, parathyroid risks.

Treatment if Toxic

- If Hashimoto's: may need β-blocker only for 3–12 weeks. Likely to cause hypothyroidism if antithyroid drugs are used.
- If subacute thyroiditis: may need β-blocker and antithyroid drugs for a few weeks but will suddenly improve, so frequent tests needed.
- If Graves': treat for a minimum of 2 years — chance of a long remission in this age group 30–40% maximum. Need to discuss ablative I^{131} for the future.
- Know evidence for I^{131} vs tablets vs surgery, risks vs benefits to discuss with family (*refer to section on treatment of thyrotoxicosis in Chapter 3, Thyroid Disorders*).

Treatment if Hypothyroid

- Hashimoto's in children often will improve spontaneously with resolution over time — may not need treatment if mild or possibly low-dose treatment only for short time.

- If child is pubertal, may need to treat until growth complete then trial off.

LONG-TERM EFFECTS AFTER CHILDHOOD CANCER

> **Boy with nasopharyngeal rhabdomyosarcoma at age 6.5 years presents at 9.5 years for endocrine assessment and advice.**

Background Knowledge

Local radiation to nasopharyngeal malignant tumours inevitably results in exposure of the hypothalamic pituitary axis to radiation scatter with a very high chance of evolving hypopituitarism.

Growth hormone deficiency is the first and most likely deficiency, occurring 1–4 years after radiation exposure followed by TSH, gonadotrophin and ACTH deficiency evolving over up to 20 years. In this particular circumstance it is likely that all hormones would eventually be lost, due to the radiation dose so close to the hypothalamic HPA.

Assessment

Assessment therefore includes the following.

- Full pituitary function testing, to be repeated at 12-monthly intervals, with appropriate replacement as required.
- Due to radiation scatter to the thyroid from the cranial component of radiation the thyroid is at increased risk for nodularity and malignancy and long-term assessment should include thyroid ultrasound every 2 years, commencing 2 years after radiation exposure.

> **An 18-year-old girl with past history of medulloblastoma at age 3; not seen by an endocrinologist previously.**

After craniospinal radiation there is a significant risk for hypopituitarism, particularly growth hormone deficiency. At age 18 with normal progress through puberty there is no possibility of altering final height. Final height will have decreased by about 10 cm, simply due to effect of spinal radiation on limiting spinal growth.

Assessment

At age 18 recurrent assessment should include:

- hypothalamic pituitary axis function: 8 am cortisol, fT_4, TSH, FSH, LH, oestradiol
- nodularity or malignancy of the thyroid due to radiation scatter from the cranial component and direct radiation from the spinal component at radiotherapy.

Although puberty may have been early, by disinhibition of the hypothalamus, followed by a period of normal function of the hypothalamic-pituitary-ovarian axis for some years, loss of menstruation, either now or in future, may indicate loss of hypothalamic cycling with *normal* oestrogen levels. This would indicate a need for HRT, for regular endometrial shedding. Gradual evolution of gonadotrophin loss with *low* oestrogen levels which would require HRT.

With evolution of gonadotrophin deficiency, secondary infertility occurs and would require treatment, if available, at the time of wanting fertility, with HRT as required in the interim.

If the past chemotherapy has caused direct gonadal damage (as reflected in extremely high gonadotrophins with a low oestrogen level), fertility is somewhat less likely. However, most chemotherapy protocols for medulloblastoma are only moderately gonadotoxic, with cyclophosphamide being the main problem. Recovery of the ovary after cyclophosphamide administration is quite common and ovarian failure, if present, might resolve at some time in the future. Nevertheless the girl will have a reduced population of ova and therefore long-term reduced fertility.

HYPOGLYCAEMIA

> Neonatal hypoglycaemia: a 4-day-old, 35-week gestation neonate with recurrent hypoglycaemia

Definition of Neonatal Hypoglycaemia

Usual clinical approach is one of 'neurophysiological safety', i.e. avoidance of levels less than 2.6 mmol/L (lab glucose). Glucometer readings do not correlate well at low BGL.

Knowledge of Neonatal Glucose Metabolism

- Basal glucose production rate 4–6 mg/kg/minute – needs to be matched by exogenous intake; may need more if increased utilisation.
- Glycogen store accumulation takes place primarily in third trimester so preterm neonates rely more on gluconeogenesis.
- Brain is major site of glucose utilisation (up to 90%) and site of greatest concern; in a term baby, the brain has ability to decrease its glucose utilisation and increase use of other substrates (ketones, lactate) as an adaptive mechanism if BGL drops; studies show that premature babies may not be able to do this – prolonged hypoglycaemia, even if mild, can have more of an effect.

Main Possibilities in This Baby

Most likely:
Depletion of glycogen stores:

- AGA (up to 15% of AGA babies have hypoglycaemia due usually to combination of decreased intake, decreased concentration of substrates and immature gluconeogenic and glycogenolytic pathways)

- **SGA** — especially if PET in mother — up to 60% have recurrent hypoglycaemic episodes; due to reduction in glycogen deposition, delay in phosphoenolpyruvate carboxykinase (PEPCK), which is the rate-limiting step in gluconeogenesis, increased utilisation of substrate etc.

Increased glucose utilisation:

- perinatal stress, asphyxia, sepsis, cold stress, cardiac failure.

Less likely:

Neonatal hyperinsulinaemic syndromes — transient or persistent. Hypoglycaemia can be quite severe:

- transient — infant of diabetic mother, small stressed babies, haemolytic disease, exchange transfusion (glucose concentration of administered blood causes increased insulin release), Beckwith—Wiedemann syndrome
- persistent hyperinsulinism — *see next scenario*.

Endocrine causes:

- GH deficiency, hypopituitarism, cortisol deficiency.

Inborn errors of metabolism:

- glycogen storage disease type 1 = glucose 6 phosphatase deficiency. AR inheritance. Hepatomegaly usually found — often present later in infancy
- fructose 1,6-diphosphatase deficiency can present first with hypoglycaemia
- galactosaemia — often jaundiced — enzymatic defect galactose 1 phosphate UDT
- disorders of FA metabolism: medium-chain and long-chain acyl-CoA dehydrogenase deficiency (carnitine/acylcarnitine profiles will help dx)
- others: MSUD, methyl-malonic acidaemia.

Perspective

- Clinical exam and history of events so far will be most important. Note: hepatomegaly may

suggest metabolic cause, e.g. glycogen storage disorder; jaundice may suggest galactosaemia, midline defects, e.g. cleft lip/palate may be associated with pituitary problems.
- Ensure intake is adequate — need 4—6 mg/kg/min CHO — if not getting it orally give by NG or IV. If requiring more than this — investigate.
- Most hypoglycaemia in babies this age is transient, related to increased metabolic requirements so important to reassess frequently.

Investigations

- Guided by clinical exam.
- Full hypoglycaemia screen should be done when lab glucose is confirmed at less than 2.6 mmol/L or after a 3—4-hour fast.
- 'Critical sample': cortisol, GH, insulin, C-peptide, pH, NH3, lactate, fatty acids, ketones, carnitine/acylcarnitine profiles, urinary organic acids and amino acids. Depending on availability, insulin is the most likely to yield a rapid diagnosis. Growth hormone may be low in an infant that is chronically stressed and cortisol levels vary widely in the neonatal period. Nevertheless, these three are the most likely to be helpful, along with ketone measurement.
- Additional: full septic work-up, LFTs, U&E, CXR and other as per clinical exam.

Treatment

- Treat the underlying cause.
- For mild/occasional hypoglycaemia in an otherwise well child, oral administration of breast milk (expressed to ensure adequate volume) with supplementation using dextrose/formula if necessary is first step.
- If hypoglycaemia persists, start parenteral infusion with continuous dextrose at ~ 6—8 mg/kg/minute concentration and increase as needed.

- Regular documentation of blood glucose – document initial recovery at 20–30 minutes and then 1–2-hourly initially, out to 3–4-hourly when more stable.
- If parenteral therapy is greater than 15 mg/kg/minute not maintaining euglycaemia, additional therapy may be needed (see subsequent clinical cases).

A term baby with birth weight 3.8 kg is now 2 weeks old and has persistent hypoglycaemia requiring continuous IV glucose at 18 mg/kg/minute.

Assessment, Investigations and Management

Perspective

Persistent hypoglycaemia despite extremely high glucose requirement is consistent with hyperinsulinism.

Assessment

Possible causes of hyperinsulinism are as follows.

1. Infant of mother with diabetes mellitus (? OGTT done in pregnancy); if there is any family history of neonatal hypoglycaemia with later onset diabetes – ? HNF4α monogenic diabetes (rare).
2. Perinatal 'stress' – birth asphyxia/sepsis/ haemolytic disease.
3. Beckwith–Wiedemann syndrome – clinical features include macrosomia, abdominal wall defects, earlobe creases/pits, organomegaly, macroglossia.
4. Genetic causes: most common are loss of function mutations of genes encoding SUR1 (ABCC8) or Kir6.2 (KCNJ11) subunits of K-ATP channel; alternatively – activating mutations of GLUD1 (glutamate

dehydrogenase) or glucokinase genes; rarer causes include hyperinsulinism in association with SCHAD or congenital disorders of glycosylation.

Given very high glucose requirements, other causes of hypoglycaemia (e.g. GH deficiency/hypopituitarism/inborn errors of metabolism) are less likely.

Investigations and Management

'Critical sample': important to verify that true (lab) glucose level is less than 2.6 mmol/L at time of sampling.
Blood:

- U&E, LFTs, NH_3
- Venous/capillary gas – HCO_3, lactate
- Blood ketones (do on bedside meter if available)
- insulin, c-peptide, GH, cortisol
- Carnitine/acylcarnitine (Guthrie card)
- Serum amino acids, FFA.

Urine (first sample after hypo episode):

- Dipstick for ketones, glucose, pH
- Organic and amino acids.

Hyperinsulinism is confirmed by presence of detectable insulin, absence of ketones and inappropriate low FFA during hypoglycaemia.

Treatment

Aim of therapy: maintenance of BGL equal to or greater than 4.0 mmol/L (3.5 mmol/L minimum) as inhibition of ketogenesis means there is no alternative substrate for brain during hypoglycaemia.

- If hyperinsulinism is confirmed, initial management includes glucagon and intravenous dextrose. These are likely to have been instigated in above baby already.
- If euglycaemia cannot be maintained with glucose, addition of *diazoxide* – 5–20 mg/kg/day in 3 divided doses.

'Response to therapy' allows weaning of IV dextrose requirement and maintenance of normoglycaemia with normal oral feeding pattern.

Infants who respond are likely to have either transient hyperinsulinism secondary to a perinatal insult or possibly a GLUD1 or glucokinase gene mutation.

- Addition of a thiazide diuretic helps minimise fluid retention (side effect of diazoxide).
- Failure to respond to diazoxide indicates likely SUR1 (ABCC8) or Kir6.2 (KCNJ11) mutation. Mutations can result in either diffuse HI (usually AR inheritance, although AD is reported) or focal HI. Focal HI arises from 'double hit' mechanism of (1) paternal uniparental disomy (loss of maternal allele) of region 11p15.5-11p15.1 and (2) paternally inherited KATP mutation.

Identification of focal vs diffuse disease can aid management; surgical resection of affected focal region is curative, whereas diffuse disease often requires near total pancreatectomy. Hyperinsulinism may persist even with minimal residual pancreatic tissue; this surgery also carries risk of subsequent diabetes mellitus.

Identification of focal disease remains problematic:

- 18FDOPA PET is only available in a few centres worldwide; where previously this was thought to be more than 90% sensitive and specific for localising a focal lesion, recent reports indicate sensitivity may be lower than previously estimated (~ 70%)
- MRI/ultrasound rarely identify a lesion — not usually helpful.

Alternative Medical Therapy

- *Octreotide*: administered subcutaneously (5–30 µg/kg/day) by intermittent injections (e.g. 6-hourly); some reports of use of continuous infusion.

- *Surgery*: if persistent hypoglycaemia despite maximal medical therapy, near total pancreatectomy may be indicated (unless clear focal lesion identifiable).

> **A 1-month-old boy with blindness and hypoglycaemia.**

Diagnosis and Approach

Most Likely Diagnosis

- *Septo-optic dysplasia* encompassing hypopituitarism, optic nerve hypoplasia +/− abnormal septum pellucidum. Hypoglycaemia results from GH +/− ACTH deficiency.

Other Possible Diagnoses

- Previous severe (possibly unrecognised) hypoglycaemia in newborn period resulting in cortical blindness (occipital lobe damage).
- TORCH infection/other severe CNS infection.

Diagnosis and Approach

History

- History of presenting features: ? symptoms of hypoglycaemia — lethargy, poor feeding, hypotonia, jitteriness, apnoea, seizures.
- History of previous episodes in newborn period.
- Other relevant history, e.g. pregnancy (TORCH) and delivery (? breech delivery increases risk of hypopituitarism).
- ? prolonged jaundice — cholestatic picture more common in hypopituitarism.
- Family history of hypopituitarism.

Examination

- Length, weight and HC centiles.

- ? other midline defects, e.g. cleft lip/palate, hypertelorism, cardiac defects, micropenis, +/− undescended testes.
- Ophthalmological exam − ? hypoplastic optic nerves (pale discs)/other associated abnormality, e.g. nystagmus, coloboma (more likely associated with CHARGE where the defect is hypogonadotrophic hypogonadism, not hypopituitarism).
- ? other neurological abnormalities, e.g. seizure activity during normoglycaemia.

Investigations

- Full 'critical sample' during hypoglycaemia (lab glucose less than 2.6 mmol/L —see previous scenario on hyperinsulinism for tests).

Particular emphasis on pituitary axis:

- during hypoglycaemia: GH, IGF1, cortisol (+/− ACTH)
- Baseline: fT_4, LH, FSH and testosterone (should still be within neonatal 'surge' period where levels are detectable), U&E and paired serum and urinary osmolalities to exclude diabetes insipidus.

In hypopituitarism causing hypoglycaemia, GH and cortisol are often undetectable. Imaging:

- Cranial ultrasound followed by MRI brain and pituitary. Note: in young infant MRI can be performed in a bean bag without need for general anaesthesia.

- SOD is associated with high incidence of malformations of cortical development (e.g. schizencephaly − associated with partial absence of septum pellucidum; or lobar holoprosencephaly − associated with complete absence of septum pellucidum).

Management

- Resuscitation if needed.

- Correction of hypoglycaemia: bolus 3−5 mL/kg 10% dextrose, followed by infusion at rate of 10 mg/kg/minute − titrate rate to BGL.

Replacement of pituitary hormones (based on deficiencies identified above) as follows.

- Hydrocortisone: start with intravenous 'stress' dose of 50−100 mg/m^2/day in 4 divided doses; maintenance therapy for presumed ACTH deficiency is 5−8 mg/m^2/day. Important to teach family regarding need for 'stress' cover during illness/other stress. Teach home BGL monitoring.
- May need thyroxine replacement − to be started only *after* hydrocortisone.
- Growth hormone therapy − if GHD confirmed, hypoglycaemia is sufficient reason to treat, do not need to wait for linear growth failure. Sometimes GH must be considered in infancy if the baby continues to be hypoglycaemic despite adequate corticosteroid.
- If micropenis, consider course of IM testosterone (e.g. 12.5−25 mg x 3 injections 4 weeks apart).
- Diabetes insipidus is uncommon in SOD, but may occur (0−20% incidence). Trial of low-dose intranasal DDAVP, e.g. 1−2 μg/dose (start low and assess response/titrate dose in 1 μg increments)
- Other issues: needs long-term follow-up − endocrine (regular assessment to ensure adequate replacement of known deficiencies and to monitor other pituitary hormones; precocious puberty occurs in small percentage), neurology (blindness +/− sequelae of hypoglycaemia) +/− community paediatrician involvement and disability services.

Aetiology

- In most cases aetiology is unclear.
- May be mutation in HESX1/Hesx1 gene (important role in forebrain, midbrain and pituitary development), although overall incidence of these mutations in SOD is rare.

CHAPTER

15

Research in Medicine: Why do we Need It and How do (should) we Do It?

Christa E. Flück, Chantal Cripe-Mamie

INTRODUCTION

During medical school and further training every future doctor reads several basic as well as specific textbooks to gain the necessary knowledge to care for patients. For ongoing education during the professional career, most medical doctors read medical journals (in print or on-line) and attend meetings where advances in their field(s) are summarised and presented in lectures and perhaps critically discussed during expert panels. Thus, good medical practice relies profoundly on up-to-date medical knowledge. On the other hand, all knowledge, not only in medicine, is based on research. Therefore, to advance medicine in any field ongoing research is crucial. Once new knowledge is generated, it needs to be critically interpreted, verified and distributed to the scientific community by means of the medical literature so that it can be finally implemented into good clinical practice.

Today the amount of available medical literature is immense; an estimated 2.5 million biomedical articles are published yearly.[1] But not every publication, be it on paper or on-line, is scientifically sound and/or clinically relevant. Therefore, it is essential that readers know how to judge good from bad medical research articles and to evaluate whether the information provided may solve relevant

Practical Pediatric Endocrinology in a Limited Resource Setting
http://dx.doi.org/10.1016/B978-0-12-407822-2.00015-3

question(s) or provide additional question(s), possibly implying a change in their own clinical practice. In order to judge and evaluate medical research, people need, first, to have access to the biomedical literature and, second, the skill to search and find relevant articles. Finally, every unsolved question should be taken as a personal motivation for considering initiating a specific research project to answer it. Therefore, if research is understood in this way, it is not meant for only an academic elite at universities but rather to be part of the professional life/career of any medical doctor.

In today's world developing countries are still underprivileged in terms of medicine. This includes not only limited availability of healthcare but also lack of specialised training for medical doctors who need unlimited access to the worldwide medical literature as well as funds for performing research tailored to their own needs and questions.

This chapter is aimed at providing some preliminary information on how to read critically and how to get started with a research project to answer an unsolved question and/or review a clinical practice.

MEDICAL LITERATURE

Biomedical literature is available in textbooks, journal articles and more and more commonly on the worldwide web. Generally, textbook knowledge is considered as firm since it is mostly written by renowned experts, who summarise published, preferentially peer-reviewed and confirmed research and thus established knowledge in a field. Disadvantages of textbooks are the price and availability and that between publication and revision, newer information may be missing. In contrast, the quality of research articles published in the broad range of biomedical journals varies profoundly. Articles may be regarded of higher quality when they have been subjected to a peer-reviewing process prior to

publication and when they are published in journals with higher impact factors in the respective field. However, it is important to realise that a high-impact factor of a journal does not always guarantee high quality of an article and that in some fields there are no high-impact-factor journals for publishing excellent, ground-breaking research results. Subscriptions to good journals are still expensive, although some journals provide free access or discounts for developing countries upon request (e.g. the journals of the BMJ Publishing Group and *Clinical Evidence*).[2] Finally, the huge amount of information which is available free on-line from all kinds of resources may need to be evaluated most critically since the vast majority of it comes unfiltered. Some quality may be implicated with information found through specific filters such as PubMed (www.ncbi.nlm.nih.gov/pubmed), BioMed Central (www.biomedcentral.com) or other filters (for a list, see http://healthlinks.washington.edu/ebp/ebptools.html#cochrane).

Overall, today's scientific community aims at supporting publications of good-quality biomedical papers in on-line journals free of charge in order to distribute knowledge worldwide (a list of such free resources is given under the link http://www.forusdocs.com/Free_Resources/Free_Medical_Journals.htm). This will certainly help physicians in developing countries to have equal access to the newest publications and become partners of the international scientific network. All a young future researcher needs (besides support from supervisors and institutions) is a working Internet connection, a computer work station, knowledge of worldwide web search tools and a critical mind to judge the quality of published literature. Some simple questions which help in critically assessing articles to evaluate the quality of presented results and conclusions are given in Table 15.1 and may also be found on-line as checklists. An additional useful (and enjoyable!) way to learn how to discriminate good from bad literature is by discussing

TABLE 15.1   Checklist for Critical Reading

1. *Source*	• Was the publication peer-reviewed?
2. *Subject*	• What is the main topic and idea of the paper? • Is there sufficient and valid background/introductory information given?
3. *Specific problem*	• What is the specific purpose or rationale for the study?
4. *Design*	• What kind of research is presented (clinical study, laboratory study, case presentation etc.)? • Who or what constituted the sample or population?
5. *Method*	• How was the study actually done? Are methods clearly described so as to be easily understood or so that others may duplicate the study?
6. *Data analysis*	• What data were collected in the study? • What statistical analyses were used? • Are they appropriate to test the study's hypotheses? • Did the researchers follow through with their hypotheses?
7. *Results*	• Do the results follow in a logical and commonsense way? • Do the results answer the specific problem? • Do they seem valid? • Does significant information seem omitted? • Do the numbers correspond to the subjects in the methods section?
8. *Discussion*	• Are the interpretations consistent with the specific problem and the design and methods of the study? • Are the results consistent with findings from similar studies? Why? • Are there any logical fallacies or errors in reasoning? • Are study weaknesses and strengths discussed?
9. *Conclusion*	• What are the conclusion(s)? • Are they sufficiently supported by the study? • What alternative conclusion(s) may be drawn?
10. *Significance*	• Can the results be applied to your research or clinical practice? • What does the knowledge gained mean to medicine, healthcare and your patient?

scientific papers with colleagues. Ideally, this may be done in so-called journal club sessions which can be supervised by more experienced physicians or scientists.

THE SCIENTIFIC PROCESS

Knowledge in medicine (and science in general) is acquired through systematic investigations on specific questions: the so-called scientific process. This process is complex and includes several steps which are depicted in Figure 15.1. However, whether planning a clinical research project or a laboratory-based project, the systematic approach remains the same and always starts with an unsolved question or a hypothesis.

In general, research comes in many forms and it is also the form that contributes to the impact of a research project when looking at it with an evidence-based medicine approach (Figure 15.2). In this perspective writing a case report will have less impact than for instance performing a prospective, controlled clinical trial. Nevertheless, both a case report and a cohort study are valuable research projects and add to our medical knowledge. Indeed, writing a report on an interesting case might be a good project for somebody who is just beginning research and may give rise to novel ideas/unsolved questions for a next-level research project.

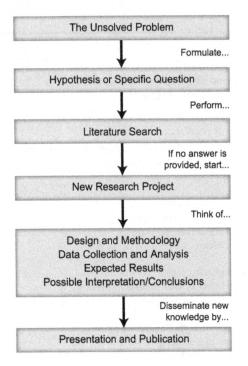

FIGURE 15.1 The scientific process and the specific steps involved.

From Research to Audit

The aim of all research is to discover and/or test a novel theory. By contrast the aim of an audit in medicine is to review how actual clinical practice compares with best recommended clinical practice (Figure 15.3).[3,4] Thus, questions of an audit are usually specific to a particular setting, motivated by local circumstances and based on firm research or consensus guidelines. Research is expected to produce generalisable theory changes which will be shared by the larger scientific community and implemented into good clinical practice. By contrast, the direct result of an audit should lead to an improvement of local quality of care. Thus in an ideal research program, audit follows research, ensuring that the results of research are being incorporated into clinical practice. The systematic process of performing an audit is similar to the scientific process of

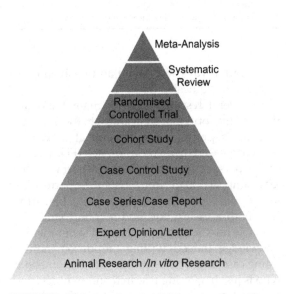

FIGURE 15.2 Levels of evidence in the primary literature.

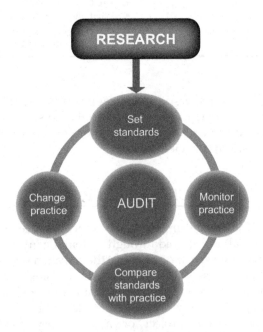

FIGURE 15.3 The process of an audit.

doing a research project. But since the audit uses mainly data which exist as part of daily clinical practice, it is easier, faster and cheaper to obtain. In addition, unlike research, audit results are often perceived to be of greater value by physicians because they relate directly to routine practice.

> **Advice:** Applying the KISS principle (coined by Kelly Johnson of Lockheed) may help — 'Keep it simple, Stupid!' or 'Keep it simple and stupid/straightforward' (http://en.wikipedia.org).

HOW DO YOU GET STARTED WITH A RESEARCH PROJECT? A STEP-BY-STEP APPROACH

Research needs to be structured and the best way to set about this is to write a protocol. It will help clarify ideas and help the investigator to organise his or her research in a logical manner; it will be the written plan for the study and it will be a useful tool in case of seeking grant funds.

Step 1: Define the Hypothesis/Specific Question

According to Isaac H Satanov, "the beginning of research is curiosity". Research is motivated by the unknown.[1] Therefore any unsolved question from daily medical practice may be considered and assessed whether it would be worth trying to solve. Good research questions may be characterised as being: (a) of general (and/or broad) and (b) significant impact to humanity; (c) novel, (d) serious and ethical; (e) able to reduce financial and/or economic burdens; and (f) of interest to biomedical sciences.

Once the topic and aim of a research project are identified, a highly specific question or hypothesis needs to be formulated which then can be tested. Generally, it is wise to solve one (at most two) questions (hypotheses) at a time. It is essential to formulate a clear question or working hypothesis in simple words.

Step 2: Search the Literature for Background Information

When the topic, the aim and the specific question/hypothesis of the project are clear, the literature search is next. The current knowledge in and around the specific field must be identified and studied. On the one hand you want to make sure that the question/hypothesis is not yet (satisfactorily) solved, tested or about to be tested (ongoing clinical studies may be registered at http://clinicaltrials.gov). On the other hand, you want to become an expert in the field so as to plan the best possible study and to be able to analyse and discuss the results and compare their significance with similar studies. Undertaking a good literature search will also help to identify areas of controversy and find ideas and validated tools for choosing adequate study design and methods. In addition, it also helps avoid frustration by minimising the risk of ending up with results which are already known or a data collection which may not be useful to answer the study's specific question because of serious flaws in the design. Finally, a broad knowledge of the literature in the field is also essential for writing a distinct and informative introduction for a future publication of your study.[5]

Step 3: Choose a Research Design and Methods to Solve the Question or Hypothesis

Research comes in many types, offering the investigator a lot of freedom to choose. This theoretical freedom is often restricted in reality by such factors as ethical considerations, funding resources or patient numbers (just to mention a few). The difficult task is to choose the right design and methods for answering the unsolved question with the highest possible level of evidence.

> **Advice**: It might be helpful to write an introduction (including the aim and references) before starting the study and have it critically reviewed by somebody (e.g. colleague, supervisor, expert in the field) to ensure the best possible starting point.

A study design may be retrospective or prospective and descriptive or analytic. Analytic studies test for either differences between groups or relationships among variables or both. They can be cross-sectional, providing a 'snapshot' of single observations at one period or case-control/cohort studies observing a defined group over a longer time period and (if possible) in comparison to a control or reference group. The study can be pre-experimental (e.g. case study or one group pre- or post-intervention study), quasi-experimental (experimental without randomisation) or experimental. Generally, a strong clinical study that will have the most impact usually consists of a true experimental design characterised by randomisation of the subjects and a control group. However, some restrictions to the design may also be given by the topic of the specific question of the study. A list providing information on what design may best fit a question of a specific field is given in Table 15.2.

Equally important to the design are all parameters of methods such as instrumentation and procedures as well as details of data collection and planned analysis. These need to be carefully defined before starting. In addition, all these parameters need to be controlled for

TABLE 15.2   Question and Design Matches

Topic of question	Suggested design/method
Therapy	Double-blind randomised controlled trial
Diagnosis	Controlled trial
Prognosis	Cohort study, case control study, case series
Aetiology/Harm	Cohort study
Prevention	Randomised controlled trial, cohort study

possible bias (errors) to eventually obtain reliable and valid results. Errors come in two forms: (1), a random error occurs by chance and will influence the outcome more heavily with small sample sizes; (2) a systematic error, which affects the true measurement by a specific inaccuracy throughout the whole series, e.g. poor measuring technique or incorrect statistical test. Reliability can be assumed when measurements are consistent. Reliability focuses on both instruments and investigators alike, assuring individual (intra-rater) as well as between-individual (inter-rater) accuracy. By contrast, validity questions the usefulness and appropriateness of the specific type of collected data.

Finally, the sample size and the inclusion and exclusion criteria for sample selection should be established before data are collected. Ideally, the sample size is small enough to save time and money, yet sufficiently large to test your research hypothesis. The three factors defining sample size are:

1. the effect size (e.g. a big effect can be investigated with a small sample size)
2. the level of significance wanted (usually 0.05 in biomedical studies)
3. the statistical power desired (usually set at 0.80, meaning that there is a 20% chance to

commit a type II beta-error incorrectly accepting a null hypothesis).

Programs for calculating sample size are found in most computerised statistical software.

In preparing the protocol one should consider a time frame during which the research should/will be conducted.

> **Advice:** Get inspired and profit from peer-reviewed literature when choosing the design and methods for your study. Many experts in the field have already thought about the optimal design and methods before those papers were published.

Step 4: Data Collection, Analysis and Presentation

As soon as you are ready to collect the data, you should be ready with an instrument for this collection. You may want to prepare a specific standardised paper form for initial data entry or enter your data directly into an electronic file which can be filled and then directly used for data analysis. When using electronic entry, it is useful to define precisely the type of entered data (Table 15.3), e.g. enter data in the right format and group them according to the planned analysis.

Overall, the type of data will determine which statistical analysis may be applied to test the data for significance. Statistical analysis of your data is necessary to summarise your findings into grouped information, to generalise from findings in your studied subjects to the larger population and to check for significant differences or relationships between groups. Choosing the right statistical test is not an easy task and, whenever possible, it is advisable to involve a statistician. It is beyond the scope of this chapter to provide further information. Some basic knowledge in medical statistics may be obtained in courses, on the web (e.g. http://lib.stat.cmu.edu/; http://onlinestatbook.com/rvls.html) or from books specifically written by experts for medical doctors. Alternatively, if there is no help available, one might try with the 'trial and error' approach using 'simple' statistic programs which help the user with in-built background information (or a handbook) deciding what tests might be applicable. Microsoft Excel is certainly the broadest available general purpose data analysis software while other more specialised statistical packages include: Minitab (www.minitab.com), SAS (www.sas.com), SPSS (www.spss.com), Mathcad (www.mathsoft.com), SigmaPlot (www.spss.com), and Design-Expert (www.statease.com).

Data can be presented either as figures or tables (preferred!) or in text form. They should be provided in a logical form related to the specific question of the study. Good presentation of results is characterised by summarising the raw data and putting them into the proper

TABLE 15.3 Data Types

Data type	Definition	Example
Nominal data	Data that categorise (non-numerical)	Sex, eye colour, race
Ordinal data	Data defined by an ordering, but the distance between the choices or values is not defined (non-numerical)	Rankings (i.e. degree of pain), preference scales
Continuous data	Data with numeric values; interval or ratio (parametric)	Numbers (height, weight)

context, indicating which initial hypotheses were supported or not after appropriate statistical calculations.

> **Advice:** Be aware that choosing the right statistical procedure to test the significance of your data is a challenge!
>
> It is preferable to present your results in graphical form rather than as text.

Step 5: Data Interpretation and Discussion

After obtaining the results of your study, you should be able to make a clear statement relating to the specific question that was initially formulated. The statement should address whether the specific question/hypothesis may be solved or not and how the research findings contribute to the understanding in the field. Often the data collected will give rise to new questions that may be contemplated in the discussions section of your article. The discussion should also include a comparison of your findings in support of prior research findings or how they contrast with previous findings, offering an explanation whenever possible. If your findings are new or in contrast to accepted scientific knowledge, you must have strong support for your interpretations and may want to suggest confirmatory studies.

> **Advice:** Do not draw conclusions that cannot be clearly supported by your results.

Step 6: Statement of Significance

At the end of a study, the overall findings may be questioned for significance. In medicine significant novel findings are defined as having an impact on good clinical practice, changing education or society or enhancing basic medical knowledge. Today a statement of significance of possible achievements of the proposed project is required in every grant application.

> **Note:** Very few studies end with ground-breaking results which advance medicine significantly.

CONCLUDING REMARKS

The scientific process (Figure 15.1) is essential for critical reading, designing a (bio)medical study, writing a research paper (or abstract) or even applying successfully for a research grant. Thus, implementing fundamental scientific principles in the process is very helpful. Every medical doctor is a scientist by training and daily uses his or her knowledge, while realising its limitations. Unsolved questions and novel hypotheses are the driving forces of research by which medical knowledge is enlarged for the sake of better medical practice. In this circle, we all can play an important role, whether we get involved in small or large research projects or perform audits. Undertaking research in developing countries is especially important as needs and questions may differ from those of first world countries and may be solved only in the specific setting of developing countries. Importantly, the impact of research projects conducted by, in and for developing countries may be bigger than studies conducted by, in and for the wealthier parts of the world.

Research is often competitive. This might be stimulating but it should never be harmful, especially not to human beings or nature in general. It is therefore a must for every researcher to know the ethical codes and comply with the common rules and standards.

If in doubt, it is the responsibility of an investigator to contact regulatory offices for information. 'Do no harm!' applies not only to study subjects but also to colleagues. Stealing ideas or results, delaying publication by unfair reviewing or copying from papers without referencing them (plagiarism) are only a few of the many observed scientific misconducts.

By contrast, doing research the proper way and sharing ideas and results with the scientific community is satisfying and rewarding.

References

1. Blessing JD. *Physician Assistant's Guide to Research and Medical Literature*. Philadelphia: F.A. Davis Company; 2006.
2. Godlee F, Horton R, Smith R, et al. Global information flow. *BMJ* 2000;**321**:776–7.
3. Proctor SJ. Why clinical research needs medical audit. *Qual Health Care* 1993;**2**:1–2.
4. Closs SJ, Cheater FM. Audit or research – what is the difference? *J Clin Nurs* 1996;**5**:249–56.
5. Zeiger M. *Essentials of Writing Biomedical Research Papers*. New York: McGraw-Hill; 2000.

Molecular Biology and Molecular Genetics in Paediatric Endocrinology

Angela Huebner, Barbara Kind, Katrin Koehler

INTRODUCTION

In the past 25 years, due to the availability of methods in molecular biology, molecular genetics and cell biology, the understanding of the molecular basis of endocrine disorders has grown exponentially. Although the genetics and pathophysiology of many monogenic disorders has been clarified, other disorders like obesity and diabetes, which have a polygenic background, are less well understood. Application of the new molecular methods to paediatric endocrine disorders has given us a lot of novel information but has also increased the complexity of scientific questions in clinical endocrinology. Therefore, understanding of the basic principles, methods and nomenclatures of molecular biology became an important basis for the understanding of aetiology, pathogenesis and therapeutic approaches of endocrine diseases.[1]

In this chapter we have summarised the most important information concerning molecular

Practical Pediatric Endocrinology in a Limited Resource Setting
http://dx.doi.org/10.1016/B978-0-12-407822-2.00016-5

biology and molecular genetics which might help with understanding of their application to paediatric endocrine disorders and scientific publications in this area.

FROM GENOME TO METABOLOME

Genetics is the science of the inheritance and variations in genetic material. In the past medical genetics has been limited to chromosomal aberrations and inherited metabolic diseases. The understanding of the molecular causes of monogenic disorders (i.e. combined pituitary hormonal deficiency) and more complex and polygenic disorders (diabetes mellitus type 2) has opened a completely new area in paediatric endocrinology which has a great impact on the diagnostics, treatment and counselling of affected families. In many complex diseases, such as diabetes mellitus type 2, hypertension and obesity, we are still just starting to identify and to understand predisposing genetic variants. In turn, the phenotype of monogenic diseases can also be modified by other genetic and environmental modifiers.

The term **genome** refers to the totality of all genes on all chromosomes in the nucleus of a cell. Alternatively, the term **genomics** stands for all the methods to analyse the genome such as chromosomal mapping, gene expression, epigenetic, DNA sequencing and others. After the human genome was decoded via the Human Genome Project in 2003, investigation of functional aspects of gene products came to the fore. Therefore we distinguish between structural and functional genomics.

The term **transcriptome** refers to the totality of the messenger RNA (mRNA) which is transcribed from the nuclear genome, whereas **transcriptomics** describes the generation of mRNA expression profiles.

The term **proteome** describes the total of proteins which are expressed by the genome of a cell. Hence **proteomics** comprises the techniques for protein separation and identification. After translation proteins usually undergo a variety of cell and tissue-specific modifications such as phosphorylation, glycosylations, acetylations, protein cleavage and others which in turn result in a tissue-specific and highly variable proteome.

Within recent years the term **metabolome** has been defined as the complement of low-molecular-weight molecules which determine the metabolic characteristics of a cell. **Metabolomics** is a quite young and emerging field which studies the contents and changes of the metabolome. The importance of this new speciality arises from the fact that each change in the genome results in a series of changes in the proteome and metabolome which determine our phenotype.

BIOINFORMATIC TOOLS

The increasing amount of biological data requires large databases in which data can be accumulated, ordered, commented and linked. Many of these databases are open and available via the Internet and can be very helpful when specific information about a gene or a protein is sought. Therefore in recent years the novel area of **bioinformatics** has been developed. A lot of databases and computer programs can be used for management of nucleotide and protein sequences, prediction of secondary and tertiary protein structures, gene and protein expression analyses, modelling of signal transduction pathways, protein interactions and networking.

In Table 16.1 some of the most frequently used databases in molecular biology and molecular genetics are summarised.

TABLE 16.1   Selected Databases for Molecular Biology, Molecular Genetics, Cell Biology and Clinical Genetics

Site	Content	Uniform Resource Locator (URL)
Basic Local Alignment Search Tool (BLAST)	Finds regions of similarity between biological sequences	*http://blast.ncbi.nlm.nih.gov/Blast.cgi*
BioGRID	Biological General Repository for Interaction Datasets	*www.thebiogrid.org/*
BioGPS	A free extensible and customisable gene annotation portal; a complete resource for learning about gene and protein function	*http://biogps.org/#goto=welcome*
Declaration of Helsinki	Declaration of Helsinki by the World Medical Association (WMA); cornerstone document of human research ethics	*www.wma.net/en/30publications/10policies/b3/index.html*
EDDNAL	European directory of DNA diagnostic laboratories	*www.eddnal.com/*
ENSEMBL	Genome databases for vertebrates and other eukaryotic species	*www.ensembl.org/index.html*
ENTREZ	Life sciences cross-database search engine for molecular genetics and molecular biology	*www.ncbi.nlm.nih.gov/sites/gquery*
European Bioinformatics Institute (EBI)	Databases of biological data including nucleic acid, protein sequences and macromolecular structures; freely available data and bioinformatics services	*www.ebi.ac.uk*
ExPASy	Bioinformatics Resource Portal, scientific databases and software tools for proteomics, genomics, phylogeny, systems biology, population genetics, transcriptomics etc.	*http://au.expasy.org/*
GeneCards	Database of human genes that provides concise genome-related information	*www.genecards.org/*
HUGO Gene Nomenclature Committee (HGNC)	Gene nomenclature and associated resources including links to genomic, proteomic and phenotypic information, as well as gene family information	*www.genenames.org/*
HUGO	Human Genome Organisation	*www.hugo-international.org/*
Human Gene Mutation Database (HGMD)	Mutation database (human inherited disease) of the Institute of Medical Genetics, Cardiff University with about 100,000 entries	*www.hgmd.cf.ac.uk/ac/index.php*
HUM-MOLGEN	International communication forum in human molecular genetics	*http://hum-molgen.de/*
Mice database	Database of the Jackson Laboratory, USA	*http://jaxmice.jax.org/index.html*
Mutation nomenclature	International nomenclature for the description of sequence variants	*www.hgvs.org/mutnomen/*

(Continued)

TABLE 16.1 Selected Databases for Molecular Biology, Molecular Genetics, Cell Biology and Clinical Genetics (*cont'd*)

Site	Content	Uniform Resource Locator (URL)
National Centre for Biotechnology Information (NCBI)	Links to different databases: UniGene, PubMed, OMIM and others	*www.ncbi.nlm.nih.gov/*
Online Mendelian Inheritance in Man (OMIM)	Compendium of human genes and genetic phenotypes; contains information on all known Mendelian disorders and over 12,000 genes	*www.ncbi.nlm.nih.gov/sites/entrez?db=omim*
Orphanet	Portal for rare diseases and orphan drugs	*www.orpha.net/consor/cgi-bin/index.php?lng=EN*
PubMed	More than 21 million citations for biomedical literature from MEDLINE, life science journals, and on-line books	*www.ncbi.nlm.nih.gov/pubmed/*
SNP database of NCBI	Database for single nucleotide polymorphisms (SNPs)	*www.ncbi.nlm.nih.gov/projects/SNP/*
Splice Site Prediction (Berkeley Drosophila Genome Project)	Splice site predictor in Human and Drosophila	*www.fruitfly.org/seq_tools/splice.html*
STRING	Known and predicted protein—protein interactions	*http://string.embl.de/*
UCSC Genome Bioinformatics	Reference sequence and working draft assemblies for a large collection of genomes; position of sequence-tagged sites (STSs) and expressed sequence tags (ESTs)	*http://genome.ucsc.edu/*
UNIGENE	A comprehensive view on the transcriptome: information on protein similarities, gene expression, cDNA clone reagents, and genomic location	*www.ncbi.nlm.nih.gov/sites/entrez?db=unigene*

STRUCTURE OF THE GENOME

Structure of the DNA

Based on structural X-ray analyses of Franklin, in 1953 Watson and Crick developed the model of the DNA double helix. This special structure is fundamentally important for the two major functions of DNA: replication and transmission of genetic information. Each DNA strand consists of a deoxyribose-phosphate polymer as the backbone with nucleotide bases which are oriented to the inner side of the helix. The four nucleotide bases are the purine bases adenine (A) and guanine (G) and the pyrimidine bases cytosine (C) and thymidine (T). RNA strands contain uracil (U) instead of thymidine. The two strands of the double helix are complementary and are connected through hydrogen bonds between adenine and thymine (uracil) as well as guanine and cytosine. The strict complementarity of both strands allows a precise replication and, in addition, provides an effective defence mechanism against DNA damage. Hence, a deletion or duplication of one base pair on one strand can be easily corrected by the complementary strand.

The existence of four nucleotides allows an amazing genetic diversity. In the protein-coding regions, the genes, the nucleotides are read as triplets (so called codons) which encode each of 20 amino acids. With the four nucleotides, 64 different codons are possible. The genetic code is degenerate. This means that all amino acids are coded by about three different triplets; hence the number of possible codons is higher than the number of amino acids. In contrast there is only one start codon (AUG) for the methionine at the first amino acid position in each protein (Tables 16.2 and 16.3).

The human haploid genome consists of about three billion base pairs (bp) which in humans are placed on 23 chromosomes. The smallest chromosome (21) consists of approximately 50 million bp whereas the longest chromosome (1) contains approximately 250 million bp. The human genome comprises 20,000–25,000 genes and is therefore much smaller than expected in the Human Genome Project (100,000 genes). At first this was surprising but its discovery allowed a completely new view of the fundamental importance of the phenomenon of alternative splicing for protein diversity.

Chromosomes

Each diploid human cell contains 46 chromosomes, comprising 22 pairs of autosomes (chromosomes 1–22) and one pair of sex

TABLE 16.2 The Genetic Code

	T		C		A		G	
	SECOND POSITION							
T	TTT	Phe	CTT	Leu	ATT	Ile	GTT	Val
	TTC	Phe	CTC	Leu	ATC	Ile	GTC	Val
	TTA	Leu	CTA	Leu	ATA	Ile	GTA	Val
	TTG	Leu	CTG	Leu	ATG	Met /*Start*	GTG	Val
C	TCT	Ser	CCT	Pro	ACT	Thr	GCT	Ala
	TCC	Ser	CCC	Pro	ACC	Thr	GCC	Ala
	TCA	Ser	CCA	Pro	ACA	Thr	GCA	Ala
	TCG	Ser	CCG	Pro	ACG	Thr	GCG	Ala
A	TAT	Tyr	CAT	His	AAT	Asn	GAT	Asp
	TAC	Tyr	CAC	His	AAC	Asn	GAC	Asp
	TAA	OCH /*Stop*	CAA	Gln	AAA	Lys	GAA	Glu
	TAG	AMB /*Stop*	CAG	Gln	AAG	Lys	GAG	Glu
G	TGT	Cys	CGT	Arg	AGT	Ser	GGT	Gly
	TGC	Cys	CGC	Arg	AGC	Ser	GGC	Gly
	TGA	OPA /*Stop*	CGA	Arg	AGA	Arg	GGA	Gly
	TGG	Trp	CGG	Arg	AGG	Arg	GGG	Gly

TABLE 16.3 Three-Letter Code and One-Letter Code of Amino Acids

Amino acid	Three-letter code	One-letter code
Alanine	Ala	A
Arginine	Arg	R
Asparagine	Asn	N
Aspartic acid	Asp	D
Cysteine	Cys	C
Glutamic acid	Glu	E
Glutamine	Gln	Q
Glycine	Gly	G
Histidine	His	H
Isoleucine	Ile	I
Leucine	Leu	L
Lysine	Lys	K
Methionine	Met	M
Phenylalanine	Phe	F
Proline	Pro	P
Serine	Ser	S
Threonine	Thr	T
Tryptophan	Trp	W
Tyrosine	Tyr	Y
Valine	Val	V
Any amino acid		Z

Stop Codes: Amber, OCHer, OPA

chromosomes (chromosomes X and Y). Female individuals carry two X chromosomes (karyotype 46,XX) whereas male individuals carry an X and a Y chromosome (karyotype 46,XY). The germ cells in the gonads carry a haploid set of chromosomes which arise through meiosis (oocyte 23,X, spermium 23,Y or 23,X). During fertilisation the homologous maternal and paternal chromosomes combine and reconstitute the diploid genome. In contrast, during mitosis of somatic cells, the chromosomes are replicated, paired and segregated into two diploid daughter cells.

The exchange of homologous paternal and maternal chromosomal segments is called recombination and is essential for genetic diversity. During meiosis each pair of chromosomes is divided in sister chromatids. At this time, a crossing over of homologous chromosomal segments occurs. The paternal and maternal chromosomes are then randomly separated into four haploid gametes. Random recombination events are the background for high genetic variability, so that each single germ cell can be seen as unique. Moreover, recombination events are the basis for so-called linkage analyses in which the inheritance of two adjacent genes or DNA marker loci can be assessed.

STRUCTURE OF A GENE

A gene consists of regulatory regions (promoter) followed by exons and introns and untranslated regions (UTR) (Figure 16.1). In the reading direction the upstream region is called the 5′ end (spoken: 'five prime' end) and the downstream region the 3′ end. The regions which regulate gene expression locate upstream (5′) of the transcription initiation site.

Exons are regions which are later spliced to the messenger RNA (mRNA).

Introns lie between the exons and are cut out. (Sometimes alternative promoters or splice sites exist so that it is possible that one single gene can create various transcripts and hence a number of isoproteins.)

The promoter region contains specific responsive elements which can bind transcription factors. These transcription factors can occur ubiquitously or may be cell-specific.

Enhancers are short sequence motifs which can specifically increase transcription of eukaryotic genes. In contrast to the promoters which are usually in close proximity to the coding

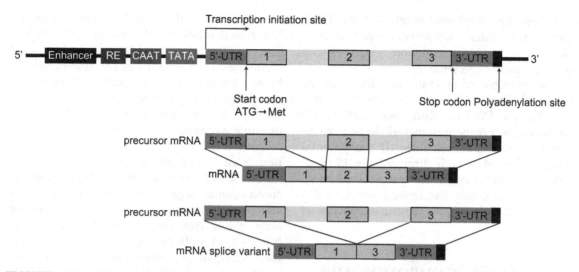

FIGURE 16.1 Structure of a gene.

Note: The regulatory region at the 5' end contains enhancer elements, responsive elements as well as CAAT and TATA boxes. The introns (light grey) are located between the coding exons (medium grey) and are spliced out. The non-coding regions (5'UTR and 3'UTR) are shown as dark grey regions. Alternative splicing causes different messenger RNA molecules (mRNA) which result in isoproteins. A − adenine, C − cytosine, G − guanine, Met − methionine, RE − responsive elements, T − thymine, UTR − untranslated region.

region, enhancers can be located far away from the gene.

Silencers are other regulatory elements which can suppress the transcription of a gene. Transcription factors are able to bind to promoters or enhancers and thereby may interact with other nuclear proteins which are called co-activators or co-repressors.

All these proteins build up larger protein complexes which finally either activate or suppress transcription.

The first step in gene expression is RNA synthesis with the help of an RNA polymerase. This process takes place in the nucleus and is termed **transcription** (Figure 16.1).

The second step, polypeptide synthesis, is called **translation** and occurs outside the nucleus, in ribosomes which are large RNA-protein complexes located in the cytoplasm. The RNA molecules which determine the polypeptide sequence are named messenger RNA (mRNA). The transcription stop (UAG) site is

located in the 3' region of a gene. A polyadenylation signal encodes the poly A tail which influences the mRNA transport from the nucleus into the cytoplasm, RNA stability and translational efficacy.

Haploinsufficiency refers to a situation in which one of the parental gene copies is deleted or mutated and the other parental copy of the gene is incapable of producing sufficient protein for a normal protein function. A mutation in both gene copies often results in a more severe phenotype. As an example, heterozygous mutations in the THOX2 gene result in transient hypothyroidism with a decreased H_2O_2 production whereas biallelic mutations in this gene lead to permanent hypothyroidism.

Epigenetic processes, for example X inactivation and imprinting mechanisms, can also influence gene expression. Genomic imprinting is a variable monoallelic gene expression which is dependent on the parental origin of the gene copy.

Different gene expression can be due to DNA methylation which usually silences gene expression, or to histone acetylation which usually activates gene expression.

One example of genomic imprinting is the Prader—Willi syndrome (PWS). The genes responsible for PWS on chromosome 15q11-q13 are activated on the paternal allele and inactivated on the maternal allele. If the paternal allele is deleted or both chromosomes 15 originate from the mother (uniparental disomy), the patient has only inactivated genes in this region which causes the typical phenotype of PWS.

ANALYSIS OF CHROMOSOMES AND DNA: METHODOLOGICAL ASPECTS

For the analysis of larger genomic alterations cytogenetic methods, fluorescence *in situ* hybridisation (FISH) or Southern blot studies are applied.

Smaller mutations are detected by polymerase chain reaction (PCR) and fragment analysis. Point mutations are detected by sequencing of PCR-amplified fragments of the gene region. In recent years novel technologies for mutation detection, gene mapping or assessment of expression profiles have been developed which rely on chip technology. With these techniques many thousands of samples can be investigated at the same time, so that it is possible to investigate not only a single gene but the whole genome in a couple of days.

In the following section we describe the most important and most frequently used molecular biologic and genetic techniques.

Cytogenetics and FISH Analysis

With fluorescence *in situ* hybridisation, chromosomal aberrations such as deletions or translocations with a size between 20 k and 1 M can be detected. FISH relies on the hybridisation of fluorescently labelled probes with chromosomes in metaphase. The sites of hybridisation are then detected with a fluorescence microscope. The staining of whole chromosomes with a mixture of probes is called 'chromosome painting'.

With the Comparative Genome Hybridisation (CGH) method, changes of DNA copy numbers (due to deletions or duplications of chromosomal regions) can be detected. The size of the changes which can be detected by array CGH can vary between a couple of hundred to millions of base pairs. For this method, equal amounts of patient and reference DNA are stained with different fluorescent dyes and are co-hybridised on a chip. Numeric changes in the genome lead to a shift of the hybridisation of patient and reference probes and hence a shift of the fluorescence signal. These changes can be automatically detected and assessed so that this method is available also for high-throughput analyses.

Nucleic Acid Hybridisation

Hybridisation of nucleotide strands relies on the fact that two complementary strands of nucleic acids bind (hybridise) to each other with high specificity. Given the complementarity of the two strands, the generation of DNA-DNA-, DNA-RNA- or RNA-RNA double helices is possible. A hybridisation probe can be a naturally occurring, cloned or an *in vitro* synthesised DNA or RNA sequence. Such probes should ideally consist of 16 or more nucleotides as such a sequence occurs with a high likelihood only once within the genome.

Southern blots are based on DNA-DNA hybridisation. They are used for analysis of restriction fragment length polymorphisms or to detect whether genomic regions have been deleted, duplicated or rearranged.

Northern blots rely on hybridisation of DNA-RNA or two RNA strands. They are used to investigate patterns and levels of gene expression in different tissues.

In contrast, **Western blots** refer to the detection of protein fragments using antibodies (see section 'Investigating gene expression and gene function' below).

In recent years, Northern blots have been replaced by more sensitive methods such as real-time/quantitative (Q) PCR (Q-PCR) or gene expression microarray analyses.

Polymerase Chain Reaction

The introduction of a cell-free method for amplification of DNA fragments (PCR) and the development of DNA sequencing methods have revolutionised molecular analysis of DNA. The PCR method provides a rapid way of selective amplification of specific DNA fragments *in vitro*. The required amount of DNA can be very small and may originate from

a cell, from tissues or from body fluids such as blood or saliva.

For a PCR the following reagents are required:

- a DNA-fragment
- two oligonucleotides (15–25 nucleotides) = primers
- a thermostable DNA polymerase
- a mix of all four nucleotides.

The two primers are complementary to the two 3′ ends of double-stranded DNA, which should be amplified. DNA synthesis is catalysed by a purified heat-stable DNA polymerase (for example from the bacterium *Thermus aquaticus*). A PCR consists of three different steps which are repeated many times (i.e. 25–35 cycles). In a first step the DNA is denatured at approximately 95°C. In the second step the primers anneal to the template DNA at a temperature of 50–65°C, and in the final third step the DNA is synthesised by DNA polymerase at a temperature of 72°C (Figure 16.2). With repeating cycles the original DNA

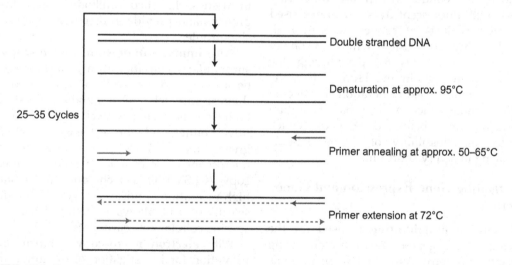

FIGURE 16.2 Principle of polymerase chain reaction (PCR).
Note: After denaturation of the double-stranded DNA, complementary synthetic oligonucleotide primers are annealed to one side of the DNA template, which has to be amplified. A thermostable DNA polymerase then extends the primers on in 5′–3′ direction and synthesises complementary strands. These steps are repeated in about 30 cycles and result in the doubling of the copies after each cycle.

fragments are amplified exponentially. The final product, referred to as amplicon, can then be subjected further to fragment analysis or sequencing.

PCR can also be used for RNA analysis. In this case, in a preceding step, the RNA is converted by reverse transcriptase (RT) into complementary DNA (cDNA). The cDNA is then amplified by PCR. The whole procedure is called RT-PCR. This analysis is often used for quantitative analyses of gene expression.

DNA Sequencing

The currently used sequencing methods are automated and are based on the chain termination method of Sanger, for which dideoxynucleotides of the four known nucleotides (A, G, C, T) are used to stop DNA polymerisation in a random manner. After separation of the differently terminated fragments using high-resolution gel or capillary electrophoresis, the sequence can be deduced. With the introduction of dideoxynucleotides which are differently labelled with fluorescent dyes, a computerised automated analysis of sequences with high throughput became possible, which was one of the main prerequisites for deciphering the human genome within the Human Genome Project. Currently, Next Generation Sequencing (NGS) methods, such as chip-based capture sequencing, are being developed, which provides the possibility of whole genome sequencing in a very short time.

Investigating Gene Expression and Gene Function

Western immunoblotting is used for the detection of the gene-encoded protein using a specific antibody. As a first step, proteins (i.e. cellular extracts) are separated according to their molecular weight/size in a one-dimensional denaturing polyacrylamide gel. Proteins of identical size will co-migrate. The

proteins are then transferred (blot) to a nitrocellulose or nylon membrane and incubated with the protein-specific antibody.

In a **2D gel electrophoresis** the proteins are separated in a first dimension according to their charge (proteins of identical size, but with different charge, will not co-migrate) and in a second dimension according to their size. This method allows for the identification of different protein bands/spots profile, between two samples obtained from the same tissue type in a control (normal) and patient (affected: tumour). The protein profile is then scanned by a computerised imaging system which enables the detection of abnormal protein spots (i.e. upregulated or down-regulated). The identity of a protein spot is then determined by mass spectrometry analysis.

In situ **hybridisation** utilises an *in vitro* synthesised single stranded DNA (ssDNA) or RNA-labelled probe to detect the expression of the gene of interest (mRNA) in cells of the investigated tissues. The method of **immunohistochemistry** is used for the detection of proteins in tissues. Labelled antibodies bind to the proteins and provide indirectly a gene expression profile.

With **immune fluorescence microscopy** the subcellular localisation of a gene product can be investigated. The cells are incubated with fluorescently labelled antibodies. These antibodies can be excited with UV light and consecutively emit light in the visible wavelength (red, green, blue, etc.) which can be observed by microscope. Confocal laser scanning microscopy (CLSM) is a technique for obtaining high-resolution optical images with depth selectivity and allows protein localisation in specific cellular compartments.

With **electron microscopy** a much higher resolution for investigation of the intracellular localisation of a gene product can be reached. The antibody is commonly labelled with electron-dense particles such as colloidal gold particles.

Animal Models for the Investigation of Human Diseases

Animal models do not only serve for the testing of novel drugs but also for investigation of the pathophysiology of inherited diseases. Animal experiments are only justified if scientific information cannot be gained by other *in vitro* experiments.

Animal models occur either spontaneously and are found through a specific phenotype or are generated by changing the genetic material of a wild animal. The latter is done, for example, with gene targeting which refers to the introduction of mutations into a gene of embryonal stem cells. The mouse plays the most important role as a model organism. However, depending on the scientific question being addressed, other species such as rats, zebra fish or drosophila are used.

MUTATIONS AND ENDOCRINE DISORDERS

Types of Mutations

DNA sequence variations are responsible for genetic diversity but also for genetic diseases. We differentiate between **mutations** (sequence variants causing a disease) and **polymorphisms** (non-pathogenic sequence variant present in less than 1% of the population). However, there are still uncertainties and the usage of these terms by scientists is not uniform.[2] Substantial discrepancies between scientific and popular usages constitute an issue of concern, because the term 'mutation' has developed a negative connotation.[3] A consistent use of the more neutral term 'sequence variant' is also difficult as it does not reflect an important dimension of the term 'mutation' (i.e. 'a change'), namely that mutation refers to a change in a former condition. In the following the term 'mutation', defined by any change in the nucleotide sequence of DNA, regardless of its functional

consequences, is used but difficulties in terminology that still exist should be acknowledged.

Mutations may include only one or a few nucleotides but can also affect larger regions of genes or chromosomes. Mutations can occur in all gene regions (regulatory regions, exons, introns) or can include the whole gene (duplications, deletions). A deletion of more than one gene within a chromosomal region can result in a so-called **contiguous gene syndrome**. One of the most frequent contiguous gene syndromes in paediatric endocrinology is a deletion on chromosome Xp22.3 that includes the adjacent genes *SHOX*, *ARSE*, *STS* and *KAL1*. Male patients with this deletion suffer from Léri−Weill dyschondrosteosis (*SHOX*), chondrodysplasia punctata (*ARSE*), ichthyosis (*STS*) and Kallmann syndrome (*KAL1*).

Mispairing of homologous sequences may lead to unequal crossovers or gene conversions. This results in a gene duplication on one chromosome and a deletion on the other chromosome.

The existence of inactive pseudogenes, with a high grade of homology to the original gene, increases the likelihood of incorrect recombinations with consecutive duplications, deletions and pathogenic mutations in the adjacent active gene. For example, in congenital adrenal hyperplasia due to recombinations between the inactive pseudogene *CYP21A1P* and the active gene *CYP21A2*, particular gene regions including mutations of the pseudogene are transferred into the active gene, thus leading to the disease.

Trinucleotide repeats are also hot spots for unequal recombination events. A small increase of the number of trinucleotide repeats may in further generations lead to a marked increase of these repeats, which clinically results in an increase of severity of the phenotype. This increase of severity from one generation to the next is called **anticipation** and can be observed, for example, in myotonic dystrophy or fragile X syndrome.

Mutations concerning only one single nucleotide are referred to as **point mutations**. A substitution of one purine (pyrimidine) base by another purine (pyrimidine) base (i.e. A>G or C>T) is called **transition**. In contrast, a change of a purine base to a pyrimidine base and the other way round (i.e. A>C or T>G) is called **transversion**.

As the genetic code is degenerated, not all mutations lead to an amino acid change. These mutations are termed **silent mutations** (e.g. TCT>TCC → serine>serine).

A **missense mutation** is a point mutation resulting in an amino acid change (e.g. TCT>TAT → serine>tyrosine).

However, if a point mutation leads to a stop codon, this mutation is called **nonsense mutation** (e.g. TGT>TGA ® cysteine>stop). Such a mutation results in the interruption of translation and a truncation of the encoded protein.

Small deletions or duplications, which do not include a multiple of a nucleotide triplet (codon), lead to a shift of the reading frame and are referred to as **frameshift mutations**. Behind this mutation a nonsense sequence is synthesised which often runs into a premature stop codon and protein truncation, causing a severe phenotype. In contrast, if deletions or duplications include a multiple of a codon, the changes are in-frame and the resulting protein is either shortened or elongated with absence of a nonsense sequence. This is often associated with a milder phenotype of the disease (Figure 16.3).

Splice mutations are mutations in introns or at highly conserved exon-intron junctions which either delete or create a splice site. Defective splicing of mRNA results either in excision of exons or leads to the interposition of an intron between two exons.

Furthermore, we differentiate between **germ cell mutations** which are present in all cells of an individual, and **somatic mutations** which arise only during embryogenesis or later and

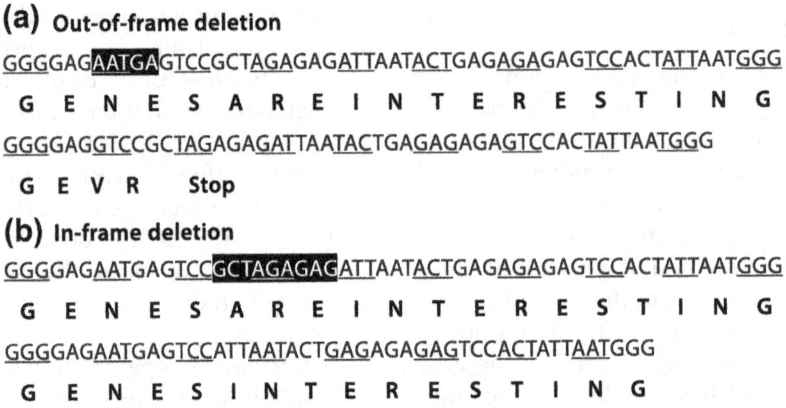

(a) Out-of-frame deletion

GGGGAGAATGAGTCCGCTAGAGAGATTAATACTGAGAGAGAGTCCACTATTAATGGG

G E N E S A R E I N T E R E S T I N G

GGGGAGGTCCGCTAGAGAGATTAATACTGAGAGAGAGTCCACTATTAATGGG

G E V R   Stop

(b) In-frame deletion

GGGGAGAATGAGTCCGCTAGAGAGATTAATACTGAGAGAGAGTCCACTATTAATGGG

G E N E S A R E I N T E R E S T I N G

GGGGAGAATGAGTCCATTAATACTGAGAGAGAGTCCACTATTAATGGG

G E N E S I N T E R E S T I N G

FIGURE 16.3 Mutation with and without a shift of the reading frame.
Note: The nucleic acid sequence (grey letters) is translated in a protein (boldfaced text). The sentence 'GENES ARE INTERESTING' stands for an easily readable protein sequence with a particular function. (a) A five bp deletion (white letters on black background) leads to an out-of-frame deletion (frameshift mutation) in which the reading frame is shifted, resulting in a nonsense protein sequence with a premature stop codon after 10 amino acids. The original sentence is not readable any more. In the translated sense a frameshift mutation results in a shortened and functionless protein causing a severe phenotype. (b) A deletion of nine bp representing exactly three codons results in deletion of three amino acids in the reading frame. The sentence 'GENES INTERESTING' is shortened but still makes some sense. In the translated sense, an in-frame deletion results in a shortened protein with residual function, causing a milder phenotype.

lead to a mosaic (i.e. a coexistence of cells with and without a mutation). An important example is McCune—Albright syndrome (MIM #174800). The underlying activating mutation of Arginine[201] of the *GNAS1* gene occurs post-zygotically so that only distinct tissues are affected. Typically affected tissues are the ovaries (resulting in a pseudo-precocious puberty), the skin (resulting in large and usually unilateral landscape-like café-au-lait spots) and the bones (resulting in fibrous bone dysplasia).

Polymorphisms are sequence variants present in more than 1% of the population and are usually not pathogenic. Examples are the previously mentioned silent mutations and so-called single nucleotide polymorphisms (SNP) which are scattered all over the genome. Despite the fact that polymorphisms do not usually cause a disease, some of them may modify mRNA stability or translation. Some combinations of SNP may play a pathogenic role in complex disease by modifying susceptibility for development of a disorder.

How to Prove Whether a Sequence Variant is a Pathogenic Mutation

The detection of an unknown sequence variant during sequencing of a candidate gene leads to the question of how to differentiate between a pathogenic mutation and a non-pathogenic polymorphism. As a first step one should search for the appropriate genomic or cDNA reference sequence by using the basic local alignment search tool function (BLAST) of the National Center for Biotechnology Information server (NCBI) (Table 16.1). With the help of SNP databases the new sequence variant can be compared with known polymorphisms.

In order to prove whether a mutation is pathogenic, different approaches should be applied. By sequencing all family members it should be shown that the mutation segregates with the disease; that is, that all affected family members

carry the mutation and all unaffected family members do not.

In addition it should be shown that the novel mutation does not occur in at least 60 control individuals (i.e. in 120 alleles).

Finally, functional analyses should be performed. This usually requires cloning of the mutation *in vitro* in an expression vector and expression of the mutated protein in cell culture. The proteins can then be analysed with different methods (e.g. binding studies, immunohistochemistry, enzyme assays, reporter gene assays and others).

Standard Nomenclature for Genes and Mutations

To translate basic research findings into clinical practice, it is essential that information about mutations and variations in the human genome are communicated easily and unequivocally. Geneticists from the Netherlands and the USA have developed a uniform and internationally generally binding nomenclature for the Human Genome Variation Society (HGVS).[4,5] In the following, the basic principles of this nomenclature are summarised.

To avoid misunderstandings between physicians and scientists it is important to use the official gene symbol of the HUGO Gene Nomenclature Committee (HGNC).[6,7] All genes and DNA markers are generally written in italics, whereas the corresponding proteins are written in roman (not italics) (e.g. *TSHR* = TSH receptor **gene** and **TSHR** = TSH receptor **protein**).

Complementary DNA (cDNA) is synthetically synthesised DNA which is complementary to mRNA and therefore corresponds to the coding parts of a gene. The generally accepted numbering of nucleotides and amino acids is based on the cDNA reference sequence and the deduced protein sequence. The cDNA reference sequence includes the full-length coding region and the non-coding 5′ and 3′

untranslated regions (UTR). The numbering of nucleotides starts at the initiation codon, so that the A of the start codon ATG refers to nucleotide number 1. Nucleotides located 5′ of the initiation codon are labelled with a '-' (i.e. -3), whereas nucleotides 3′ of the stop codon carry a '*' (i.e. *3). The start codon encodes for a methionine, which is number 1 of the amino acids in the protein. Depending on the reference sequence used, the mutations take different prefixes: 'c.' for the cDNA-, 'g.' for a genomic, 'm.' for a mitochondrial, 'r.' for a RNA- and 'p.' for a protein sequence.

A simple **exchange of a nucleotide** is shown with the symbol '>', and the number of the nucleotide precedes the base change (e.g. c.55G>A) (Figure 16.4).

In contrast, when showing an **amino acid change**, the number of the amino acid stands between the exchanged amino acids. For amino acids either the three-letter or the one-letter amino acid code can be used (e.g. p.Gly19Arg or p.G19R). A change of an amino acid by a stop codon is depicted by an X (e.g. p.Thr11X). To avoid confusion it is generally recommended to cite the source of the reference sequence used when describing

a mutation (e.g. NM_000492.3: c.350G>A, p.Arg117His).

Other sequence variants are shown as follows.

- **Deletions**: two examples: c.250delA or c.250_254delATTCG
- **Duplications**: two examples: c.250dupA or c.250_254dupATTCG
- **Insertions**: two examples: c.250_251insT or c.250_251insGCGTGA

In the **SNP** database of the NCBI[8] the name and the localisation of the SNP in different reference sequences can be found (e.g. rs2306220:A>G).

Compound heterozygous mutations are shown in angled brackets and combined with a '+' (e.g. c. [250A>G]+[1598insC]).

Frameshift mutations are described on the protein level and usually the short form is sufficient (e.g. p.Ser56fs). A more detailed description (e.g. p.Ser56ArgfsX21) consists of the number of the first amino acid changed, its position in the protein, the first changed amino acid followed by fs (frameshift) and the length of nonsense amino acid sequence until the next stop codon X.

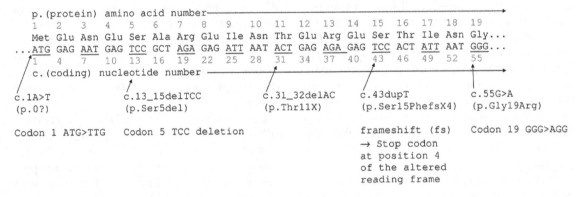

FIGURE 16.4 Example of the standard mutation nomenclature on the basis of a cDNA sequence. Note: The amino acid change for 'c.1A>T' is described as p.0 because amino acid changes secondary to codon 1 mutations are frequently unpredictable. *Source: Modified from Ogino et al 2007,[4] with approval of the American Society for Investigative Pathology.*

Intronic mutations should be shown on the basis of both the genomic reference sequence, which refers to the sequence of the genome including introns, and the cDNA sequence (e.g. AJ574942.1: g.2410G>T and NM_000492.3: c.489-1G>T). The change in the cDNA reference sequence describes the relation of the intronic mutation to the adjacent exon. In the given example the G is a non-coding intronic nucleotide which lies one position before the coding nucleotide 489. This information is of clinical relevance as it allows conclusions to be drawn concerning the pathogenetic effect of the mutation.

Functional Consequences of Mutations

Mutations can be generally classified as **gain-of-function (activating)** and **loss-of-function (inactivating)** mutations. Whereas activating mutations are mainly dominantly inherited, inactivating mutations mainly follow a recessive mode of inheritance.

Mutation of one allele may lead to **haploinsufficiency**, a situation in which one normal allele is not enough to ensure normal function of the gene and gene product. Haploinsufficiency is often found in connection with mutations of transcription factors. For example, a heterozygous mutation of the *PAX8* gene leads to congenital hypothyroidism.

Monoallelic mutations may also have a **dominant negative effect** and thereby lead to a loss of protein function. In these cases the mutated protein interferes with the wild-type gene product by one of the following mechanisms:

- incorrect protein–protein interactions (e.g. osteogenesis imperfecta type III)
- dysfunction of mutated proteins during transcription (e.g. thyroid hormone resistance)
- cytotoxic effects (e.g. familial autosomal-dominant diabetes insipidus).

A change of the **gene dosage** can also be pathogenic. For example, duplications of the *NROB1* (*DAX1*) gene may result in a dosage-sensitive sex reversal.

Genotype and Phenotype

The term **phenotype** refers to the totality of characteristics which can be observed in an individual. The genetic information responsible for the phenotype is referred to as **genotype**.

Alternative variants of a gene or a genetic marker at the same gene locus are termed **alleles**, which may be mutations or polymorphisms. As each healthy individual has two copies of each autosomal chromosome, each individual can only hold two alleles. However, within a population, more alleles of the same gene may exist. The commonly occurring allele is called the **wild-type** allele.

If an individual carries two identical alleles, the term **homozygosity** is used. In consanguineous families homozygous alleles usually have a founder and the homozygous allele is 'identical by descent'. In this case the term **autozygosity** is used. If two alleles of an individual differ, the individual is **heterozygous** for the respective gene locus.

In an autosomal recessive disease, **compound heterozygosity** may occur: in this case the patient has inherited two mutated alleles from his or her parents which are, however, not identical. **Hemizygosity** describes the situation in which the phenotype is determined by the existence of only one allele of a gene in an individual. This may occur in X-linked disorders or through a loss of one allele and a mutation on the corresponding second allele.

A **haplotype** is a group of adjacent alleles in a certain chromosomal region. Haplotype analyses are, for example, used to investigate segregation of a certain gene allele with the alleles of flanking DNA markers.

Penetrance and **expressivity** are two different but related concepts that are often confused. Penetrance is a qualitative notion, designating whether a phenotype is expressed for a particular genotype.

Expressivity is a quantitative concept, describing the degree to which a phenotype is expressed. It is used to describe the phenotypic spectrum in individuals with a particular disorder. Thus, expressivity is dependent on penetrance.[1] Complete penetrance means that all individuals bearing a particular mutation show the phenotype. In contrast penetrance is incomplete if some mutation-positive individuals do not show the typical phenotype. This can happen in particular in autosomal dominant diseases where sometimes one generation does not show the features of a disease.

HOW TO APPROACH A PATIENT WITH A GENETIC ENDOCRINE DISEASE

A detailed patient history, a thorough clinical investigation and biochemical evaluation are the most crucial prerequisites to uncover the aetiology of a genetic disease. Special emphasis should be placed on the family history as this information can already provide pivotal clues concerning the mode of inheritance and the phenotype.

When taking a family history, one should go through the following steps:

- drawing of the pedigree
- actively asking about the affected status and age of onset in any available family member
- asking for any written medical reports of any affected family members
- ascertainment of the causes of death of deceased family members.

As penetrance and expressivity of a genetic disorder may be age-dependent, the family history should be repeated after a while, if appropriate. Increase in family size or numbers also mandates a review of family history periodically.

If the data point to a genetic disorder, the first database which could be approached is the Online Mendelian Inheritance in Man (OMIM) database,[9] which is freely available on-line and comprises information, which can be grasped quickly, concerning thousands of genetic disorders. In this database the following information can be called up in a couple of minutes:

- clinical synopsis of the phenotype
- gene names and molecular genetic data of the gene locus
- chromosomal localisation of the gene
- information about allelic variants
- information about gene and protein function
- availability of animal models for the disorder.

Moreover, the OMIM database is linked to a series of other electronic databases such as GenBank, UniGene, nucleotide and protein databases and Medline and therefore provides very valuable tools for obtaining all relevant information concerning the suspected disorder.

Selection of appropriate samples for molecular genetic analyses is highly important for the expected result. To look for germ cell mutations, the purified DNA of a 3–10 mL EDTA blood sample is sufficient. However, somatic mutations can only be detected in affected tissues. In McCune–Albright syndrome, for example, the activating *GNAS1* mutation is only to be found in DNA of leukocytes of severely affected individuals but can be detected in ovarian tissue and occasionally in pigmented areas of the skin.

If a molecular genetic diagnosis in a patient seems possible, the physician has to take into account basic ethical rules for medical research involving human subjects. These have been summarised in the World Medical Association Declaration of Helsinki (59th WMA General Assembly, October 2008), which is also available via the Internet.

GENETIC COUNSELLING

The human genome is a primary element of personal and familial integrity. In contrast to many other medical investigations, results of genetic analyses may have profound impact on psychosocial well-being and family planning. Therefore special attention should be directed to a competent and detailed counselling of patients, before and after genetic testing. When planning molecular genetic diagnosis in patients with paediatric endocrine disorders one should therefore closely collaborate with medical or human geneticists.

Before taking a blood or tissue sample for molecular analyses, patients and/or parents should be thoroughly informed about possible consequences of the result for the patient and for the entire family.

Genetic counselling requires appropriate time and competence. Hence it is desirable to perform the counselling together with a clinical geneticist. The transmission of genetic results via telephone should be avoided as results can be misunderstood or misinterpreted. Children and teenagers should be informed in a manner appropriate to their age and to their capability to cope with the information. For example, genetic counselling of parents of a girl with Ullrich—Turner syndrome should also include age-based counselling for the growing girl, to ensure understanding of diagnostic and therapeutic procedures. As children get older, the patient counselling should be repeated from time to time, at a level suitable for their comprehension.

Besides a diagnostic aspect for the patients, for some genetic endocrine disorders prenatal molecular diagnostics can be considered. This should be done with special care and parents and the attending physician have to carefully balance whether knowledge about a disorder of the fetus is really necessary and helpful for family planning.

OVERVIEW OF GENETIC DISORDERS IN PAEDIATRIC ENDOCRINOLOGY[1]

In the following section selected genetic disorders which are of relevance for paediatric endocrinology are summarised (Tables 16.4A—4L).

TABLE 16.4A Selected Chromosomal Disorders with Endocrine Manifestations

Disorder/phenotype	Chromosomal defect	OMIM
Klinefelter syndrome Hypogonadism, tall stature	47,XXY and variants	
Ullrich—Turner syndrome Ovarian failure, short stature, autoimmune thyroid disease	45,XO and variants	
Down syndrome Autoimmune thyroid disease, diabetes mellitus type I, mental retardation, stunted growth	Trisomie 21, Mosaicism	190685
Prader—Willi syndrome Short stature, obesity, hypogonadism	del15q11-13 (paternal copy), maternal uniparental disomy	176270
Williams—Beuren syndrome Hypercalcemia, supravalvular aortic stenosis, mental impairment, growth retardation	del7q11.23 (contiguous gene syndrome), mutations in ELN (elastin) gene	194050
DiGeorge syndrome Hypoparathyroidism, thymus hypoplasia, cardiac defects	del22q11.2, mutations in TBX1 gene	188400

Note: OMIM = Online Medlian Inheritance in Man.

TABLE 16.4B   Selected Hypothalamic and Pituitary Disorders

Disorder/phenotype	Gene	Inheritance	OMIM
CPHD (GH, PRL, TSH, LH, FSH)	PROP1	AR	601538
CPHD (GH, PRL, TSH)	POU1F1 (PIT1)	AR, AD	173110
CPHD (GH, PRL, TSH, LH, FSH) with rigid spine	LHX3	AR	600577
CPHD (GH, PRL, TSH, LH, FSH) cerebellar and rhombencephalic defects	LHX4	AD	602146
CPHD with septo-optic dysplasia, agenesis of corpus callosum	HESX1	AR	601802
CPHD with various constellations of pituitary hormone deficiencies	HESX1	Monoallelic mutations	601802
Kallmann syndrome 1: hypogonadotropic hypogonadism, anosmia, renal agenesis	KAL1	X	308700
Kallmann syndrome 2: hypogonadotropic hypogonadism, anosmia	FGFR1	AD	136350
Kallmann syndrome 3	PROKR2	AR	607123
Kallmann syndrome 4	PROK2	AR	607002
Kallmann syndrome 5	CHD7	AD	608892
Kallmann syndrome 6	FGF8	AD	600483
Hypogonadotropic hypogonadism, delayed puberty	GNRHR	AR	138850
Hypogonadotropic hypogonadism, adrenal insufficiency	NROB1 (DAX1)	X	300473
Hypogonadotropic hypogonadism	FSHB	AR	136530
Hypogonadotropic hypogonadism	LHB	AR	152780
Obesity	LEPR	AR	601007
Obesity	MC4R	AR	155541
Obesity, adrenal insufficiency, red hair	POMC	AR	176830
Central adrenal insufficiency, CRH deficiency	CRH	AR	122560
Central adrenal insufficiency, ACTH deficiency	TBX19	AR	604614
Short stature	GHRHR	AR	139191
Short stature	GH1	AR, AD	139250
Central hypothyroidism	TRHR	AR	188545
Central hypothyroidism	TSHB	AR	188540
Neurohypophyseal diabetes insipidus	AVP-NPII	AD, AR	192340

Notes: AD = autosomal dominant, AR = autosomal recessive, CPHD = combined pituitary hormone deficiency, FSH = follicle stimulating hormone, GH = growth hormone, LH = luteinising hormone, OMIM = Online Mendelian Inheritance in Man, PRL = prolactin, S = sporadic, TSH = thyrotropin, X = X-chromosomal, Y = Y-chromosomal.

TABLE 16.4C Selected Defects in Thyroid Development, Thyroid Hormone Synthesis, Transport, and Action

Disorder/phenotype	Gene	Inheritance	OMIM
Congenital hypothyroidism, thyroid hypoplasia	PAX8	AD	167415
Congenital hypothyroidism, thyroid hypoplasia	TSHR	AR (inactivating mutations)	603372
Bamforth–Lazarus syndrome: congenital hypothyroidism, cleft palate, curly hair	FOXE1 (TTF2)	AR	602617
Congenital hypothyroidism with impaired iodine uptake	SLC5A5 (NIS)	AR	601843
Congenital hypothyroidism with impaired organification	TPO	AR	606765
Congenital hypothyroidism with impaired organification	DUOX2 (THOX2)	AR	606759
Transient congenital hypothyroidism, impaired H_2O_2 formation	DUOX2 (THOX2)	Monoallelic mutations	606759
Pendred syndrome: sensorineural deafness, organification defect	SLC26A4	AR	605646
Congenital hypothyroidism, thyroglobulin defects	TG	AR	188450
Thyroid dysfunction, respiratory distress, choreoathetosis	NKX2-1 (TTF1)	Monoallelic deletions or mutations	600635
Congenital non-autoimmune hyperthyroidism	TSHR	AD (activating mutations)	603372
Resistance to thyroid hormone	THRB	AD, (AR)	190160
Allan–Herndon–Dudley syndrome, elevated T3, decreased T4, quadriplegia, hypotonia	SLC16A2 (MCT8)	X	300095
Consumptive hypothyroidism due to overexpression of deiodinase type III in haemangiomas	DIO3	S	601038
Familial dysalbuminaemic hyperthyroxinaemia	ALB	AD	103600
Euthyroid hyperthyroxinaemia	TBG	X	314200
Euthyroid hyperthyroxinaemia, amyloid polyneuropathy	TTR	AD	176300

Notes: AD = autosomal dominant, AR = autosomal recessive, OMIM = Online Medelian Inheritance in Man, S = sporadic, X = X-chromosomal.

TABLE 16.4D   Selected Parathyroid and Bone Disorders

Disorder/phenotype	Gene	Inheritance	OMIM
Familial hypoparathyroidism	CASR	AD	601199
Familial hypoparathyroidism	PTH	AD, AR	168450
Hyperparathyroidism with jaw fibromas	HRPT2	AD	607393
Hyperparathyroidism	Fusion of the regulatory region of PTH with CCND1	Somatic mutation (PRAD1-rearrangement)	168461
Albright's hereditary osteodystrophy	GNAS1	AD	139320
Familial benign hypocalciuric hypercalcemia	CASR	AD	601199
Severe neonatal hyperparathyroidism	CASR	AR (AD)	601199
Vitamin D-dependent rickets type I	CYP27B1	AR	609506
Vitamin D-dependent rickets type II: vitamin D resistance	VDR	AR	601769
Hypophosphataemic rickets	PHEX	X	300550
Hypophosphataemic rickets	FGF23	AD	605380
Jansen metaphyseal chondrodysplasia	PTHR1	AD	168468

Notes: AD = autosomal dominant, AR = autosomal recessive, OMIM = Online Medelian Inheritance in Man, X = X-chromosomal.

TABLE 16.4E   Selected Disorders of Adrenal Hormone Synthesis and Action

Disorder/phenotype	Gene	Inheritance	OMIM
Congenital adrenal hypoplasia, hypogonadism	NROB1 (DAX1)	X	300200
Lipoid adrenal hyperplasia, adrenal insufficiency, ambiguous genitalia	STAR	AR	201710
Congenital hypoaldosteronism, adrenal insufficiency	CYP11B2	AR	606984
X-linked adrenoleukodystrophy	ABCD1	X	300100
Neonatal adrenoleukodystrophy	PEX1, PEX5 (PXR1), PEX10, PEX13, PEX26		202370
Congenital adrenal hyperplasia, 3b-dehydrogenase II	HSD3B2	AR	201810
Congenital adrenal hyperplasia, 11b-hydroxylase	CYP11B1	AR	202010
Congenital adrenal hyperplasia, 17-Hydroxylase	CYP17A1	AR	202110

TABLE 16.4E   Selected Disorders of Adrenal Hormone Synthesis and Action (*cont'd*)

Disorder/phenotype	Gene	Inheritance	OMIM
Congenital adrenal hyperplasia, 21-Hydroxylase	CYP21	AR	201910
Glucocorticoid-remediable aldosteronism	CYP11B2-CYP11B1 fusion gene	AD	103900
Familial glucocorticoid deficiency 1; FGD1	MC2R	AR	202200
Familial glucocorticoid deficiency 2; FGD2	MRAP	AR	607398
Familial glucocorticoid deficiency 3; FGD3	STAR	AR	600617
Triple A syndrome	AAAS	AR	231550
Glucocorticoid resistance	GCCR	AD	138040
Aldosterone resistance (pseudohypoaldosteronism)	NR3C2 (MR)	AD	177735

Notes: AD = autosomal dominant, AR = autosomal recessive, OMIM = Online Medelian Inheritance in Man, X = X-chromosomal.

TABLE 16.4F   Selected Disorders of β-cell Dysfunction and Pancreas Development

Disorder/phenotype	Gene	Inheritance	OMIM
MODY 1	HNF4a	AD	125850
MODY 2	GCK	AD (inactivating mutations)	125851
MODY 3	HNF1a	AD	600496
MODY 4, renal cysts	IPF1	AD	606392
MODY 5	HNF1ß	AD	137920
MODY 6	NEUROD1	AD	606394
Pancreas agenesis	IPF1	AR	260370
Rabson–Mendenhall syndrome	INSR	AR	262190
Leprechaunism	INSR	AR	246200
Familial hyperinsulinaemic hypoglycaemia 1; HHF1	ABCC8 (SUR1)	AR/AD	256450
Familial hyperinsulinaemic hypoglycaemia 2; HHF2	KCNJ11	AR	601820
Familial hyperinsulinaemic hypoglycaemia 3; HHF3	GCK	AD (activating mutations)	602485
Hyperproinsulinaemia	INS	AD	176730

Notes: AD = autosomal dominant, AR = autosomal recessive, OMIM = Online Medelian Inheritance in Man.

TABLE 16.4G   Selected Disorders of Gonadal Development, Hormone Synthesis and Action

Disorder/phenotype	Gene	Inheritance	OMIM
Persistent Müllerian duct	AMH	AR	261550/600957
Persistent Müllerian duct	AMHR2	AR	261550/600956
XY sex reversal, adrenal failure	NR5A1 (SF1)	AD, AR	612965/184757
Androgen insensitivity, androgen receptor inactivation	AR	AR	300068/313700
Androgen insensitivity, 5α-reductase deficiency	SRD5A2	AR	264600/607306
Azoospermia	DAZ	Y	400003
Estrogen resistance	ESR1 (ER)	AR	133430
Leydig cell hypoplasia, 46XY,DSD	LHCGR	AR (inactivating mutations)	238320/152790
Male-limited precocious puberty	LHCGR	AD (activating mutations)	176410/152790
Premature ovarian failure	FSHR	AR	233300/136435
Aromatase deficiency, female genitalia with masculinisation during puberty	CYP19A1	AR	107910
Frasier syndrome: 46,XY DSD streak gonads	WT1	AD	136680
46,XX DSD (male phenotype)	SRY translocation	X	278850/480000
46,XY DSD (female phenotype)	SRY mutations	Y	400044/480000

Notes: AD = autosomal dominant, AR = autosomal recessive, DSD = disorders of sex development, OMIM = Online Medelian Inheritance in Man, X = X-chromosomal, Y = Y-chromosomal.

TABLE 16.4H   Selected Disorders of Water and Salt Metabolism

Disorder/phenotype	Gene	Inheritance	OMIM
Nephrogenic diabetes insipidus	AVPR2	X	304800
Nephrogenic diabetes insipidus	AQP2	AR, AD	125800
Liddle syndrome: hypokalaemic metabolic acidosis, hypertension	SCNN1B or SCNN1G	AD	177200
Gitelman syndrome: hypokalaemic metabolic alkalosis, hypocalciuria, hypomagnesaemia	SLC12A3	AR	263800
Bartter syndrome: hypokalaemic metabolic alkalosis, hypocalciuria, hypovolaemia	SLC12A1, KCNJ1, CLCNKB, BSND	AR	601678 241200 607364 602522

Notes: AD = autosomal dominant, AR = autosomal recessive, OMIM = Online Medelian Inheritance in Man, X = X-chromosomal.

TABLE 16.4I Selected Defects in Fat Metabolism

Disorder/phenotype	Gene	Inheritance	OMIM
Obesity	LEP	AR	164160
Familial hypercholesterolaemia	LDLR	AD	606945
Familial hypobetalipoproteinaemia	APOB	AD	107730
Congenital generalised lipodystrophy types 1–3	AGPAT2 BSCL2 CAV1	AR	603100 606158 601047

Notes: AD = autosomal dominant, AR = autosomal recessive, OMIM = Online Medelian Inheritance in Man.

TABLE 16.4J Tumour Syndromes with Endocrine Manifestations

Disorder/phenotype	Gene	Inheritance	OMIM
Multiple endocrine neoplasia 1: parathyroid adenoma Pituitary adenoma, pancreas tumours	MEN1	AD	131100
Multiple endocrine neoplasia 2A: medullary thyroid cancer, phaeochromocytoma, parathyroid hyperplasia	RET	AD	171400
Multiple endocrine neoplasia 2B: medullary thyroid cancer, phaeochromocytoma ganglioneuromas	RET	AD	162300
Familial medullary thyroid cancer	RET	AD	155240
Cowden syndrome: multiple hamartomas, thyroid tumours	PTEN	AD	158350
Gardner syndrome: familial colon polyposis, papillary thyroid carcinoma, adrenal cancer	APC	AD	175100
Carney complex: lentigines, pituitary adenomas, pigmented nodular adrenocortical disease with atypical Cushing syndrome	PRKAR1A	AD	160980
Peutz–Jeghers syndrome: mucosal pigmentation, gastrointestinal cancers, thyroid and Leydig cell tumours, other malignancies	STKII	AD	175200
Von Hippel–Lindau disease: renal carcinomas, phaeochromocytomas, other tumours	VHL	AD	193300

Notes: AD = autosomal dominant, OMIM = Online Medelian Inheritance in Man.

TABLE 16.4K Syndromes with Complex Endocrine Manifestations

Disorder/phenotype	Gene	Inheritance	OMIM
Autoimmune polyglandular syndrome type I: adrenal insufficiency, hypoparathyroidism, candidiasis	AIRE	AR	240300
McCune—Albright syndrome: precocious puberty, fibrous dysplasia, café-au-lait spots, hyperthyroidism	GNAS1	Mosaic mutations	174800
Pseudohypoparathyroidism 1A: Albright's hereditary osteodystrophy, hypoparathyroidism, hypothyroidism, hypogonadism	GNAS1	Inactivating mutations in maternal allele	103580
Cystic fibrosis: pulmonary obstruction, exocrine and endocrine pancreas dysfunction, infertility, congenital aplasia of vas deferens	CFTR	AR	219700

Notes: AR = autosomal recessive, OMIM = Online Medelian Inheritance in Man.

TABLE 16.4L Selected Endocrine Disorders with a Polygenic/Multifactorial Aetiology

Disorder/phenotype	Genes/loci	OMIM
Diabetes mellitus type I	HLA DR3/4-DQ201/0302, HLA DR4/4-DQ0300/03022, HLA DR3/3-DQ0201/0201 Insulin VNTR, NEUROD, CTLA4, multiple others	222100
Diabetes mellitus type II	CPN10, PPARgINS, SUR1, IPF1, IRS-1, multiple others	125853
Hashimoto thyroiditis	HLA DR3, HLA DR4, HLA DR5, CTLA4, TG, others	140300
Autoimmune polyglandular syndrome type II: adrenal insufficiency, autoimmune thyroid disease, diabetes mellitus type I, other autoimmune disorders	HLA DR3-DQ2, HLA DR4-DQ8, others	269200

Notes: OMIM = Online Medelian Inheritance in Man.

References and Further Reading

1. Kopp P. Genetics, genomics, proteomics and bio-informatics. In: Brooks C, Clayton P, Brown R editors. *Brook's Clinical Pediatric Endocrinology*, 5th ed. Oxford: Blackwell, 2005:18—44.
2. Condit CM, Achter PJ, Lauer I, Sefcovic E. The changing meanings of 'mutation': a contextualized study of public discourse. *Hum Mutat* 2002;19:69—75.
3. Cotton RGH. Communicating 'mutation': modern meanings and connotations. *Hum Mutat* 2002;19:69—75.
4. Ogino S, Gulley ML, den Dunnen JT, Wilson RB, and the Association for Molecular Pathology Training and Education Committees. Standard mutation nomenclature in molecular diagnostics. *J Mol Diagn* 2002;9:1—6.
5. HGVS (Human Genome Variation Society) (2007) Nomenclature for the description of sequence variations. [On-line] [Accessed 5 August 2011] Available at URL: www.HGVS.org/mutnomen/
6. HGNC (HUGO Gene Nomenclature Committees) (2009) HUGO Gene Nomenclature Committees. [On-line] [Accessed 5 August 2011] Available at URL: www.genenames.org/
7. HUGO (Human Genome Organisation) (2007) Human Genome Organisation. [On-line] [Accessed 5 August 2011] Available at URL: www.hugo-international.org/
8. NCBI (National Centre for Biotechnology Information) (2009) Single nucleotide polymorphism. [On-line] [Accessed 5 August 2011] Available at URL: www.ncbi.nlm.nih.gov/projects/SNP
9. OMIM (Online Mendelian Inheritance in Man) (2009) OMIM – Online Mendelian inheritance in man. [On-line] [Accessed 5 August 2011] Available at URL: www.ncbi.nlm.nih.gov/sites/entrez?db=omim

Index

type III, 211–212
  clinical features, 211
  treatment, 211–212
type IV, 212–213
  clinical findings, 212–213
  differential diagnosis, 213
type V, 213
  clinical features, 213
  management, 213
types of, 207t
Osteomalacia, 171, 173–174
Osteoporosis, 219–220. *See also* Bone
    health
  infantile, 219–220
  juvenile, 220
Ovarian cysts, 230
Ovarian failure, 50
Overt hypothyroidism, 71

P

Paediatric gynaecology, 223–224.
    See also Adolescent
    gynaecology
  abnormal genital appearance
      with no visible vagina,
      223–224
    management, 223–224
  vulvovaginitis, 224
    management, 224
Pamidronate, 208
Pancreas tumours, 377t
Panhypopituitarism, 19
Papillary thyroid carcinoma, 377t
Paragangliomata, 119
Paramesonephric ducts, 129–132
Parathyroid adenoma, 377t
Parathyroid disorders, 374t
Parathyroid hormone (PTH), 159,
    162–164
  blood sample for, 168b
  in bone, 163
  in kidney, 163–164
  related peptide (PTHrP), 164
Parathyroid hyperplasia, 377t
  congenital, 357t–358t
Parental height, 11, 31–32
Partial androgen insensitivity
    syndrome (PAIS), 47, 54, 64
Pathogenic mutation, sequence
    variant, 367
Pendred syndrome, 73–74, 373t
Pendrin, 70, 74
Penetrance, 370

Percentiles, 2
  and standard deviation, relationship
      between, 3
Perchlorate discharge test, 76
Peripheral precocious puberty (PPP),
    57–58
Permanent neonatal
    hyperthyroidism, 91
Persistent Müllerian duct syndrome,
    376t
Peutz–Jeghers syndrome, 377t
Phaeochromocytoma, 118–120, 377t
  clinical features, 118
  family history, 118–119
  management, 120
  physical examination, 119–120
Phenothiazine, 64
Phenoxybenzamine, 120
Phenylalanine, 360t
Phenytoin, 64
Phosphate and alkali solutions
    composition, 182t
Phosphaturia, 182–184
Phosphorus
  deficiency, 172–173
  metabolism, 161–162
  sources, 162
Phosphorus deficiency type of
    rickets, 183
Physical activity, for obesity, 148–149
Pigmented nodular adrenocortical
    disease, with atypical
    Cushing syndrome, 147
Pituitary adenoma, 377t
  increased TSH production from, 81
Pituitary disorders, 372t
Pituitary hormone deficiencies, 18
Plasma urea and electrolytes, 18
Pleiotropic obesity syndromes,
    140t–142t
Point mutations, 366
Polycystic ovarian syndrome
    (PCOS), 226–228, 246–247
  early onset, 108
Polycythaemic babies, 234
Polymerase chain reaction (PCR), 35,
    362–364
  principle of, 363f
Polymorphisms, 367
Polyuria, 198–199, 306b. *See also*
    Diabetes insipidus
Positron emission tomography
    (PET), 118

Poverty-related nutrition issues, 268
Prader orchidometer, 58
Prader–Willi syndrome (PWS), 23,
    362, 371t
  clinical features of, 23
  genetics of, 23
  management of, 23
Precocious puberty, 25, 55–57, 378t
  causes of, 59t
  clinical setting, 58
  diagnosis, 60–62
    in boys, 60–61
    in girls, 60
  examination, 59–60
  history, 58–59
  investigations, 61
    biochemical, 61
    imaging, 61
  management, 62–63
    acute, 62–63
      expected outcomes, 63
      GnRH agonist, 62–63
      long-term, 63
      progestogen, 63
      rationale for, 61–62
  pathophysiology, 57–62
  and tall stature, 25
Prednisolone, 89, 113, 217, 236
Premarin, 41, 51–52, 229
Premature adrenarche, 55–56
Premature pubarche, 55–56
Premature thelarche, 56–57, 63
Preterm babies, 234
Preterm hyperthyroidism, 91
Primary adrenal insufficiency, 101,
    110–113
  clinical presentation, 111
  diagnostic approach, 110–111
  family history, 111
  investigations, 112
    with minimal resources, 112
    with optimal resources, 112
  management, 112–113
    acute management, 112–113
    emergency management plan,
      113
    long-term, 113
  pertinent past history, 111–112
  physical signs, 112
Primary amenorrhoea, 224–226
  normal pubertal progression
    increased pubic and axillary
      hair, 225–226

Printed in the United States
By Bookmasters